This book is due for return on or before the last date shown below.

ATLAS OF CATARACT SURGERY

FRONT COVER

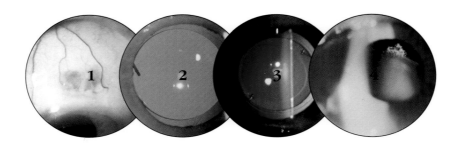

1 Postoperative scleral melting from nylon suture toxicity. (Courtesy of Samuel Masket MD.)
2 Postoperative view of Memory Lens. (Courtesy of Dott. Matteo Piovella.)
3 Postoperative view of Acrysof Lens. (Courtesy of Samuel Masket MD.)
4 Subluxated cataract with pseudoexfoliation noted on zonules. (Courtesy of Roger Furlong MD.)

ATLAS OF CATARACT SURGERY

Edited by

Samuel Masket MD

Clinical Professor of Ophthalmology
Jules Stein Eye Institute
UCLA, Center for Health Sciences
Los Angeles, CA
USA

Alan S Crandall MD

Professor of Ophthalmology
John A Moran Eye Center
Department of Ophthalmology
University of Utah School of Medicine
Salt Lake City, UT
USA

MARTIN DUNITZ

© Martin Dunitz Ltd 1999

First published in the United Kingdom in 1999 by

Martin Dunitz Ltd
The Livery House
7–9 Pratt Street
London NW1 0AE

A CIP catalogue record for this book is available from the British Library.

ISBN 1-85317-557–9

Distributed in the United States by:
Blackwell Science Inc.
Commerce Place, 350 Main Street
Malden, MA 02148, USA
Tel: 1-800-215-1000

Distributed in Canada by:
Login Brothers Book Company
324 Salteaux Crescent
Winnipeg, Manitoba, R3J 3T2
Canada
Tel: 204-224-4068

Distributed in Brazil by:
Ernesto Reichmann Distribuidora de Livros, Ltda
Rua Coronel Marques 335, Tatuape 03440-000
Sao Paulo
Brazil

Composition by Scribe Design, Gillingham, Kent
Printed and bound in Hong Kong by Imago

Contents

Contributors

Aziz Y Anis MD
Anis Eye Institute
Nebraska Eye Surgical Center
The Bryan Medical Plaza, Suite 610
1500 South 48th Street
Lincoln, NE 68506
USA

Graham D Barrett MD
Lions Eye Institute
2 Verdun Street
2nd floor, A Block
Nedlands 6009, WA
AUSTRALIA

Surendra Basti MD
Research Associate
Division of Ophthalmology
Box 70
Children's Memorial Hospital
2300 N, Children's Plaza Chicago, IL 60614
USA

Oswaldo M Brasil MD
Instituto Brasiliero de Oftalmologia Ltda
Ave N.S. de Copacabana
1052 Copacabana
Rio de Janeiro
BRASIL 22060-000

Fabrizio I Camesasca MD
Instituto Clinico Humanitas
Milano
ITALY

Robert J Cionni MD
Cincinnati Eye Institute
10494 Montgomery Road
Cincinnati, OH 45242-5214
USA

D Michael Colvard MD
Director, Centre for Ophthalmic Surgery
5363 Balboa Blvd. #545
Encino, CA 91416-2809
USA

Leif Corydon MD PhD
Director, Department of Ophthalmology
Vejle Hospital
Kabbeltoft 25
DK-7100 Vejle
DENMARK

James A Davison MD FACS
Assistant Clinical Professor
University of Utah and Wolfe Clinic, PC
309E Church Street
Marshalltown, IA 50158
USA

David M Dillman MD
Medical Director
Dillman Eye Care Associates
600 N Logan Avenue
Danville, IL 61832-4321
USA

I Howard Fine MD
Clinical Associate Professor of Ophthalmology
Oregon Health Science University
Portland, Oregon and
Oregon Eye Institute
1550 Oak Street
Suite 5
Eugene, OR 97401
USA

Luther L Fry MD
Fry Eye Associates, P.A./Ophthalmology
310 E. Walnut
Garden City, KS 67846
USA

Albert J Galand MD
Centre Hospitalier Universitaire
Service D'Opthalmologie
Liège 4000
BELGIUM

Almir Ghiaroni MD
Clinica e Cirurgia de Olhos
Rua General Venancio Flores 305 Sala 309
Rio de Janerio – RJ
CEP 22441-090
BRASIL

James P Gills MD
Clinical Professor of Ophthalmology
University of South Florida and
Director, St Luke's Cataract & Laser Institute
43309 US Hwy 19 N
PO Box 5000
Tarpon Springs, FL 34688-5000
USA

Richard S Hoffman MD
Oregon Eye Institute
1550 Oak Street
Suite 5
Eugene, OR 97401
USA

Jack T Holladay MD MSEE FACS
McNeese Professor of Ophthalmology
University of Texas Medical School at Houston
Houston, TX
USA

Markus J Koch MD
Zentrum für Augenheilkunde
Johann Wolgang Goethe-University
Department of Ophthalmology
Theodor-Stern-Kai 7
60590 Frankfurt am Main
GERMANY

Thomas Kohnen MD
Zentrum für Augenheilkunde
Johann Wolfgang Goethe-University
Department of Ophthalmology
Theodor-Stern-Kai 7
60590 Frankfurt am Main
GERMANY

Susanne Krag MD
Consultant, Aarhus Kommunehospital
Department of Ophthalmology
Nørrebrogade 44
DK 8000 Aarhus C
DENMARK

Richard P Kratz MD
5363 Balboa Blvd. #545
Encino, CA 91416-2809
USA

Brian Leonard MD
Director, Vitreoretinal Service
University of Ottawa Eye Institute
Ottawa General Hospital
501 Smyth Road, 3rd floor
Ottawa, ON K1H 8L6
CANADA

Arthur SM Lim FRCS
Clinical Professor and Head,
Dept of Ophthalmology
National University of Singapore
Medical Director, Singapore National Eye Center
SINGAPORE

William F Maloney MD
Eye Surgery Associates
2023 West Vista Way, Suite A
Vista, CA 92083
USA

Samuel Masket MD
Advanced Vision Care
7320 Woodlake Avenue
Suite 380 West Hills, CA 91307
USA

David J McIntyre MD FACS
Medical Director
McIntyre Eye Clinic and Surgical Center
1920 116th Ave NE
Bellevue, WA 98004-3012
USA

Kevin M Miller MD
Associate Professor of Clinical Ophthalmology
University of California, Los Angeles
School of Medicine and
Jules Stein Eye Institute
100 Stein Plaza, UCLA
Los Angeles, CA 90095-7002
USA

Soheila Mirhashemi PhD
Bausch & Lomb Surgical, Inc
555 West Arrow Highway
Claremont, CA 91711
USA

Michael Mittelstein PhD
Bausch & Lomb Surgical, Inc
555 West Arrow Highway
Claremont, CA 91711
USA

Joaquim Neto Murta MD PhD
Associate Professor of Ophthalmology
Ophthalmology Department
University Hospital of Coimbra
3049 Coimbra Codex
PORTUGAL

Kunihiro B Nagahara MD
President, Santa Maria Eye Clinic
2-1-39 Muromachi
Sakaide City
Kagawa 762-0007
JAPAN

Tobias H Neuhann MD
Medical Director
AAM - Augenklinik am Marienplatz
Marienplatz 18–19
80331 München
GERMANY

Okihiro Nishi MD
Director, Jinshikai Medical Foundation
Nishi Eye Hospital
4-14-26 Nakamichi
Higashinari-ku
Osaka 537-0025
JAPAN

Matteo Piovella MD
Centro Microchirurgia Ambulatoriale srl
Via Donizetti 24
20052 Monza
ITALY

Maria J Quadrado MD
Serviço de Oftalmologia
Hospitais da Universidade
3049 Coimbra Codex
PORTUGAL

Barry S Seibel MD
Clinical Assistant Professor of Ophthalmology
University of California at Los Angeles Medical
School and
1515 Vermont Avenue
7th Floor, Station C
Los Angeles, CA 90027
USA

Kimiya Shimizu MD
Professor and Chairman
Kitasato University, School of Medicine
1-15-1 Kitasato, Sagamihara
Kanagawa 228-0829
JAPAN

Bradford J Shingleton MD FACS
Ophthalmic Consultants of Boston
Center for Eye Research
50 Staniford Street
Boston, MA 02114
USA

John T Sorensen ScD
Bausch & Lomb Surgical, Inc
555 West Arrow Highway
Claremont, CA 91711
USA

Christian J Spaleck MD
Pfahlstr. 27
85072 Eichstätt
GERMANY

Kirsten Thim MD
Consultant, Vejle Hospital
Department of Ophthalmology
Kabbeltoft 25
DK-7100 Vejle
DENMARK

Abhay Vasavada MS FRCS
Director, Iladevi Cataract & Intraocular Lens
Research Center & Raghudeep Eye Clinic
Gurukul Road
Memnagar, Ahmedabad 380052
INDIA

Richard P Wilson MD
Attending Surgeon
Wills Eye Hospital
Glaucoma Service
900 Walnut Street
Philadelphia, PA 19107
USA

Ronald LS Yeoh FRCS
Senior Consultant Ophthalmologist
Singapore National Eye Centre
SINGAPORE

Preface

Remarkable changes have occurred in cataract rehabilitation during the past decade. It is commonplace for people to present for surgery and return to their full and complete lifestyle with good vision within hours. Optical and physical rehabilitation are rapid. The postoperative needs of the patient require little beyond self-reliance. The dramatic improvements for patients with visually disabling cataract are the product of the marriage of surgical skill and engineering technology.

Given that cataract microsurgery lends itself to video recording and live transmission, skill transfer has been facilitated to all corners of the world. As a result, contributions to our current state-of-the-art have not been limited to any specific geographic region. The *Atlas of Cataract Surgery* recognizes the global nature of cataract surgical technology. Its ecumenical concept brings contributions from all five continents. This book is not intended to be a comprehensive text for the novice cataract surgeon. Rather, it tells us where we are and where we might be heading in the near future. The Editors are very grateful to all those who contributed their knowledge and expertise, and to Alan Burgess and Clive Lawson at Martin Dunitz Ltd.

Samuel Masket
Alan S Crandall

This book is dedicated to our families whose sacrifices have enabled us to share information with our colleagues.

Chapter 1 Preoperative evaluation of the patient with visually significant cataract

Samuel Masket

As in the case of many medical conditions, advanced cataract formation produces a characteristic symptom, profound visual loss, which may be deduced from the patient's medical history. Likewise, the physical findings of a well-developed cataract can be determined during a basic ocular examination, which includes simple tests of visual function. Cataracts in earlier stages or in eyes with concomitant disease, however, require a greater degree of diagnostic skill and clinical investigation to determine the visual significance of the cataract and how to best advise and treat (assuming treatment is advantageous) the patient in question.

Until recently, the only device employed to assess the loss of visual function associated with cataract formation was Snellen acuity testing developed by Dr Hermann Snellen during the middle of the 19th century. Snellen testing employs high-contrast familiar letter optotypes. As such, it is a measure of the optical resolving power of the ocular system. Moreover, Snellen testing is performed under the controlled lighting conditions (generally darkened) of the refracting lane and therefore does not simulate the varied visual challenges of daily life. Patients with certain types of cataract in relatively early stages often note diminished visual function, although good Snellen acuity may be maintained.[1–4]

Given that 'real-life' conditions present a far more complex series of visual clues to interpret than does Snellen testing, there has been an interest in and a need for the development of additional methods for testing visual function. Such devices have been referred to as tests of 'functional vision', which are designed to simulate the visual disability induced by ocular disease and its impact on the visual tasks presented under conditions of daily life. Two general categories of functional vision testing devices have been developed; one system tests for glare disability, or the diminution of vision induced by ambient light,

and the other evaluates contrast sensitivity function (CSF), which tests visual recognition of various target sizes against backgrounds of differing contrasts. Although the two testing systems have significant overlaps, and a reduction in one function often leads to a diminution of the other, they are distinctly different, but vital, aspects of functional vision evaluation. They are useful in assessing the visual loss attributed to cataract and other ocular diseases when good Snellen acuity is noted despite significant visual complaints offered by the patient. Tests of functional vision are designed to aid in the determination of the visual significance of cataract formation; they are not intended to be used as screening devices or to induce patients without functional complaints to have surgery.

Preoperative evaluation of the patient with cataract additionally requires an appreciation of the visual prognosis for surgery, or potential visual acuity. This is particularly valuable for patients with ocular disease occurring in association with cataract formation. Several methods are available to help determine the potential postoperative vision.

Recently, the Agency for Health Care Policy and Research, an arm of the Department of Health and Human Services, performed a comprehensive review of cataract care and issued a set of guidelines outlining suggested preoperative, intraoperative and postoperative management of the adult with cataract.[5] Although these guidelines are somewhat controversial and have not been met with wide acceptance among ophthalmologists, they serve as a framework upon which to construct a paradigm (see further on) for the evaluation of the adult with cataract. Included in the guidelines, among other material, is a review of the ophthalmic literature regarding preoperative functional vision testing. It should be mentioned that the guidelines recognize that functional vision loss may be noted with certain cataract types and good Snellen acuity. Yet, on the basis of the rigid criteria for the literature review, there was no recognition of the value of any specific test of glare disability, CSF, or potential visual acuity. Nevertheless, clinicians often find that tests for these parameters are useful in evaluating patients with cataracts that have not reached maturity. A 1989 random survey of members of the American Society of Cataract and Refractive Surgery indicated that 65% of the respondent members employed either glare disability testing or CSF in evaluating the patient with cataract.[6]

In contrast, advanced cataracts, those that prohibit adequate ophthalmoscopy, require evaluation for the potential visual benefit of their removal, since the integrity of the retina and optic nerve cannot be assessed by routine means.

GLARE DISABILITY

Glare may be considered a subjective visual response to light. In the absence of significant ocular disease, bright light may induce *discomfort glare* prior to retinal photic adaptation; visual function, however, is unimpaired by discomfort glare. Conversely, *disability glare* implies that there is reduction in visual function caused by the scattering of incoming light by inhomogeneity of the ocular media. As in other ocular diseases that induce partial opacification of the ocular media, cataracts disperse incoming light, creating forward light scatter and a 'veiling luminance' that interferes with the perception of the visual object of regard. More commonly, this phenomenon is referred to as *glare disability*.[3] In general, opacities of the anterior segment (cataract being the most typical) are associated with glare disorders, whereas posterior segment abnormalities are less likely to induce disabling glare. The closer

the media opacity is to the retinal image plane, the less the geometric opportunity for light scattering and obscuring of the image. Therefore, corneal edema is a more likely source of glare than is macular edema.[7] Cataracts disperse incoming light and are anterior in the path of light. Therefore, patients with cataracts may exhibit marked disability glare while retaining good visual acuity under favorable lighting conditions, such as the darkened refracting lane. Cortical and posterior subcapsular cataracts generally cause daytime glare more readily than do nuclear cataracts, which are more prone to cause nighttime glare.[4,8] Glare disability, therefore, is a common cataract-related symptom, and testing for glare should be sufficiently sensitive to correlate well with patient complaints and adequately specific to avoid confusion with posterior segment disorders.

Several useful devices for determining and measuring glare disability are employed in current clinical practice (Table 1.1). These devices are generally designed to test a function of vision with and without the addition of an offending light or glare source. The difference in visual function with and without the glare source is attributed to glare disability. However, each testing system uses a different glare source (central or peripheral point light sources, diffuse background illumination, and so on) and test of visual function (letter optotypes, sine wave gratings, Landolt ring, and so on). The Brightness Acuity Tester (BAT)[9] is in common use because it is readily portable, compact, and relatively inexpensive, and may be used in conjunction with the Snellen chart of the refracting lane. The BAT offers three levels of background illumination in a small hemispheric bowl held near the eye. As a result, one possible source of error is pupil constriction by the illuminator; certain patients with cataract will perform better with pupil constriction, thereby giving a false-negative test. Conversely, the third level of brightness is dazzling,

Table 1.1
Automated instruments for measuring glare disability.

Instrument	Manufacturer	Test format	Glare light
BAT	Mentor	Letter acuity	Background
Eye Con 5	Eye Con	Letters	Background
IRAS GT	Randwal Instrument Co	Sine wave acuity	4-point
MCT 8000	Vistech	Sine wave contrast	Points or background
Miller–Nadler	Titmus Optical	Landolt C contrast	Background
TVA	Innomed	Letter acuity	Point

From *Ocular Surgery News*, Slack, Inc., Thorofare, NJ.

inducing false-positive results. Moreover, because no point source of light is used, the BAT does not simulate night-driving conditions.

Another popular device is the Miller-Nadler glare-testing device.[10] This unit relies upon a modified table-top slide projector to provide diffuse background illumination against which the patient views one of a series of 20/400-sized Landolt rings that sit upon a constant-contrast background circle. The rings vary in contrast to the background. Since the Miller-Nadler system employs background glare with a contrast test, it may be useful in simulating daytime glare disability but has been faulted for offering only one object size.[11]

As noted in Table 1.1, other automated devices have been developed and marketed. Moreover, simple, albeit non-calibrated, methods may also be used to assess glare disability. One simple means is to measure Snellen acuity indoors and then retest the patient outdoors with the chart positioned in front of the direct sunlight. Another method is to direct a penlight obliquely towards the pupillary margin while Snellen testing is under way; the difference between the Snellen acuity with and without the penlight is attributed to glare disability.[12]

No uniform standards have been established for glare-testing devices, a fact that limits their acceptance by rigidly scientific criteria. Nevertheless, it appears that measurement of disabling glare is most useful because it correlates well with cataract symptomatology and is reversible with successful cataract surgery.[13–15]

CONTRAST SENSITIVITY

Activities of daily living, such as driving a car, confront the individual with an ever-changing set of visual targets, luminances, and contrasts that require rapid visual interpretation. CSF evaluates the patient's ability to perceive a variety of coarse, intermediate or fine details at differing contrasts relative to the background. In such fashion, contrast testing seeks to objectively assess the equivalent of the patient's visual function in daily life.

Contrast sensitivity testing is somewhat analogous to audiometry, which measures hearing threshold sensitivity to audible tones of differing intensities and audio frequencies. Snellen testing of visual acuity, which is performed only at high contrast, is similar to audiometry performed at only one volume, or much like listening to music in which all notes are played at the same loudness. Therefore, contrast sensitivity testing is

a much more complete form of vision analysis than is Snellen testing.[16] Nevertheless, because different object sizes are tested in both systems, there is a clear relationship between visual acuity and contrast sensitivity. The 20/20 'E' optotype subtends a total of 5' arc on the retina, with each arm and each space accounting for 1'. A contrast grating pattern correlates to the arm and space of the letter 'E'. One dark and one light bar together equal one cycle. Thirty cycles per 1 degree (or 60') of retinal arch, therefore, corresponds to the spacing of a 20/20 optotype. It follows then, that just one point, 30 cycles per degree, on a contrast sensitivity curve at high contrast corresponds to the 20/20 line of Snellen testing. The typical human contrast sensitivity curve reveals that the peak contrast sensitivity of the visual system occurs at image sizes near six cycles per degree as subtended on the retina. An object that subtends six cycles per degree on the retina corresponds in size to a 20/100 optotype. This indicates that the human visual system requires higher contrast for perception at higher spatial frequencies. Therefore, it is possible that the eye may perceive small target sizes at high contrast while not recognizing larger objects at reduced contrast levels. This concept offers an explanation for the visual complaints of patients who retain reasonably good Snellen acuity yet express difficulty in 'real-life' visual function.

Given that CSF is analogous to a greatly expanded form of Snellen testing, it stands to reason that reduced contrast function will occur at high spatial frequencies when visual acuity is reduced for any reason, including uncorrected refractive errors and a number of anterior segment abnormalities, e.g. keratoconus and pterygium.[17] CSF, therefore, is quite sensitive but not as specific as is disability glare testing when evaluating symptomatic cataract.[18] It has been reported that early cataracts reduce contrast sensitivity primarily at high and intermediate frequencies,[19,20] whereas optic neuropathies are purported to reduce contrast sensitivity at low frequencies. As one might deduce, reduced CSF has also been noted and reported in a host of posterior segment disorders, including macular degeneration and diabetic retinopathy.[17]

Recently, interest has centered on the effect of monocular cataract on binocular visual function. By means of CSF testing, it has been established that at high spatial frequencies, binocular contrast sensitivity decreases to a level below that of the cataractous eye alone. This demonstrates binocular visual inhibition and indicates that a patient with one cataract may suffer significant visual disability, even when the non-cataractous eye has normal monocular vision.[21,22] Furthermore, this information suggests that correcting only one eye in a patient with binocular cataracts may not fully improve functional vision; often, the second eye will require surgery for the patient to gain the benefits of cataract rehabilitation. Moreover, a patient's perceived visual disability with cataract may correlate better with tests of binocular contrast sensitivity than with any of the monocular tests of visual function.[23]

MEASUREMENT OF CONTRAST SENSITIVITY FUNCTION

The determination of a CSF curve for the eye requires measurement of two separate functions: (1) the perceived contrast threshold between the object and the background and (2) the target size of the object subtended on the retina and measured in cycles per degree. Originally used as a research tool in the evaluation of ocular and neural diseases, early contrast testing systems used a series of sinusoidal (sine wave) grating patterns. Currently, the familiar letter optotype contrast charts (Table 1.2) designed by Terry, Pelli-Robson and Regan are used as clinical

alternatives to sine wave gratings, and CSF is often measured in a fashion similar to Snellen testing, with the subject reading letter charts of differing contrasts. The Regan charts each employ log MAR optotypes between 20/200 and 20/20 at varying contrasts of 96%, 50%, 25%, 11% and 4%. The 25% and 11% Regan contrast charts have been found particularly useful in evaluating cataract patients.[24] Since the Regan charts present letter targets of differing sizes at varied contrasts, they can be used to establish a true CSF curve for the eye. In contrast, the Pelli-Robson and Terry charts each offer only one size of letter targets. Both attempt to evaluate the most sensitive part of the contrast sensitivity curve, near six cycles per degree. Without targets of varied sizes, a complete contrast curve for the eye cannot be determined.

When measuring contrast sensitivity with letter charts, it is essential that the room and chart illumination be standardized. Self-contained tabletop vision testing devices offer the possible advantage of uniform internal illumination for enhanced reproducibility. Table 1.3 lists the available automated devices for evaluating CSF. Unfortunately, as in the case of glare disability testing, there is as yet no consensus on the appropriate standards for contrast

Table 1.2
Letter optotype charts for contrast sensitivity testing.

	Pelli-Robson	*Regan*	*Terry*
Contrast range	1–100%	4%, 11%, 25%, 50%, 96%	2.5–80%
Letter sizes	20/80	20/20–20/200	20/70
Testing distance	10 ft	10 ft	10 ft

Table 1.3
Contrast sensitivity testing devices.

Device	*Manufacturer*	*Format*	*Target type*
B-VAT II	Mentor	Computer screen	Sine wave
CSV 1000	Vector Vision	Illuminated wall chart	Sine wave
Eye Con 5	Eye Con	Computer screen	Letters
MCT 8000	Vistech	Tabletop view box	Sine wave
Optech 1000	Stereo Optical	Tabletop view box	Sine wave
Optech 2000			
TVA	Innomed	Computer screen	Square wave
VCTS	Vistech	Near-far charts	Sine wave

From *Ocular Surgery News*, Slack, Inc., Thorofare, NJ.

sensitivity testing, and a number of devices are available to determine CSF, with each of them employing a somewhat different method.

COMBINATION OF GLARE AND CONTRAST SENSITIVITY TESTING

It has been well established that glare disability reduces the contrast sensitivity of the visual system.[25] Therefore, certain glare-testing systems, such as the Miller–Nadler Glare Tester, evaluate the effect of a glare source on contrast targets to determine glare disability. Testing of CSF or low-contrast visual acuity in the presence of glare is superior to the testing of disability glare with high-contrast targets in assessing cataract patients with essentially normal neuroretinal function.[26] Most recently, it has become common practice to evaluate visual function when combining the BAT as a glare source with the Regan or Pelli-Robson contrast sensitivity charts.[23] This form of testing has been adopted by the United States Food and Drug Administration as requisite for determining visual function after placement of multifocal lens implants. Conversely, separate glare or contrast tests may have specific value for assessing other neurovisual conditions.[11] Given that high-contrast testing alone is of limited value in simulating the visual complaints of the patient with cataracts, it is likely that clinicians will accept into daily practice the combination of low-contrast visual acuity testing with an added glare source as the most effective means to quantify cataract-induced visual symptoms. A simple and gross system employs a penlight as a glare source in combination with Pelli-Robson contrast charts.[27] Hopefully, standard means for combining glare and contrast testing for the evaluation of patients with symptomatic cataract will soon be established and widely accepted among academicians, clinical practitioners, and regulating organizations.

ASSESSMENT OF POTENTIAL VISUAL FUNCTION FOLLOWING CATARACT REMOVAL

Patients with symptomatic cataract formation and otherwise normal ocular examinations can anticipate amelioration of their diminished vision with success-ful cataract removal. However, patients with cataract and concomitant ocular disease, e.g. macular degeneration, may present a dilemma in management, since ophthalmoscopy may be misleading or particularly difficult with advanced cataracts. Often, patient and surgeon are reluctant to consider cataract surgery when the prognosis for return of visual function is limited. Nevertheless, in some cases of multiple ocular disease, cataract rehabilitation may prove significantly beneficial to the patient. Determination of the expected visual improvement after surgery may allow the patient to arrive at an appropriate decision for or against surgery. Toward that end, a few devices for the determination of potential retinal function or visual return have been brought to the clinical arena (Tables 1.4 and 1.5).

Testing devices for the determination of potential visual acuity attempt to project visible targets through the cataract to reach the retina for subjective interpretation. Two basic target forms have been employed. One system, the Guyton–Minkowski Potential Acuity Meter (PAM),[28] is temporarily attached to a slit lamp and uses a reduced Snellen chart that is projected through a pinhole aperture onto the macular region; refractive errors may be

Table 1.4
Devices for determination of potential visual acuity.

Guyton-Minkowski Potential Acuity Meter (Mentor)	Reduced Snellen chart
Lotmar Visometer (Hagg–Streit)	Laser interferometer
Rodenstock (Rodenstock)	Laser interferometer
IRAS interferometer (Randwal)	Laser interferometer

Table 1.5
Methods for determination of retinal function integrity.

Blue-field entoptoscopy (Mira)	Foveal capillary net
Visual evoked potential	Evoked cortical responses
Electroretinography	Electroretinography
B-scan ultrasonography	Imaging
Pinhole acuity	Potential acuity
Penlight entoptic phenomena	Purkinje images
Maddox rod	Gross macular function
Two-point discrimination	Gross retinal function
Color perception	Gross macular function

compensated for by the apparatus. The second type of potential acuity apparatus uses laser-generated interference stripes or fringes that are projected onto the retinal surface through the ocular media; the width of the fringes, corresponding to acuity, is variable.[29–32] Refractive errors need not be corrected with interferometry testing, since projection of the laser images on the retina is not affected by ametropia.

The potential acuity devices, whether the Snellen chart or the PAM or the interferometry fringes, are subjective methods that require an alert and cooperative patient in addition to a skilled and compassionate examiner. Moreover, these tests are of greatest value when the cataract has not advanced past the 20/200 level because very dense lens opacities may yield false-negative results. A clinical rule of thumb indicates that a predicted improvement of four lines of vision by the acuity tester suggests a good prognosis for cataract surgery. Typically, then, if a patient's best-corrected visual acuity is recorded at 20/70, a 20/30 potential acuity response is considered indicative of significant visual improvement with surgery. Caution must be exercised in interpreting the results of potential acuity testing because some cases of maculopathy may yield a false-positive response, whereas extremely dense cataracts may produce false-negative results.

Additionally, simple and less expensive clinical tools may be useful in determining the visual prognosis after cataract removal in cases of suspected macular disease. One method is the yellow filter test suggested by Koch.[33] In this system, when a transparent yellow filter is placed over reading material, it is noted to worsen vision in the presence of a significant cataract but might be noted to improve vision if the macular degenerative process is more significant than the cataract. A simple pinhole device may also yield useful information about potential recovery of vision following surgery. A pinhole, in combination with a brightly lit chart, can simulate a potential acuity evaluation.

Occasionally, a cataract or other media opacity may be sufficiently dense to preclude any view of the posterior segment; in such cases, the prognosis for return of vision cannot be assessed by means of laser interferometry or the PAM. A number of alternative means to determine gross potential acuity in patients with markedly advanced cataracts have been developed over time and may be useful. Two-point discrimination, penlight-generated entoptoscopy, gross color perception, blue-field entoptoscopy and Maddox rod testing are among the available tests of

certain value (Table 1.5). Standard B-scan ultrasonographic imaging and electrophysiologic studies, such as electroretinography and the visual evoked potential, may provide useful information when considering an eye with totally opaque media, but these methods may be too costly for routine use in determining the indication for cataract surgery.

Two-point discrimination testing employs two light sources of equal intensity that are held about 25 inches (or 62 cm) from the patient. If the patient can correctly identify the two lights, retinal function is assumed to be grossly intact. No information is learned about macular potential. This test is most useful in cases of fully mature cataracts or otherwise dense ocular media. Similarly, gross color perception may be useful as a tool to establish general retinal integrity; the cobalt blue light source or the green filter (red-free source) of the slit lamp may be useful for this purpose.

Tests of entoptic phenomena have also been used to assess the function of the retina. A penlight of transilluminator may be placed over the closed lid directly on the globe to stimulate perception of the Purkinje vascular tree images. Although some patients may observe and describe the retinal vasculature, optic nerve and macular region accurately, other patients, even with intact retinas, cannot observe the Purkinje images. The test, therefore, is most useful in comparing the two eyes of one patient, assuming that one eye is normal and the involved eye has opaque media. In patients with one normal eye and one eye with densely opaque media, testing for an afferent pupillary defect may also be beneficial because at virtually all stages of development, cataracts do not induce abnormal pupillary reactions.

Blue-field entoptoscopy is more specific for macular function and is based upon the ability of the patient to observe the flow of white blood cells in the parafoveal capillaries. Blue light is absorbed by the red blood cells but not the white blood cells. As a result, with proper filters and an appropriate bright light source, the patient can observe 'flying corpuscles' or white blood cells if the fovea is functionally intact. Unfortunately, the test requires special apparatus, relies on a carefully discerning patient as observer, and may yield false-negative results with dense cataracts.

A Maddox rod may be used as a simple test of macular function in patients in whom the ocular media is not totally opaque. The Maddox rod is held in front of the eye to be tested and a light source is held approximately 14 inches (or 35 cm) away. If the

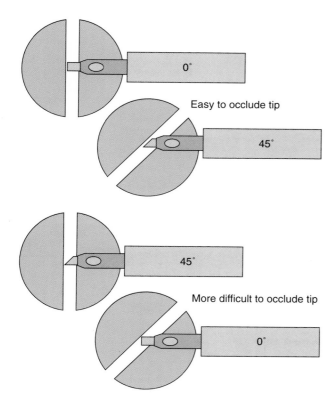

Figure 2.13. *Correct apposition of the needle bevel and the surface to be impaled is far more important than the angle of the bevel.*

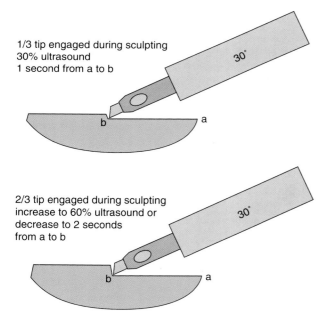

Figure 2.14. *The correct amount of phaco power is related to the linear speed of sculpting as well as the degree of tip enlargement.*

In order to appropriately adjust the machine parameters for various stages of surgery, it is necessary to analyze the function of those parameters for a given stage. For example, sculpting requires titration of ultrasound power as described in the previous paragraph. Furthermore, it requires enough flow to clear the anterior chamber of the emulsate produced by ultrasound as well as sufficient flow to cool the phaco tip; a modest flow of 18 ml/min is usually adequate for these functions. There is little need for vacuum during sculpting; there are not yet any fragments which need to be impaled and gripped. Furthermore, vacuum is not needed to counteract the repulsive action of ultrasound, since the nucleus is held stationary by the capsule, zonules, and its intact structure at this point. Therefore, a low vacuum is adequate for sculpting. Although 0 mmHg is advocated by some surgeons, a slightly higher level of 15–30 mmHg still provides significant safety (in cases of contraincisional peripheral epinuclear or capsule incarceration) while decreasing the likelihood of a clogged aspiration line.

Once the nucleus is debulked or grooved, it then needs manipulation such as rotation or cracking. These maneuvers should be performed in pedal position 1, so that the chamber will be pressurized without any pump action which might inadvertently aspirate unwanted material. Once the nucleus is debulked or cracked into fragments, machine parameters need to adapt to the needs of emulsifying these fragments. Ultrasound power requirements are lower at this stage relative to sculpting, because of the increased efficiency of phacoaspiration with complete or almost complete tip occlusion. Even with only moderate ultrasound levels, though, flow rate and vacuum must usually be increased from their sculpting levels in order to overcome the repulsive action of ultrasound at the axially vibrating needle tip. Although 26 ml/min flow rate and 120 mmHg vacuum are reasonable baseline values at this stage, these parameters should ideally be linearly titrated intraoperatively to a given ultrasound level and nuclear density. This level of control has only recently been available to the surgeon with the advent of the dual-linear pedal as previously described.

Chopping maneuvers often require further manipulation of parameters. The actual chop may require only moderate vacuum because the nucleus is mechanically fixated between the phaco tip and the chopper. However, higher vacuum levels of 200–250 mmHg can be used advantageously to grip and manipulate the nucleus. For example, the gripped nucleus can be displaced so that the chopper is more centrally located

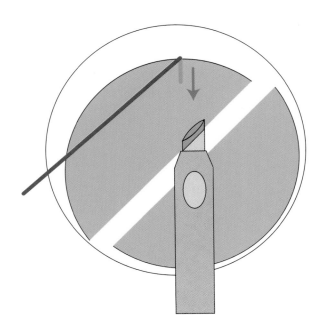

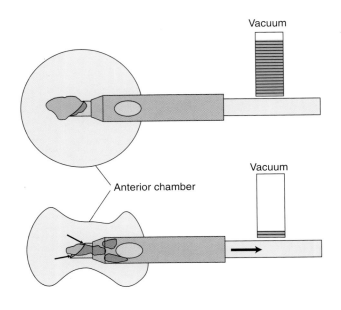

Figure 2.15. *Step and Chop Technique (Koch) with vacuum used to grip and centrally displace heminucleus for enhanced safety when starting chop.*

Figure 2.16. *Surge phenomenon.*

when engaging the nuclear periphery. This maneuver is especially effective if the nucleus was previously grooved and hemisected, as has been described by Koch and Stasiuk (Fig. 2.15). If a flow pump is used, 26 ml/min is a useful compromise between a reasonably rapid rise time and a reasonable safety margin against surge. If a vacuum pump is used at 200–250 mmHg, the surge potential is especially high. When the chop is completed and the occlusion breaks, the subsequent induced flow with a standard needle would be over 60 ml/min. A MicroFlow or similar needle with a reduced inner diameter (and therefore increased fluidic resistance) reduces this flow by about 40% to a safer level. The safest technique, though, would be to use the high vacuum level during the actual manipulation and chop when gripping the nucleus and then to dynamically decrease the vacuum with pedal control just as the chop is completed to minimize the surge potential.

Surge, as has been discussed, occurs when an occluded fragment is held by high vacuum and is then abruptly aspirated (i.e. with a burst of ultrasound); fluid tends to rush into the tip to equilibrate the built-up vacuum in the aspiration line, with, potentially, consequent shallowing or collapse of the anterior chamber (Fig. 2.16). In addition to the preventive

measures mentioned in the previous paragraph, phaco machines employ a variety of methods to combat surge. Fluidic circuits are engineered with minimal compliance which will still allow adequate ergonomic manipulation of the tubing as well as functioning of the pump mechanism, the latter being primarily important for peristaltic pumps. Small-bore aspiration line tubing, utilized by Allergan and Alcon, provides increased fluidic resistance which obtunds surges in a manner similar to that of the MicroFlow needle previously discussed. The Surgical Designs machine incorporates a second, higher irrigating bottle whose fluidic circuit is engaged upon detection of a surge. While all of these designs are helpful, it is ultimately up to the surgeon to set parameters which optimize a given machine for a given patient with regard to surge prevention.

The parameter of bottle height has a constant function during all phases of surgery: to keep the chamber safely formed without overpressurization which might stress zonules, misdirect aqueous into the vitreous, or cause excessive incisional leakage. Approximately 10 mmHg hydrostatic pressure is produced intraocularly for every 15 cm of bottle height above the eye. However, it is vital that the appropriate bottle height be set hydrodynamically

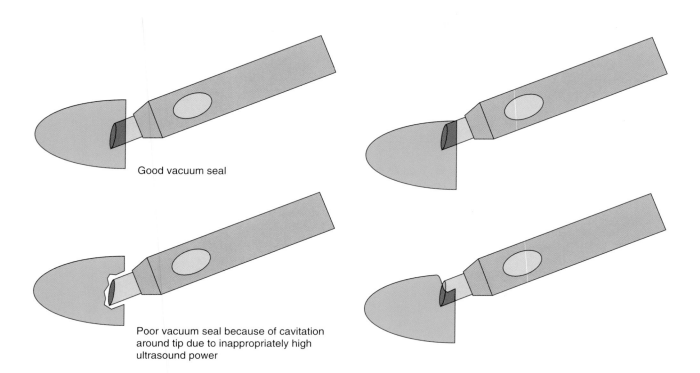

Good vacuum seal

Poor vacuum seal because of cavitation
around tip due to inappropriately high
ultrasound power

Figure 2.17. *A vacuum seal must be achieved in order for the pump to produce a grip of an occluding fragment efficiently.*

Figure 2.18. *This phaco needle is too anterior for an effective seal.*

with the pump operating (pedal position 2 or 3) and the tip unoccluded so that an adequate pressure head will be established to keep up with the induced aspiration outflow from the eye.

This chapter has stressed the importance of appropriate machine parameter settings. It should also be stressed, of course, that surgical technique is not only just as important, but is, moreover, integrally related. For example, if a surgeon wishes to grip and pull a heminucleus in preparation for chopping, but finds that the tip instead pulls away from the lens material, the tendency might be to increase the vacuum parameter to give a stronger grip. However, it is critical to remember that the full preset vacuum can be produced at the phaco tip only with complete tip occlusion regardless of whether a flow pump or a vacuum pump is employed. Therefore, if an adequate vacuum seal is not obtained, the preset value will not be reached. Increasing the vacuum preset will not affect the clinical performance in the absence of a

good vacuum seal, which is obtained by embedding the phaco tip at least 1–1.5 mm with light ultrasound energy so as to avoid excessive cavitation (Fig. 2.17). The tip is also embedded in the central densest nucleus as opposed to more peripheral, softer material which might irregularly aspirate, again causing a loss of the vacuum seal (Fig. 2.18). This subtle attention to technique pays off with the machine being used to its most effective potential.

In summary, modern phaco machines offer unprecedented levels of control and safety. In order to fully exploit these values, a thorough understanding of the principles by which the machines operate is essential. In particular, the surgeon must appropriately adjust flow rate, vacuum, ultrasound power and bottle height as necessary for a given patient and for a given stage in the operation. This vigilance and attention, coupled with meticulous technique designed to optimize the machine's performance, will result in the safest, most efficient phaco surgery.

Chapter 3 Intraocular irrigating solutions with cataract surgery

James P Gills

Optimal cataract surgery is characterized by a minimal level of anesthesia, the absence of discomfort, minimal postoperative inflammation and near-immediate visual recovery with no complications. Cataract surgical techniques have changed over the past decade to achieve these goals, and so has the composition and method of delivery of our pharmaceutical armamentarium. The goal is to use ocular pharmaceuticals during surgery that are highly effective and very specific in their effects, thus producing minimal side-effects. During the past few years, the main areas of change regarding intraoperative medication routines for cataract surgical patients have been in: (1) prevention of infection, (2) anesthesia, and (3) inflammation control and early physical and visual recovery. Delivery of appropriate pharmaceuticals for these indications has changed from systemic to more specific intraocular delivery. Use of the irrigating solution during phacoemulsification to deliver these medications intracamerally has proven effective.

PROPHYLACTIC ANTIBIOTIC TREATMENT

Delivery of antibiotics in the irrigating solution was initiated over 20 years ago. Our transition into this method of antibiotic delivery came after a series of infections when we first began implanting intraocular lenses (IOLs). These particular infections in the early 1970s were possibly related to foreign contaminants within the IOL or to the solutions we were using at that time. There were many changes in extracapsular surgical technique, and IOL designs and manufacturing quality were in transition. We had noted with interest that retinal surgeons, among them Gholam Peyman and Bob Machemer, were reporting the use of antibiotics in the surgical irrigating solution.[1] We initiated a similar regimen using the smallest effective dose possible of gentamicin sulfate and vancomycin. This was our first use of antibiotics in the irrigation solution. Since then we have made alterations to our regimens, using different antibiotics and trying both intracameral injection and delivery through the irrigation solution. Our goal has been to use the smallest possible doses of the most effective drugs. Choice of antibiotic is made to cover both Gram-positive and Gram-negative bacterial strains effectively while minimizing risk of retinal toxicity.

A very important aspect of irrigation solution and infection control is the practice of filtering the irrigation solution. The following section summarizes our history of infection control and intraocular antibiotics, through the filtered irrigation solution and by intracameral injection.

ENDOPHTHALMITIS AND INTRAOCULAR ANTIBIOTICS

Even with sterile surgical technique, infection can occur from many sources. In 1983, an epidemic of infectious endophthalmitis occurred which was traced back to commercially prepared balanced salt irrigating solution contaminated with *Candida parapsilosis*.[2] Prior to the manufacturer's recall, 110 of our patients were exposed.

None of these patients developed any sign of infection.[3] We attribute this outcome directly to our use of filtered irrigating solution. We had long been filtering our irrigating solution through a 0.2-μm millipore filter (Fig. 3.1). Prior to filtration, our incidence of endophthalmitis was 1–2 per 1000, which was the same as the national average. After filtration, our overall incidence dropped to 1 in 8000 to 10 000, but in a small series of eight cases performed without filtration, we experienced a case of endophthalmitis. Neumann et al. found particulate matter in all randomly chosen samples of balanced salt solution (BSS) from seven different manufacturers, with as

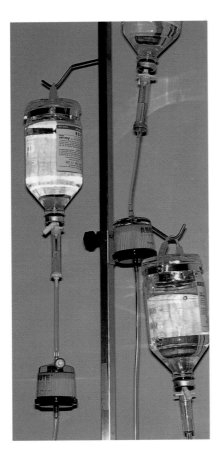

Figure 3.1. *The use of a 0.22-μm micropore filter as a prophylactic measure against postoperative endophthalmitis.*

many as 2400 particles per millimeter.[2] Thus he had recommended filtration of all intraocular solutions, corroborating our practice.

Individual studies of endophthalmitis have reported rates between 0.05% and 0.5% during the 1980s.[4-12] A 'pooled' rate of endophthalmitis was estimated by Powe et al.[13] using a series of studies evaluating cases operated during that period. They reported the pooled incidence to be 0.13%, with a 95% confidence interval of 0.09–0.17. The decrease in rates of endophthalmitis, when compared with levels earlier in the century (as high as 10%) and mid-century (up to 1.0%), has been attributed to better aseptic technique, smaller incisions, the switch to extracapsular surgery with an intact posterior capsule, decreased operative time, etc.[9] Nevertheless, the current average rate of 5–10 cases per 10 000 procedures (0.05–0.10%) results in over a thousand cases of endophthalmitis per year in this country. While rare, this complication is associated with a high rate of ocular morbidity, often leaving the patient with severely compromised vision despite rigorous treatment.

In the mid-1980s, I initiated the use of antibiotics in the irrigating solution.[3] My protocol at that time was to use gentamicin sulfate (Garamycin) solution (0.008 g/ml) filtered through a 0.2-μm millipore filter. During this period I modified the antibiotic protocol by adding vancomycin (0.1 ml at 100 mg/ml in each 500-ml bottle of BSS) to provide protection against Gram-positive bacteria, which are the most prevalent organisms cultured in endophthalmitis cases (75–90% of positive cultures).[9,10,14,15] In a series of 27 000 cases of planned extracapsular operations with limbal-based flaps using filtered solution with antibiotic, we had no incidence of endophthalmitis.[3] Sterile hypopyons, which had been prevalent at a rate of 1 per 400 before the use of antibiotics, no longer occurred.[16] The positive effect of the antibiotic use combined with filtering of the infusate caused me to conclude that some transient hypopyons may be a form of mild infection. Currently, our rate of endophthalmitis is less than 1 in every 10 000 cases. Thus we have reduced our rate to about a tenth of what it had been by use of the prophylactic treatment.

The value of prophylactic antibiotics administered both topically and by subconjunctival injection has been documented.[5,6,8,17] Past studies have shown that the incidence of endophthalmitis can be further reduced when both the topical and subconjunctival prophylactic measures are taken together. Our work demonstrates a high level of efficacy of prophylactic use of antibiotics in the irrigating solution. Clearly, the use of all available routes of prophylactic treatment should be considered. All methods we have used to deliver intracameral antibiotics have been effective in

Table 3.1

Irrigating solution.

Supplies
    Heparin 1000 units/ml
    Adrenaline 1 : 1000
    Vancomycin 50 mg/ml
    500-ml bottle BSS

Preparation
    To 500-ml bottle BSS add:
        0.8 ml heparin (800 units)
        0.5 ml adrenaline (1 : 1000)
        0.2 ml vancomycin (10 mg)

A 0.22-mm micropore filter is used to filter all irrigation solutions lidocaine has been shown to be an effective adjunct to topical anesthesia.[36]

SUMMARY

Delivery of various intraocular pharmaceuticals via the phacoemulsification fluid or by intracameral injection provides highly specific, safe and efficacious results, particularly the use of intracameral prophylactic antibiotics and intraocular lidocaine. Modern microsurgical techniques combined with topical anesthesia, intraocular lidocaine and efficient medication regimens provide the patient with a highly comfortable experience and a very safe procedure. Rigorous prophylactic measures protect against endophthalmitis and optimize safety.

REFERENCES

1 Peyman GA, May DR, Ericson ES, Apple D. Intraocular injection of gentamicin: toxic effects of clearance. *Arch Ophthalmol* 1974; **92**: 42–7.

2 Neumann AC, Dzelzkalns JJ, Bessinger DJ. Endophthalmitis investigative protocol: a plan for source identification and patient protection. *J Cataract Refract Surg* 1991; **17**: 353–8.

3 Gills JP. Prevention of endophthalmitis by intraocular solution filtration and antibiotics. *J Am Intraocul Implant Soc* 1985; **11**: 185–6.

4 Stark WJ, Worthen DM, Holladay JT, et al. The FDA report on intraocular lenses. *Ophthalmology* 1983; **90**: 311–17.

5 Christy NE, Lall P. A randomized controlled comparison of anterior and posterior periocular injection of antibiotic in the prevention of postoperative endophthalmitis. *Ophthalmic Surg* 1986; **17**: 715–18.

6 Christy NE, Lall P. Postoperative endophthalmitis following cataract surgery: effects of subconjunctival antibiotics and other factors. *Arch Ophthalmol* 1973; **90**: 361–6.

7 Allen HF, Mangiaracine AB. Bacterial endophthalmitis after cataract extraction: a study of 22 infections in 20,000 operations. *Arch Ophthalmol* 1964; **72**: 454–62.

8 Allen HF, Mangiaracine AB. Bacterial endophthalmitis after cataract extraction. II. Incidence in 36,000 consecutive operations with special reference to preoperative topical antibiotics. *Arch Ophthalmol* 1974; **91**: 3–7.

9 Novak MA, Rice TA. The realities of endophthalmitis. In: Weinstock FJ, ed. *Management and Care of the Cataract Patient* (Cambridge MA: Blackwell Scientific Publications Inc., 1992) 238–62.

10 Mamalis N. Postcataract inflammation and endophthalmitis: diagnosis, prevention, and management. In: Weinstock FJ, ed. *Management and Care of the Cataract Patient* (Cambridge MA: Blackwell Scientific Publications Inc., 1992) 222–37.

11 Kattan HM, Flynn HW, Pflugfelder SC, et al. Nosocomial endophthalmitis survey—current incidence of infection after intraocular surgery. *Ophthalmology* 1991; **98**: 227–38.

12 Javitt JC, Vitale S, Canner JK. National outcomes of cataract extraction—endophthalmitis following inpatient surgery. *Arch Ophthalmol* 1991; **109**: 1085–9.

13 Powe NR, Schein OD, Gieser SC, et al. Synthesis of the literature on visual acuity and complications following cataract extraction with intraocular lens implantation. *Arch Ophthalmol* 1994; **112**: 239–52.

14 Gills JP. Antibiotics in irrigating solutions. *J Cataract Refract Surg* 1987; **13**: 344.

15 Gills JP. Filters and antibiotics in irrigating solution for cataract surgery. *J Cataract Refract Surg* 1991; **17**: 385.

16 Gills JP. Sterile hypopyon. *J Cataract Refract Surg* 1992; **18**: 203.

17 Christy NE, Sommer A. Antibiotic prophylaxis of postoperative endophthalmitis. *Ann Ophthalmol* 1979; **11**: 1261–5.

18 Leaming DV. Practice styles and preferences of ASCRS members—1996 survey. *J Cataract Refract Surg* 1997; **23**: 527–35.

19 Alfonso EC, Flynn HW. Controversies in endophthalmitis prevention. *Arch Ophthalmol* 1995; **113**: 1369–70.

20 Donnenfeld E. Should we use antibiotics in the infusion bottle? No. They're ineffective and dangerous. *Rev Ophthalmol* 1997; **4**: 132–4.

21 Fiscella RG. Vancomycin use in ophthalmology. *Arch Ophthalmol* 1995; **113**: 353–4.

22 Masket S. ASCRS endophthalmitis survey. Presented at the 1997 annual meeting of the ASCRS, Boston, MA.

23 Hospital Infection Control Practices Advisory Committee. Recommendations for preventing the spread of vancomycin resistance. *Infect Control Hosp Epidemiol* 1995; **16**: 105–13.

24 Freeman J, Freeman J. Should we use antibiotics in the infusion bottle? Yes. It is best to cover our bases. *Rev Ophthalmol* 1997; **4**: 133–7.

25 Ferro JF, de-Pablos M, Logrono MJ, et al. Postoperative contamination after using vancomycin and gentamicin during phacoemulsification. *Arch Ophthalmol* 1997; **115**: 165–70.

26 Kraff MC, Sanders DR, Jampol LM, et al. Prophylaxis of pseudophakic cystoid macular edema with topical indomethacin. *Ophthalmology* 1982; **89**: 885–90.

27 Flach AJ, Stegman RC, Graham J, Kruger LP. Prophylaxis of aphakic cystoid macular edema without corticosteroids: a paired comparison. *Ophthalmology* 1990; **97**: 1253–8.

28 Miyake K, Sakamura S, Miura H. Longterm follow-up study on the prevention of aphakic cystoid macular oedema by topical indomethacin. *Br J Ophthalmol* 1980; **64**: 324–8.

29 Yannuzi LA, Landau AN, Turtz AI. Incidence of aphakic cystoid macular edema with the use of optical indomethacin. *Ophthalmology* 1981; **88**: 947–54.

30 Sanders DR, Kraff M. Steroidal and non-steroidal anti-inflammatory agents: effect on post-surgical inflammation and blood aqueous humor barrier breakdown. *Arch Ophthalmol* 1984; **102**: 1453–6.

31 Kraff MC, Sanders DR, McGuigan L, Raanan MG. Inhibition of blood aqueous humor barrier breakdown with diclofenac: a fluorophotometric study. *Arch Ophthalmol* 1990; **108**: 380–3.

32 Flach AJ, Kraff MC, Sanders DR, Tannenbaum L. The quantitative effect of 0.5% ketorolac tromethamine solution and 0.1% dexamethasone sodium phosphate solution on postsurgical blood–aqueous barrier. *Arch Ophthalmol* 1988; **106**: 480–3.

33 Gimbel HV. The effect of treatment with topical nonsteroidal anti-inflammatory drugs with and without epinephrine on the maintenance of mydriasis during cataract surgery. *Ophthalmology* 1989; **97**: 585–8.

34 Keates RH, McGowan KA. The effect of topical indomethacin ophthalmic solution in maintaining mydriasis during cataract surgery. *Ann Ophthalmol* 1984; **16**: 1116–21.

35 Keates RH, McGowan KA. Clinical trial of flurbiprofen to maintain pupillary dilation during cataract surgery. *Ann Ophthalmol* 1984; **16**: 919–21.

36 Gills JP, Cherchio M, Raanan MG. Unpreserved lidocaine to control discomfort during cataract surgery using topical anesthesia. *J Cataract Refract Surg* 1997; **23**: 545–50.

37 Fichman RA. Topical anesthesia. In: Fine IH, Fichman RA, Grabow HB, eds. *Clear Cornea Cataract Surgery and Topical Anesthesia* (Thorofare, New Jersey: Slack, Inc., 1993) 97–162.

Chapter 4 Phaco chop — development and recent advances

Kunihiro B Nagahara

BIRTH OF PHACO CHOP

The phaco chop technique was born out of need on 23 November 1992. On that day I had 10 cataract operations and half of them were hard and mature. Since 1989, my routine cataract surgery technique had been the divide and conquer (D&C) technique, described by Gimbel. However, a Morganian cataract required that phaco chop be used for the first time. Regarding the Morganian cataract, the nucleus is freely mobile in the liquified cortex and one cannot make a trough to perform the D&C technique. I therefore tried to hold the nucleus with a hook and a phacoemulsification (phaco) tip. After I caught the nucleus, it cracked into two pieces. This was the first phaco chop (Fig. 4.1). After this, the residual nucleus fragments were cracked in the same manner and removed from the capsular bag. From this surgery, I understood the nature of the nucleus to be cracked, and my operation technique gradually changed from D&C to the phaco chop. Phaco chop is so-called because the method of cracking the nucleus is similar to chopping wood. I used the Sinsky hook for a while, but it was not effective for some cases because the point of the hook was short. I therefore modified and improved the Sinsky hook and made the phaco chopper.

MECHANISM OF THE PHACO CHOP

A substance with a lamella structure can easily be cracked along the direction of its fibers. Wood is broken simply in the direction of the fibers with an axe and a chopping block, and the phaco chop applies this principle (Fig. 4.2). The crystalline lens fiber runs from one side of the equator towards the opposite side through the center of the nucleus, if we do not consider the

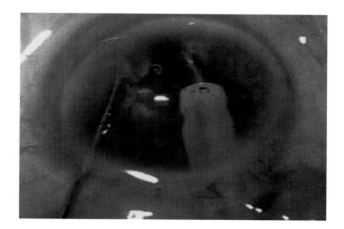

Figure 4.1. *First phaco chop.*

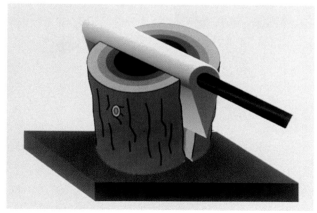

Figure 4.2. *Wood chopping. Phaco chop applies this mechanism*

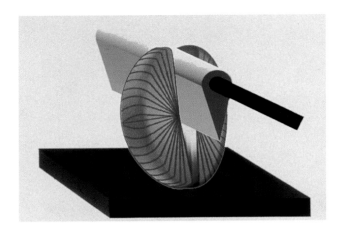

Figure 4.3. *Image of the phaco chop.*

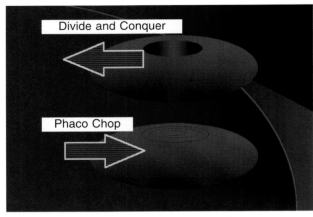

Figure 4.4. *Difference between phaco chop and D & C.*

complex anatomy of a Y-suture. Therefore, the human crystalline lens nucleus is also cracked in the direction of the lens fibers (Fig. 4.3). In the phaco chop technique, the phaco chopper is an axe and the phaco tip is a chopping block. It is hard to crack a new and soft wood, but an old and hard wood is easy to crack with an axe. In the same way, a hard nucleus can easily be cracked, and the phaco chop technique is more effective for a hard nucleus than a soft one.

DIFFERENCE BETWEEN PHACO CHOP AND D&C

The distinct difference between phaco chop and D&C is the cracking direction of the nucleus. In the phaco chop technique, the cracking direction is from the equator to the center. In the D&C technique, it is from the center to the equator. Therefore, in the D&C technique we need to sculpt the center of the nucleus to make a trough or a crater to start the cracking from the center. But in the phaco chop we do not have to make a trough or crater, because the cracking starts from the equator (Fig. 4.4). Instead, we need to stick the phaco tip into the nucleus and insert the phaco chopper into the space between equator and capsule at the 6 o'clock position (Fig. 4.5). Then, the phaco chopper is drawn to the phaco tip to crack the nucleus (Fig. 4.6). We need no sculpting during the procedure, so we can reduce the phaco energy compared to the other phaco technique. Sculpting is the easiest and safest step of the operation, but there is no sculpting in the phaco chop.

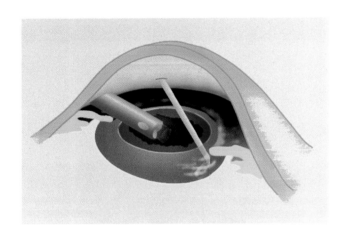

Figure 4.5. *Key point of the phaco chop. Phaco tip holds the nucleus and phaco chopper on the equator.*

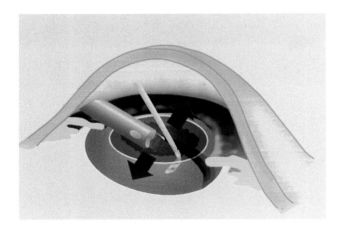

Figure 4.6. *First chop.*

PEA AND PAE

When we remove the nucleus from the eye, the efficiency of the procedure is different in two situations, phacoemulsification aspiration (PEA) and phacoaspiration emulsification (PAE). In PEA, the phaco tip port is opened and the nucleus is emulsified and then aspirated afterwards so the power available to break and remove the nucleus is phaco energy only. But in PAE, the port is closed first with the aspirated nucleus and then emulsified, so the power available to break and remove the nucleus fragment comprises the phaco energy and the aspiration vacuum (Fig. 4.7). As a result, in PAE we can use less phaco energy than with PEA. This enables us to cut the operation time, leading to less wound and endothelial damage. In the phaco chop technique, all of the procedure is PAE, so we are able to remove the nucleus by low energy and more effectively.

PHACO CHOPPER

The phaco chopper is necessary when we perform the phaco chop. When I started using the phaco chop, I used the Sinsky hook as a second instrument. However, I experienced some difficulty with this, so I improved the Sinsky hook and made the phaco chopper. In a trial, I made phaco choppers of three lengths (length of tip: 1.25 mm, 1.5 mm, 1.75 mm). After many operations, we recognized that the phaco chopper with a length of 1.5 mm was best. After deciding what the best length was, I improved the shape of the point and made a wedge-shaped one to enable easy chopping of the hard nucleus. We can chop a soft nucleus with a short-point Sinsky hook, but for the hard nucleus the wedge-shaped-point phaco chopper is very effective (Fig. 4.8).

ZERO TIP

The bevel of a phaco tip is prepared in order to shave (sculpt) a nucleus. In the phaco chop technique, there is no need to shave a nucleus. Therefore, the bevel is not needed for this technique, so I eliminated the bevel of the phaco tip and made the zero tip. The zero tip which I designed has no bevel but it has a sharp inside cutting edge (Fig. 4.9). Therefore, the

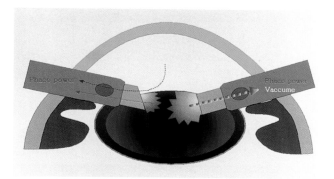

Figure 4.7. *PAE is more effective than PEA.*

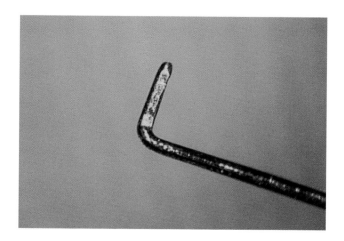

Figure 4.8. *Wedge-shaped phaco chopper.*

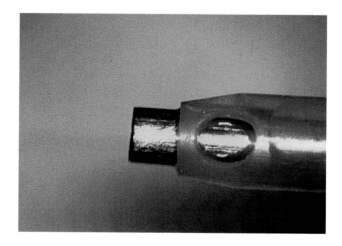

Figure 4.9. *Zero tip.*

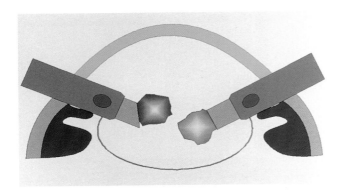

Figure 4.10. *Zero tip catches the nucleus in the capsular bag.*

All of these machines are equipped with the zero tip, but the Diplomat is the only machine that has the inside cutting edge zero tip. The Legacy, with a specially designed tubing cassette, can be used at a high-vacuum setting without any surge, so we can perform high-vacuum PAE and reduce the phaco energy much more than with the other machines.

PHACO CHOP TECHNIQUE

As in other operations, continuous curvilinear capsulo-rhexis (CCC) and hydrodissection are important and necessary in this technique. After the hydrodissection is completed, the phaco tip is inserted into the anterior chamber and the epinucleus inside the CCC is aspirated with use of weak phaco energy. If the epinucleus cannot be removed, the phaco chop technique becomes difficult, because the phaco tip cannot reach to the center of the nucleus. However, removing the epinucleus is not necessary for a dense cataract with a small epinucleus. The phaco chopper is introduced into the anterior chamber through the side-port incision before the phaco tip starts to stick the nucleus. The nucleus is slightly dislocated to the 6 o'clock position with the phaco chopper and then the phaco tip is driven into the nucleus (Fig. 4.11). We have to pay careful attention when sticking the soft nucleus, because the zero tip will penetrate the nucleus easily with the use of high vacuum and high phaco energy. When the phaco tip holds the nucleus exactly, pull and dislocate it with the phaco tip a little towards 12 o'clock and make a space between the nucleus equator and the capsule at 6 o'clock. Insert the phaco chopper there (Fig. 4.12). When an anterior capsulotomy is small, we have to take care not to injure it. It is easy to insert the phaco chopper when the equator of the nucleus is moved inside the CCC. I draw the chopper towards the

zero tip has the same shaving capability as a 45° phaco tip and more aspiration power. With use of the zero tip, the vacuum power is utilized effectively, and ultrasound (US) energy can therefore be reduced. The zero tip always catches the nucleus fragments at the tip end (Fig. 4.10), but the beveled US tip catches them on the bevel, so the location of the phaco is far from the corneal endothelium with the zero tip compared to the beveled tip. This also contributes to there being less corneal endothelial damage.

MACHINE SETTING

I use three phaco machines in my routine cataract surgery. These machines are Diplomat (Allergan), Legacy (Alcon), and Protégé (Storz). My settings for each machine during phaco are as shown in Table 4.1.

Table 4.1.
Phaco machines.

Machine	Type of pump	US control	US power (%)	US vacuum (mmHg)	US flow rate (ml/min)	US tip
Diplomat	Peristaltic	Linear	70	110	24	0
Legacy	Peristaltic	Linear	60	300–400	25	0
Protégé	Venturi	Linear	50	150	—	0

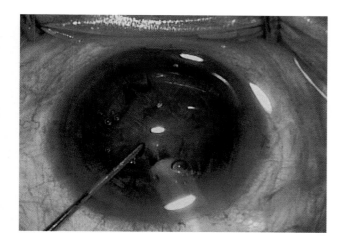

Figure 4.11. *Phaco tip driving into nucleus.*

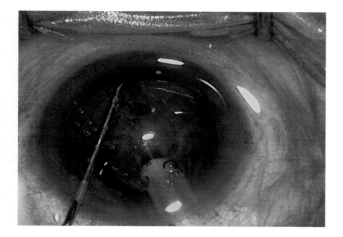

Figure 4.12. *Phaco chopper insertion.*

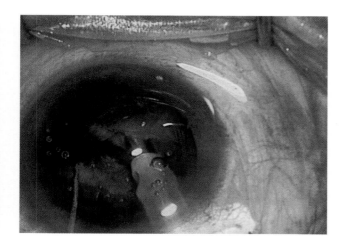

Figure 4.13. *Phaco chop.*

phaco tip and chop the nucleus into two pieces (Fig. 4.13). After the first chop is completed, the nucleus is rotated 90° and the inferior half-piece is chopped into quadrants. The two quadrant pieces are gently aspirated and phacoemulsified in the capsular bag. Then, the superior half-fragment is rotated 180° and divided. The steps of emulsification are accomplished in the center of the capsular bag to prevent corneal endothelial damage and posterior capsule rupture. Generally, I chop the soft lens nucleus into four pieces, but in the case of a hard nucleus I make eight or more pieces, because the residual small fragments after emulsification of the large piece come easily into the anterior chamber and injure the corneal endothelium; it is therefore safer to make small nucleus pieces in the case of a hard nucleus cataract.

KARATE PHACO CHOP

Karate phaco chop reinforces a weak point of the phaco chop. In the phaco chop technique, the phaco chopper has to be inserted under the anterior capsule and needs to go to the equator. When mydriasis is bad, we have to insert the phaco chopper under the iris blindly. This is a very dangerous and difficult procedure. The karate phaco chop technique overcomes this weak point. In this technique, the whole procedure is completed within a pupil or CCC. The power to crack the nucleus with the phaco chop goes from the equator to the center, but with the karate phaco chop it goes from the anterior pole to the posterior pole of the crystalline lens (Fig. 4.14).

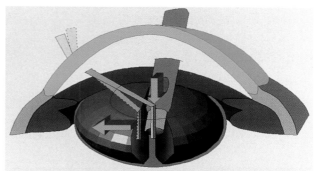

Figure 4.14. *Cracking direction of the karate phaco chop.*

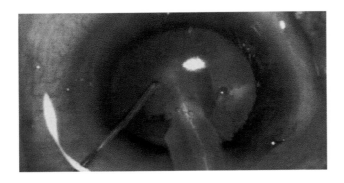

Figure 4.15. *Smoke from the nucleus.*

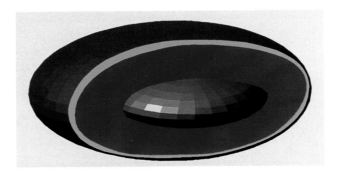

Figure 4.16. *Dual structure of the hard nucleus.*

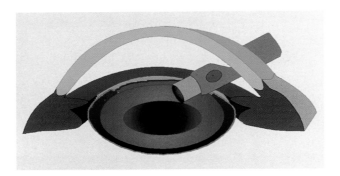

Figure 4.17. *Phaco tip cannot catch the core without sculpting.*

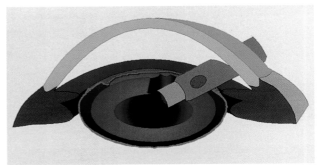

Figure 4.18. *Crater phaco chop. Phaco tip can catch the core.*

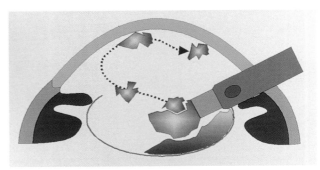

Figure 4.19. *Endothelial damage by nucleus fragments.*

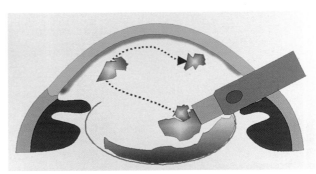

Figure 4.20. *Low molecular weight viscoelastics protect endothelium.*

There is therefore no need to take the phaco chopper to the equator of the crystalline lens, and the cracking procedure is performed within visible range. This is effective for a small pupil and a small CCC. However, this technique is not very suitable for a soft nucleus. In cases with good mydriasis and a soft nucleus, it is better to perform the usual phaco chop technique. The karate phaco chop technique is effective for a nucleus with hardness grade 3 or more. During an operation, if lens smoke is emitted when the phaco tip is driven into a nucleus (Fig. 4.15), this is a sign that the karate phaco chop is effective and a nucleus is hard.

CRATER PHACO CHOP

The epinucleus of a hard nucleus is thin, and a hard nucleus has a dual structure, consisting of an outer soft and inner hard nucleus (core) (Fig. 4.16). Moreover, a hard nucleus is thicker than a soft nucleus, and the posterior pole part is harder and more elastic. With nuclei of grade 4 or 5 (brown or black cataract), the phaco chop is not completed easily. The phaco tip has to catch the core of the nucleus, and a point of the chopper should go over the equator and arrive at the posterior pole side. It is not difficult to take a point of the phaco chopper over the equator, but it is difficult to catch the core of the nucleus with the phaco tip. Even if the phaco tip is driven to the nucleus after the thin epinucleus has been removed, a core cannot be caught (Fig. 4.17). Therefore, it is essential to shave and make a crater in the outer layer in order to stick the phaco tip into the nucleus (Fig. 4.18). After a crater is made, the phaco tip is driven towards the wall of it. The best depth of the crater depends on the hardness of each nucleus, but we need more than the width of the phaco tip. In my routine surgery of a hard nucleus cataract, sometimes the first chopping procedure does not go well and fails. In such cases, the phaco chopper tip is moved to a deep place of a crevasse and the nucleus is divided again. Even if this does not go well, a crater should be deepened more, and an attempt made to catch a core of a nucleus.

In the case of a divided hard nucleus, the side rim becomes sharp, especially the apex of the wedge-shaped nucleus. We may therefore break the posterior capsule with a mobile nucleus. In such cases, it is important to catch the sharp apex of the wedge-shaped fragment first, so that this does not harm the posterior capsule.

VISCOSURGERY

A weak point of the phaco chop technique is that large nucleus fragments are mobile in the eye, and a mobile nucleus can move into the anterior chamber and damage the corneal endothelium (Fig. 4.19). There are two ways to prevent this. The first is to divide a hard nucleus into small fragments and try to handle a nucleus below the anterior capsule. Small nucleus fragments are aspirated and emulsified with the phaco tip at the same time, so there is less chance of the fragment coming into the anterior chamber. If the nucleus is soft, it will be divided into four quadrants. The second way is to use low molecular weight viscoelastic material. High molecular weight viscoelastic material can remain in the deep anterior chamber and the capsular bag when an intraocular lens is implanted, but it leaves the eye with irrigating solution during phaco, so there is a chance of the corneal endothelium being damaged. Low molecular weight viscoelastic material stays in the anterior chamber during phaco and protects the corneal endothelium, so this also reinforces the weak points of the phaco chop technique (Fig. 4.20).

Chapter 5 Advanced technology for phacoemulsification

I Howard Fine and Richard S Hoffman

Dramatic improvements in phacoemulsification (phaco) technology involving every aspect of phaco systems have been occurring over recent years. Improvements in the generation of ultrasonic power, fluidics, user interfaces, and tips and handpieces have been extremely advantageous to the cataract surgeon. It is because of these innovations that phaco continues to evolve as a safe and effective technique and has rapidly become the primary extraction technique in many parts of the developing world, despite the challenges of harder, darker nuclei.

ULTRASONICS

Advances in the generation of ultrasonic power stem from improvements in both the quality and quantity of crystals in the piezoelectric crystal configuration in systems such as the Alcon Series 20,000 Legacy. The ultrasonic driver in the Legacy is controlled by a dedicated microprocessor which allows for exact control of ultrasonic power at all power levels. The turbosonic handpiece utilizes a four-crystal transducer design which is capable of producing a much more standard and reproducible stroke length at each power setting regardless of the load (mass and density of nuclear material) at the phaco tip. Since the load is continually changing, the system must be able to adjust or else the cutting efficiency will be compromised. The Legacy is able to maximize efficiency by utilizing a new complex control system, 'constant admittance tuning', which matches the driving frequency of the console to the operating frequency at the phaco handpiece, maintaining optimal power regardless of lens density.[1]

The new Mentor SIStem uses similar feedback technology, utilizing AutoScan Digital Harmonic Tuning, which assesses subtle differences in individual handpieces and locks onto the optimum resonant frequency for each. Throughout phaco, digital software maintains optimum performance by constantly fine-tuning the ultrasonic driver to compensate for variations in lens density. This results in smooth, precise energy transfer at all power levels.

Some of the other advances affecting the ultrasonic generation of energy for phaco involve technology that harnesses options for judicious application of power, such as the power modulations available on the AMO Diplomax System. Among these modulations are autopulse phaco, burst-mode phaco, and occlusion-mode phaco.

In autopulse phaco, the phaco handpiece will run in continuous power mode at high phaco powers and will automatically change to pulsed power when the foot pedal is eased into lower powers. This setting is useful for grooving the central nucleus at higher powers in continuous mode while using the more delicate control of pulsed phaco at lower powers for extending the groove out of the periphery if desired. Burst-mode phaco produces bursts of 40-, 60- or 80-ms duration at preset ultrasound power levels when the foot pedal is placed in position 3. This mode is helpful for impaling the nucleus for chopping techniques and in quadrant removal, where vacuum accompanied by intermittent bursts of power is commonly utilized. Finally, occlusion-mode phaco allows for power modulation of the phaco handpiece in continuous, pulse, autopulse, burst, or power-off modes, depending on whether the phaco tip is occluded or unoccluded (Table 32.1). This setting allows for the judicious use of phaco power with programmable vacuum levels and aspiration rates.[2] All of these modulations allow for programmable changes in ultrasound energy delivered to the eye, so that inappropriate energy that can result in

Table 5.1

Ultrasonic modes available in occluded and unoccluded states. In this example, sculpting occurs in continuous mode prior to tip occlusion. Once occlusion takes place, the ultrasonic energy switches to pulse mode.

High Vacuum Tubing Phaco Power Mode (Sculpting - Phaco 1)	
Unoccluded	*Occluded*
Continuous	Continuous
Pulse 33%	**Pulse 33%**
Pulse 50%	Pulse 50%
Pulse 66%	Pulse 66%
Autopulse	Autopulse
Burst 40 ms	Burst 40 ms
Burst 60 ms	Burst 60 ms
Burst 80 ms	Burst 80 ms
Power OFF	Power OFF

increased chatter and less purchase of nuclear material can be avoided.

PHACOTMESIS

Other energy sources have been combined with ultrasound with the hope of achieving enhanced efficiency; however, it is difficult to foresee whether these new technologies will find a market niche. Phacotmesis combines high-speed mechanical rotatory power with ultrasonic linear oscillation, with the achievement of some added safety for the iris, corneal endothelium, and posterior capsule. The tmesis tip is covered by the irrigating silicone sleeve, so there is no sharp oscillating or rotating tip exposed to touch or damage vital intraocular tissues. The tmesis tip creates a pulverizing effect on the nucleus at a small distance just in front of the tip without the need for actual contact. In addition, the rotating tip creates a circular fluid current which, combined with the aspiration flow, causes a microscopic whirlpool effect that maintains the followability of the lens fragments within the pulverizing aspiration zone.[3] Although there is added safety from phacotmesis, this may be at the expense of efficiency.

LASER

In the constant search for improvements in cataract extraction, surgeons have begun to investigate laser energy as an alternative energy source to ultrasound. Four ultraviolet (excimer) laser wavelengths have been investigated, including 193 nm (argon fluoride), 248 nm (krypton fluoride), 308 nm (xenon chloride), and 351 nm (xenon fluoride). Use of the excimer laser for cataract removal appears to be hampered by limitations in fiber optic technology and safety concerns regarding possible injury to the surgeon and patient from ultraviolet excimer laser energy.[4]

Concern regarding the safety of ultraviolet wavelengths has led to the investigation of the infrared wavelengths as potential energy sources for cataract removal. The Nd:YLF 1053-nm picosecond laser has been shown to be effective in softening the lens and cortex by external ablation followed by internal standard irrigation and aspiration. The main disadvantage of this technique is that it requires a two-stage procedure, since no intraocular device using this wavelength currently exists.[4]

Premier Laser Systems, in conjunction with Dr D Michael Colvard, has designed and manufactured an erbium:YAG laser for cataract extraction which offers many advantages compared to ultrasound energy. The erbium laser uses non-ultraviolet radiation and can be delivered through a fiber optic delivery system, so that cataract extraction can be performed with a one-stage intraocular technique. In addition, the erbium laser can be used to perform a continuous curvilinear capsulotomy and ablates tissue without thermal injury. This laser offers a substantially gentler lens-cutting mechanism with a shorter learning curve than ultrasonic phaco, potentially making small-incision cataract surgery more accessible to a greater number of surgeons around the world.[5]

The Nd:YAG laser, the energy source most commonly associated with intraocular applications, has been the most studied of all energy sources and is presently in clinical use as part of an FDA-sponsored study in the USA and in studies in other countries. The laser developed by Paradigm Medical Industries uses a solid-state pulsed Nd:YAG 1064-nm laser whose energy can be delivered through a fiber optic intraocular delivery system. In this system, a columnated beam allows for a high energy density for efficient emulsification while permitting the beam to be confined within a metal-walled chamber.[6]

A Nd:YAG 1064-nm laser developed by Dr Jack Dodick differs from the Paradigm laser in that the lens is not ablated by applying laser energy directly to the lens. In his system, the lens is disrupted by shock waves created by the laser striking a titanium target within the probe. The use of a titanium target greatly reduces the threshold needed for optical breakdown of lens material, allowing for much lower energy use compared to the quantity of energy required without a target. In addition, the titanium target shields the surrounding intraocular structures as well as the eyes of the surgeon from direct laser light.[4]

Although these lasers are still restricted except under FDA-approved clinical trials, eventual approval for widespread clinical use by cataract surgeons worldwide has the potential of replacing ultrasonic phaco with a safer, more efficient, laser energy source.

HOT WATER

Dr Mark Andrew has patented a process in which pulsed hot water is used to dissolve cataracts while simultaneously killing lens epithelial cells. The procedure does not damage either the lens capsule or the corneal endothelium. By destruction of the lens epithelial cells, it is hoped that posterior capsular fibrosis, anterior capsule phimosis and instances of lens decentration will be markedly reduced. The process is being developed into prototypes by Alcon Surgical (personal communication).

FLUIDICS

The most important recent advance in phaco fluidics involves high-vacuum cassettes and tubing which allow use of much higher vacuums than were previously considered safe in an intraocular environment. These cassettes have resulted in the ability to utilize vacuum as an extractive instrument, with a reduced need for the application of ultrasound energy. With high-vacuum cassettes, ultrasound is utilized mainly for fashioning segments of nuclear material in such a way that they continuously occlude the tip for evacuation by the vacuum. New pump systems make the achievement of vacuum smoother and more precise, and microprocessor controls help to achieve stabilization of the anterior chamber. High-vacuum tubing is generally thicker-walled and has a narrower bore than standard tubing, resulting in some restriction of movement of

fluid through it. As a result, there is an inherent increase in safety resulting from downsized tips and vacuum tubing, so that, with loss of occlusion at the tip, the added resistance to flow prevents fluid from moving rapidly through the tip and the tubing. This added resistance markedly reduces collapse of the anterior chamber and vaulting of the posterior capsule.

In addition to high-vacuum cassettes and the ability to utilize vacuum in extraction techniques, one of the more important changes in fluidics has been the programmable vacuum rise times available on several machines, such as the AMO Diplomax, Surgical Design Ocusystem II, and the Mentor SIStem. In systems which utilize a peristaltic pump, the speed of vacuum rise following occlusion of the tip is directly proportional to the aspiration rate. Thus, a low aspiration rate will produce a slow vacuum rise time, and a high aspiration rate will produce a fast vacuum rise time.

With occlusion-mode phaco, the AMO Diplomax has the ability to program an occluded aspiration rate that is independent of the aspiration rate in the non-occluded state. With this ability, the surgeon can program a low aspiration rate setting in the non-occluded state with a slow or fast vacuum rise time once occlusion occurs, or a high aspiration rate setting in the non-occluded state followed by a slow or fast vacuum rise time in the occluded state.[2]

This feature allows the surgeon to customize flow and vacuum rise times for each stage in the phaco procedure. For instance, sculpting can occur with a low aspiration rate and slow vacuum rise time, allowing the surgeon adequate time to react if undesired occlusion takes place. During nuclear quadrant removal, a low aspiration rate with a fast vacuum rise time allows the quadrant to be seized under low flow without aspiration of the surrounding epinucleus. Then, once occlusion occurs, the vacuum will rise quickly, allowing the quadrant to be extracted efficiently for emulsification. Finally, a high aspiration rate and slow vacuum rise time can be programmed for safe and efficient removal of the epinucleus. This is performed by allowing the high flow rate to attract the epinucleus towards the tip without having to extend the tip out towards the periphery; once occlusion takes place, a slow vacuum rise time will aspirate the epinucleus in a slower, more controlled, environment which is less likely to rupture the posterior capsule.[2] The sophistication of the AMO Diplomax allows the surgeon the option of choosing from any one of a number of power modulations of vacuum and aspiration flow rates in the non-occluded state and a wide variety of other parameters in the occluded state, all during the same step within the cataract procedure.

Two additional innovations with respect to fluidics involve reverse-flow phaco, first described by Kelman. In this system, the standard sources of irrigation and aspiration are reversed—gravity-fed fluid from the irrigation bottle is directed through the phaco needle, and aspiration fluid exits the eye through the side-ports in the silicone sleeve. Reverse-flow sculpting allows the phaco tip to safely sculpt very deeply without the risk of capturing and rupturing the posterior capsule, since it is always being repulsed by the fluid flowing from the phaco tip.[7] Singer's 'phaco unplugged' utilizes a similar mechanism, with appropriate placement of valves between the lines in the OcuSystem II.

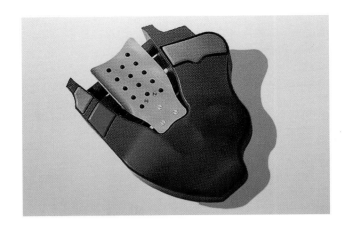

Figure 5.1. *Storz Millennium dual-linear foot controller.*

USER INTERFACE

Improvements and changes in user interfaces have simplified the surgeon's life in the operating room and made phaco more efficient. Most new systems have multiple programmable features. The most sophisticated utilization of these systems allows separate programs to be set up for multiple surgeons in any one facility, different grades of nuclei for each surgeon, and different steps by any particular surgeon during the same procedure. A variety of graphics and clearly recognizable icons are available in many of the systems, expediting the programmable features of these machines.

The Alcon Legacy System and Storz Millennium have voice confirmation of changes in phaco programs, freeing the surgeon to respond once the program has changed without having to wait for a nurse or technicians's confirmation. The new Mentor SIStem has three distinct volume-controlled, dual-channel tones which provide stereo feedback of flow rate, vacuum level and phaco power, to alert surgeons to changes in parameters throughout the procedure. The foot pedal of the AMO Diplomax has a control for the program changes, so that a kick to the right takes the machine to a second program, and another kick to a third program, and a kick to the left moves back one program. This frees the surgeon from having to communicate with the operating room staff and wait for confirmation of the change.

Many of the machines have complete set-up programs that, through graphical and icon representation, enable the technician to automatically prime the machine and confirm its readiness. In addition, there are trouble-shooting programs which allow one to rapidly search for sources of trouble.

Perhaps the most sophisticated user interface exists in the foot controller of the new Storz Millenium (Fig. 5.1). The foot controller allows the surgeon to control most of the functions contained within the microsurgical system. The most innovative aspect of the new controller is the dual-linear feature, which allows the surgeon to control both ultrasound power and vacuum in a linear fashion, using two different planes of movement in the foot pedal, both pitch and yaw. In the dual-linear mode, up and down movement of the pedal (pitch) linearly controls vacuum levels within programmable ranges, while outward side movement of the pedal (yaw) linearly controls ultrasound power. Using this dual-linear mode, the surgeon can simultaneously control both power and vacuum levels, enabling exquisite control of these functions. The pedal can also be used in traditional single-linear mode for linear control of ultrasound power, aspiration, or bipolar coagulation in the standard up and down direction. The foot controller also enables the surgeon to change preprogrammed numerical ranges for ultrasound power or vacuum using a rocker switch. All of these features allow the surgeon to function more independently of the operating room staff, with more control over every aspect of the surgical procedure.

PHACO TIPS AND HANDPIECES

Probably the most widely expanding area in phaco instrumentation involves improvements in phaco tips.

Increasingly there has been an attempt to down-size tips and modify sleeves so that they are easier to insert through the incision. In addition, much thought has been given to designing tips which will reduce the incidence of incisional burns and increase cutting efficiency.

Several phaco tips have been designed specifically to reduce incision burns. These include the MicroSeal tip, the MicroFlow tip, the Martin Quadraflow tip (Mastel Instruments), the Alcon Aspiration Bypass, and the spiral-sleeved Cobra tip (Surgical Design).

The MicroSeal tip (Mackool system) contains a central titanium needle, surrounded by a Teflon fluid jacket (Fig. 5.2), both of which are surrounded by a soft silicone sleeve (Fig. 5.3). The soft outer silicone sleeve is designed to deform to the shape of the incision, preventing incisional outflow. The inner

rigid Teflon jacket acts as a heat insulator and a cooling jacket. It prevents the silicone sleeve from being compressed against the titanium ultrasonic needle by the incision, thus preventing heat transfer from the vibrating needle to the incisional tissue. The MicroSeal tip has an added benefit in that it allows for a large expansion of the anterior segment space and dramatically reduces the total volume traveling through the eye during a procedure. At the same time, it enhances followability because all fluid exits the eye through the phaco needle, rather than turbulence being created by competing currents passing through the phaco needle and through the incision.[8]

The MicroFlow tip, designed by Dr Graham Barrett, has spiral grooves in the outer wall of the phaco needle against which the silicone sleeve cannot be fully compressed (Figs. 5.4 and 5.5). As a

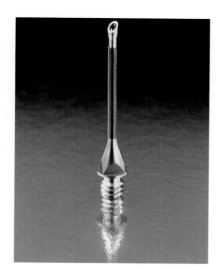

Figure 5.2. *The MicroSeal phaco tip.*

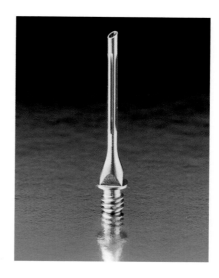

Figure 5.4. *The MicroFlow phaco tip.*

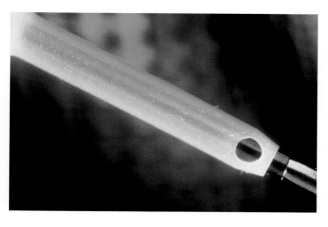

Figure 5.3. *Silicone infusion sleeve surrounding the MicroSeal tip.*

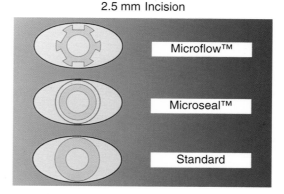

Figure 5.5. *Profiles of the MicroFlow, MicroSeal and conventional phaco tips within a small incision.*

Martin Quadraflo

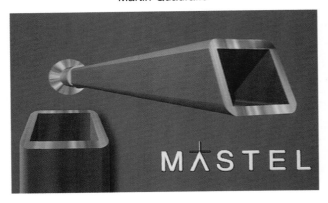

Figure 5.6. *Mastel Instruments' Martin Quadroflow phaco tip.*

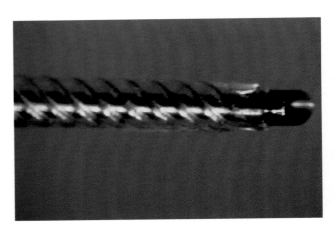

Figure 5.7. *Surgical Design Cobra tip surrounded by a non-compressible spiral-ridged polysulfone sleeve.*

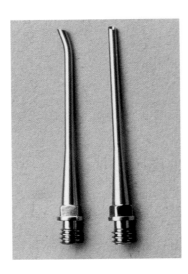

Figure 5.8. *Comparison of the standard tubosonic tip (left) and the Kelman tip with a 30° bevel (right).*

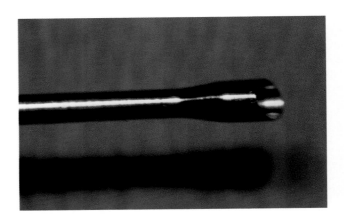

Figure 5.9. *Surgical Design Cobra tip, wide distally, narrow proximally, with a funnel-shaped acoustic orifice.*

result, there is always some cooling fluid flowing around the needle in the grooves, even during instances when the incision may be compressing the sleeve against the needle.

In a similar fashion, the Martin Quadraflow tip (Fig. 5.6) was designed to allow greater amounts of fluid to flow around the vibrating needle because of its square configuration. This particular tip is useful for grooving because it allows for very precise narrow grooves. It is also helpful for chopping, because of the flat angle of contact between the nuclear material and the tip. The Alcon aspiration bypass tip has a small opening in it to prevent complete occlusion of the tip. Since there is always some outflow through the tip, there is always some inflow around the tip—

this protects against thermal injury to the incision but necessitates higher flow and vacuum settings. Finally, the spiral sleeve of Surgical Design's Cobra tip (Fig. 5.7) is designed to avoid complete occlusion of inflow around a tight incision, thus lowering the possibility of incision heating.

Innovations for the phaco tip are also related to increasing cutting efficiency. The Kelman tip (Fig. 5.8), which has a 30° downward bend at the front portion of the needle, achieves increased non-axial vibration, which produces considerable enhancement of the cavitational energy at the tip. This results in a greatly improved ability to cut or groove nuclear material in advance or in front of the tip without a need for contact of the nuclear material with the tip

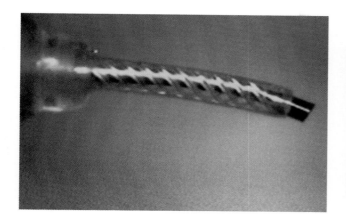

Figure 5.10. *Surgical Design Curved Cobra tip.*

Superior Standard

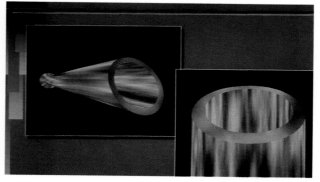

Figure 5.11. *Mastel Instruments' Superior Standard phaco tip.*

Power Chisel

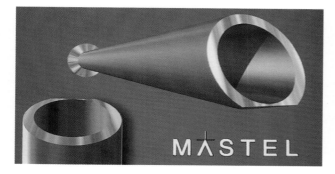

Figure 5.12. *Mastel Instruments' Power Chisel phaco tip with sharpened inferior edge.*

Shepherd Improved Cylinder

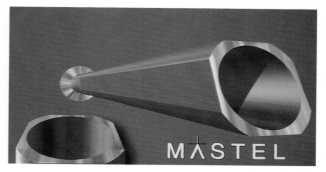

Figure 5.13. *Mastel Instruments' Shepherd Improved Cylinder phaco tip.*

itself. In very hard nuclei, one can actually create grooving without any downward or forward force on the nucleus by the tip, which is obviously a great advantage in cases of weakened zonules, zonular dialysis, pseudoexfoliation, postvitrectomy, and traumatic cataracts.[1]

Surgical Design has created a unique innovation for phaco needles which it has named the Cobra tip. While most conventional phaco tips have a uniform thickness throughout their length, the Cobra tip is widened distally and narrowed proximally, with an inner bell configuration at the tip (Fig. 5.9). This bell or funnel configuration creates much more surface area than conventional tips for acoustic wave generation, in addition to focusing the ultrasonic energy to

a more localized area. This innovation allows for lower energy settings to be used, reducing potential damage to the corneal endothelium.[9] Surgical Design has subsequently added a curve to the Cobra tip (Fig. 5.10), which allows for automatic cracking of the nucleus as it is lollipopped, as described by Singer.

Mastel Precision Instruments has worked with a variety of other changes in tip conformation, size and finish in an attempt to improve performance. Mastel has produced several tips to enhance cutting as a result of the addition of a sharper edge. These include the Superior Standard (Fig. 5.11), the Power Chisel (Fig. 5.12), the Shepherd Improved Cylinder (Fig. 5.13), and the Martin Diamond Pentium (Fig. 5.14). The superior Standard tip has a sharper edge

Martin Diamond Pentium

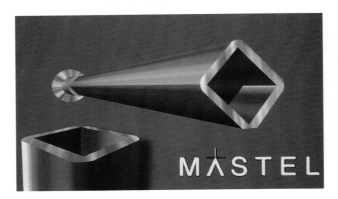

Figure 5.14. *Mastel Instruments' Martin Diamond Pentium phaco tip.*

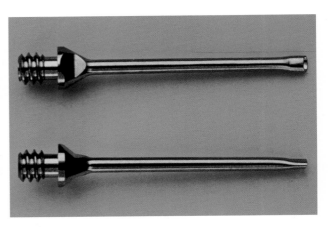

Figure 5.15. *Superior (above) and side (below) views of Microsurgical Technology Seibel flat head phaco tip.*

because of the angulation at the bottom of the tip. The Power Chisel tip has a single sharpened facet at its leading edge at the bottom of the bevel. The Improved Cylinder has four chiseled facets on the leading edge, allowing for enhanced cutting. The Martin Diamond Pentium has a chiseled front at the bottom of a diamond-shaped tip, which enhances the ability to create a narrow grooved valley when sculpting the nuclear material. In addition to these changes in tip shape, there is some feeling that changing the finish from highly polished to matte may result in an enhancement in cavitational energy.

With the advent of chopping techniques for cataract extraction, there has been increasing interest in the development of zero-degree tips. The fine details of the shape and size of these tips are undergoing continued evaluation by many companies. There is no question that chopping procedures are facilitated by zero-degree tips, where good control requires adequate lollipopping of the nucleus by the phaco tip. High cavitational energy tips tend to be associated with a widening of the tunnel as one tries to drive the needle in to lollipop the nucleus, resulting in a less firm hold on nuclear material. Mastel has designed a zero-degree square chisel tip which appears to facilitate lollipopping for chopping techniques. In addition, Microsurgical Technology has designed a unique tip called the Seibel flat head phaco tip, which is claimed to perform more rapid grooving and enhanced lollipopping of the nucleus for chopping procedures, especially in the presence of softer nuclei, because of the broader angle of

contact between the tip and the nuclear material (Fig. 5.15).

With the aim of continuing to improve the comfort of the phaco handpiece, Masket has designed an 'ergonomic tip'. This tip is bent near the hub in such a way that the hand is in a more comfortable position above the plane of the needle during the course of phaco (Fig. 5.16). Handpieces themselves are also undergoing change. These changes are mostly directed towards lighter weight and slimmer models, with a variety of contours on the surface that enable easy manipulation by the surgeon. There is also a tendency for companies to internalize the irrigation and aspiration lines within the handpiece in order to decrease the overall bulk created by externalized lines along the length of the handpiece.

CONCLUSION

As techniques for cataract removal have changed, phaco systems have also evolved in order to improve the safety and efficacy of modern cataract surgery. Concurrently, advances in phaco systems have allowed for advances to be made in lens extraction techniques. Improvements in the generation and judicious use of ultrasonic power in addition to the potential benefits of other energy sources allow for less traumatic removal of lens material, with lower energy requirements. Likewise,

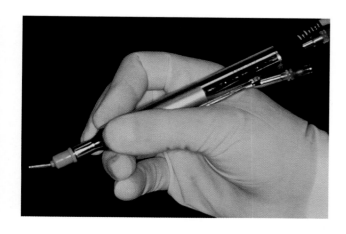

Figure 5.16. *The AMO Diplomax phaco handpiece with angled phaco tip (Masket Ergo tip).*

sophisticated fluidic programmability with high-vacuum cassettes and tubing allows phaco to be performed with more efficient use of energy under a more controlled intraocular environment than has ever been available in the past. Improvements in user interfaces have simplified the utilization of these machines by both the surgeon and support staff. Finally, design changes for tips and handpieces have improved efficiency and comfort while potentially decreasing the incidence of serious wound complications such as incisional burns in clear corneal tissue. These advances and future improvements in phaco systems will probably result in increasing use of phaco as the primary technique for cataract extraction throughout the world as the procedure becomes even safer and easier to master.

ACKNOWLEDGMENT

This is an expansion of our previously published chapter 'Recent advances in phacoemulsification systems' in *Cataract Surgery: The State of the Art*, with permission from Slack, Inc.

REFERENCES

1 Fine IH. Alcon Series 2000 Legacy phacoemulsification system. In: Fine IH, ed. *Phacoemulsification: New Technology and Clinical Application* (Thorofare, NJ: Slack, 1996) 19–36.
2 Masket S, Thorlakson R. The OMS Diplomax in endolenticular phacoemulsification. In: Fine IH, ed. *Phacoemulsification: New Technology and Clinical Application* (Thorofare, NJ: Slack, 1996) 67–80.
3 Anis A. Phacotmesis. In: Fine IH, ed. *Phacoemulsification: New Technology and Clinical Application* (Thorofare, NJ: Slack, 1996) 131–43.
4 Dodick JM, Sperber LTD. Current techniques in laser cataract surgery. In: Fine IH, ed. *Phacoemulsification: New Technology and Clinical Application* (Thorofare, NJ: Slack, 1996) 146–53.
5 Colvard DM, Kratz RP. Cataract surgery utilizing the erbium laser. In: Fine IH, ed. *Phacoemulsification: New Technology and Clinical Application* (Thorofare, NJ: Slack, 1996) 162–80.
6 Eichenbaum DM, Paradigm system: a laser probe for cataract removal. In: Fine IH, ed. *Phacoemulsification: New Technology and Clinical Application* (Thorofare, NJ: Slack, 1996) 155–8.
7 Kelman CD. Reverse-flow phaco technique for safe nucleus sculpting. Presented at the Fourth Annual Ocular Surgery News Symposium, Cataract and Refractive Surgery, New York, 1995.
8 Mackool RJ. Storz Premiere/MicroSeal System description. In: Fine IH, ed. *Phacoemulsification: New Technology and Clinical Application* (Thorofare, NJ: Slack, 1996) 83–100.
9 Grabow HB. The Surgical Design Ocusystem II[ART]. In: Fine IH, ed. *Phacoemulsification: New Technology and Clinical Application* (Thorofare, NJ: Slack, 1996) 104–28.

Chapter 6   **Endocapsular phaco quick chop**

David Dillman

INTRODUCTION

Phaco quick chop is a phacoemulsification technique that was introduced by Vladimir Pfeifer of Slovania. Pfeifer calls his technique 'phaco crack'. However, Maloney and I felt a need to identify a name that we felt might better describe what actually takes place. Since it is a chopping technique (not a cracking technique) and since it happens so quickly, Maloney suggested 'phaco quick chop'.

Phaco quick chop can be done via an endocapsular approach or just as well with the supracapsular approach.

ENDOCAPSULAR TECHNIQUE

The main difference between phaco chop and phaco quick chop is subtle, and yet makes a great deal of difference; it deals with the placement of the chopper itself. With traditional phaco chop, once the phaco tip is buried in the center of the lens, the chopper is placed under the inferior anterior capsule and then advanced peripherally until it reaches the equator of the lens (Fig. 6.1). The chopper is then pulled towards the buried phaco tip in a near-horizontal movement (Fig. 6.2). However, in my hands the maneuver was not easy to execute. On at least two occasions that I recall, I thought I had the chopper under the anterior capsule when, in fact, I was on top of the anterior capsule. When I attempted the actual chop, I succeeded in creating a huge rent in the anterior capsule which quickly wrapped around to include the posterior capsule early in the case.

On reviewing Pfeifer's technique, I was happy to see that he ignored the anterior capsule altogether. He simply placed the chopper on top of the buried phaco tip, pretty much at the center of the lens (well away from the anterior capsule) and initiated the chop with a near-vertical movement (Fig. 6.3). This provides the efficiency of phaco chop, but with what I perceived to be considerably greater safety.

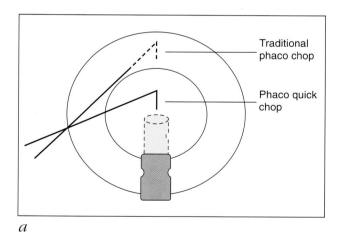

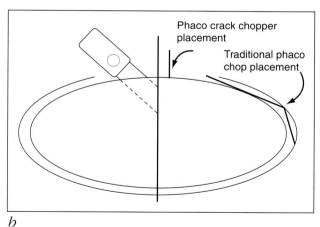

a   *b*

Figure 6.1. *Top view (a) and side view (b) of the contrasting locations for the placement of the chopping instrument for phaco quick chop versus traditional phaco chop.*

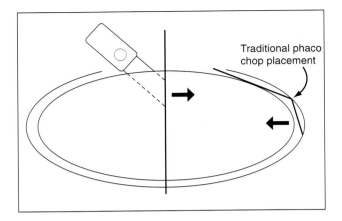

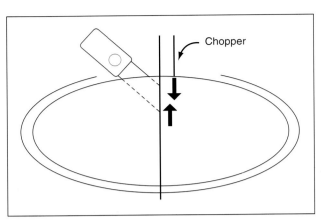

Figure 6.2. *In traditional phaco chop, the chopper is pulled towards the buried phaco needle in a near-horizontal fashion.*

Figure 6.3. *In phaco quick chop, the chopper is moved straight downwards and the buried phaco tip is moved straight upwards, resulting in a 'vertical' chopping maneuver. Contrast this with the 'horizontal' chopping maneuver of traditional phaco chop (Fig. 6.2).*

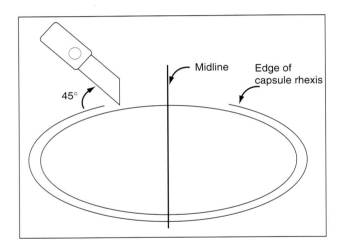

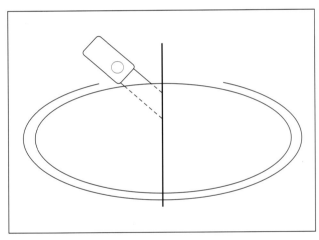

Figure 6.4. *The angle with which the phaco needle contacts the surface of the lens is determined by the size of the capsulorhexis. A smaller capsulorhexis will demand a steeper angle, whereas a larger capsulorhexis will allow for a flatter angle. In general, aim for approximately a 45° angle.*

Figure 6.5. *With the use of short, interrupted bursts of ultrasound, the phaco needle is buried into the center of the lens. Please note that the buried tip does not come anywhere close to the posterior capsule.*

TECHNIQUE

Phaco quick chop should be preceded by a good capsulorhexis and excellent hydrodissection. By excellent hydrodissection, I am referring to the ability to easily rotate the lens within the confines of the capsular bag with your hydrodissection cannula.

Following capsulorhexis and hydrodissection, the phaco needle is introduced into the eye through the phaco incision and then the chopper is introduced into the eye through the side-port incision. The phaco needle is placed on the surface of the lens just in front of the edge of the capsulorhexis nearest you (Fig. 6.4). The phaco needle is then buried, aiming it

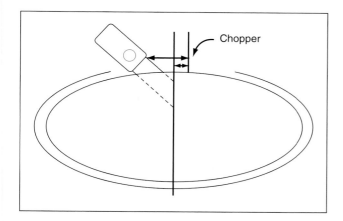

Figure 6.6. *The chopper is placed anywhere from right on top of the end of the buried phaco needle to a millimeter in front of it.*

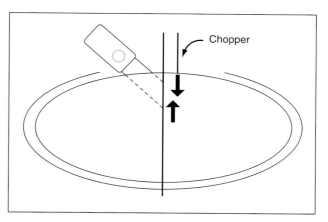

Figure 6.7. *The first chop is initiated by vigorously moving the chopper in a downward fashion while gently moving the buried phaco tip in an upward fashion.*

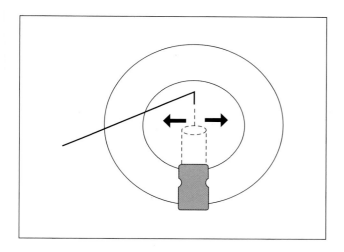

Figure 6.8. *The central chop is propagated out to the periphery by laterally separating the buried chopper and buried phaco needle.*

towards the dead center of the lens (Fig. 6.5). Since this means that you will be very quickly working with a totally occluded phaco needle, and since a totally occluded phaco needle carries a high risk of corneal/scleral burn, I would suggest that this burying process be done with three or four short (foot-pulsed) bursts of phaco (foot position three) as opposed to a single continuous, uninterrupted one. Once the needle is buried, remain in foot position two (aspiration).

The chopper is now lightly placed on the surface of the lens, either directly above the end of the buried phaco needle or as much as a millimeter or two in front of it (Fig. 6.6). You are now ready to make the first chop. Simultaneously, the chopper is moved downwards while the buried phaco needle is moved upwards (Fig. 6.7). For a long time, I thought that 50% of the effort was devoted to the downward movement of the chopper and 50% to the upward movement of the buried phaco needle. More recently, I have decided that the chopper is actually doing most of the work—probably a more accurate ratio would be 90% chopper/10% buried phaco tip. The important point here is to be very aggressive with the chopper. From my observations, I am convinced that nothing bad can happen from a definitive downward chopping motion. This 'vertical' maneuver initiates the division of the lens centrally. However, the peripheral propagation of the division is accomplished by yet a third maneuver that virtually follows on the heels of the first two. Once the chopper and buried phaco needle have come into very near contact (or they can even come into actual contact), they are laterally separated (Fig. 6.8). This triad of maneuvers—chopper down, buried phaco needle up, and lateral separation—should smoothly flow into what might well be perceived to be a single movement by a first-time observer.

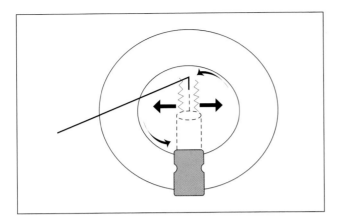

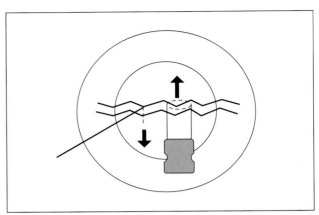

Figure 6.9. *Because excellent hydrodissection is a quick chop prerequisite, it is easy to rotate the lens into a position that puts the two halves in a 'horizontal' position.*

Figure 6.10. *As with any chopping or cracking technique, it is crucial to ensure complete separation of individual pieces. Therefore, before proceeding beyond the initial chop, use the phaco needle and chopper to 'work the split' until you are convinced there has been a complete chop.*

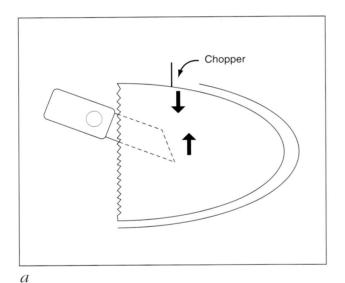

a

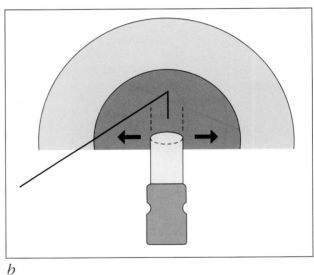

b

Figure 6.11. *Further chops are made in a near-identical fashion to the initial chop. (a) The phaco needle is buried in the lens, the chopper is placed on top, and a vertical chopping maneuver is carried out. (b) This is followed by lateral separation.*

Because excellent hydrodissection precedes this initial chop (and, therefore, good mobility of the lens within the capsular bag is certain), the lateral separation maneuver might well be accompanied by a spinning of the lens within the bag. This is not a problem, because the next intended maneuver is to spin it anyway. Rotate the lens (clockwise or counterclockwise, as you choose) so that the split in

the lens is in the horizontal position from your perspective (i.e. the split in the lens is parallel to the phaco incision) (Fig. 6.9).

It is prudent at this point to take a moment to ensure that this first chop is truly complete, i.e. both posterior and peripheral nuclear plates are completely severed. This is easily accomplished by placing both the phaco needle (you are now in foot position one, irrigation only) and chopper within the split, and then pushing the inferior one-half of the lens away from you with the phaco needle while simultaneously pulling the superior one-half towards you with the chopper (Fig. 6.10).

Now that you have two completely separated halves, there are a variety of ways in which to proceed but, for sake of simplicity, I am here going to follow the quartering approach. The phaco needle is now buried into the center of the inferior one-half (foot position three). Once again, I recommend doing this with two or three short bursts of ultrasound as opposed to one continuous burst. The chopping of this half into quarters is accomplished in exactly the same fashion as the initial chop. The chopper is lightly placed on the surface of the lens, essentially on top of the end of the buried phaco needle (which is now in foot position two) and in front of the edge of the capsulorhexis.

The aforementioned triad of maneuvers is then carried out: (1) chopper down (90% of the effort); (2) buried phaco tip up (10% of the effort); and (3) lateral separation (Fig. 6.11). I would strongly recommend ensuring that this second chop is also complete, both posteriorly and peripherally. Although there are a variety of ways to do this, my personal approach is to support the left, inferior quadrant with the phaco needle (foot position one or two) and to push the right, inferior quadrant away from it by bringing the chopper over the phaco needle and using it to push the right inferior quadrant away in a cross-action fashion (Fig. 6.12).

With the first half quartered, a whole myriad of options now present themselves. The density of the lens, plus your surgical preferences, will probably dictate how you decide to proceed. But, by way of example, here are a few possible avenues: (1) remove both quarters; (2) chop one quarter into eighths, remove each eighth, chop the second quarter into eighths, and remove them; (3) leave both quarters alone, spin the lens 180° so as to bring the other half into the inferior capsular bag, and chop it into quarters.

IMPORTANT POINTS

It would be unfair and inappropriate to deny the fact that there is definitely a learning curve to phaco quick chop. However, it should be a fairly painless one. Hopefully, in an effort to smooth out some potential bumps along the way, let me now share with you a few observations regarding phaco quick chop that may not be immediately obvious.

The first two deal with the initial chop. The tendency is to be much too tentative, both in burying the tip and using the chopper. Let us start with the phaco needle. This must be buried in the substance of the lens. In order to facilitate this, I retract the silicone sleeve approximately double the amount I would normally do for a divide and conquer technique (Fig. 6.13).

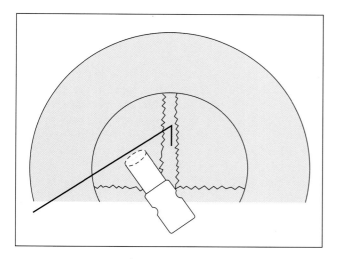

Figure 6.12. *Use both instruments (phaco needle and chopper) to constantly 'work the chops' to ensure they are complete, both posteriorly and peripherally.*

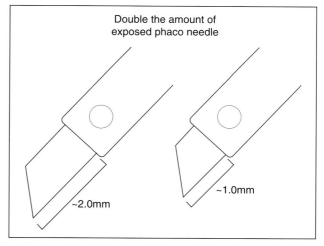

Figure 6.13. *If you are like me, you will be too tentative in burying the phaco tip at first. Exposing more of the titanium needle facilitates burying. Just be careful not to overdo it and have the irrigating sleeve out of the eye.*

There may be a concern that this extra technique could lead to the posterior capsule being broken. Since the center thickness of the human lens is some 3.5–4.0 mm and we have exposed 2 mm of the titanium tip, the silicone sleeve will act as a physical barrier to further advancement of the tip. If we approached the center of the lens at a 90° angle and went straight down, we would only reach the middle of the lens, well away from the central posterior capsule. But, in reality, we are not going to approach the lens at a 90° angle; we will be much closer to 45° (Fig. 6.4). Therefore, the actual penetration of the centrally buried tip will actually be less than 50%.

Once the phaco needle is well buried, keep in mind that it is the action of the chopper that most determines the success or failure of the initial chop. Therefore, use it with controlled aggression. Sink the chopper into the substance of the lens and push down with authority.

If, for whatever reason, the initial chop is not successful, you can either immediately abort phaco quick chop and convert to your divide and conquer technique, or you can spin the lens 90° or so and try again. If it does not work the second time, you could choose to convert to your standard technique or you could spin it another 90° or so and try again.

Do not be frightened or concerned if your initial chop does not result in a lens split perfectly down the middle. It might well be that you will not have two absolutely equal-sized halves. You might end up with a one-third/two-thirds split. All this means is that the bigger piece will need more further chopping than the smaller piece.

A point that I feel is worth re-emphasizing is that just because you see a chop, do not assume that it is a complete chop. Be very active with both the chopper and the phaco needle. Use them to poke and pry, and push and pull. Incomplete chops in phaco quick chop are every bit as bothersome (and dangerous) as incomplete cracks in a divide and conquer technique.

Lastly, I do the following prior to the initial burying of the phaco needle. In foot position number two (aspiration), I use the phaco needle to vacuum away much of the central cortex and epinucleus. This 'cleans things up a bit' and facilitates better visualization for the initial chop.

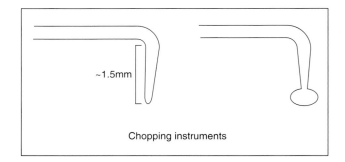

Figure 6.14. *Although phaco quick chop can be done with a Sinskey hook (Pfeifer does so), I feel it is much easier to do with an instrument designed for chopping. I personally believe it should be at least 1.5 mm long and have a non-bulbous ending.*

INSTRUMENTS

The chopper that I am currently using is the Koch chopper (Storz #E0713, St Louis) (Fig. 6.14). It belongs in the family of the modified Sinskey hook-type choppers. In addition, you should be aware that several of the choppers on the market have rounded or bulbous endings. For traditional phaco chop, this facilitates getting under the anterior capsule. And, in addition, for traditional phaco chop, it is less likely to split the anterior capsule if, indeed, you are on top of it when you thought you were underneath it. However, it is my feeling that a rounded or bulbous ending is counterproductive to phaco quick chop, and I would advise against it.

I would advise you to retract the silicone sleeve on the phaco needle in such a fashion as to leave approximately 2 mm of the titanium tip exposed. This is probably considerably more than you would expose for a traditional divide and conquer technique. I suggest this because the very strong tendency at first is to be tentative in burying the phaco tip. By retracting the silicone sleeve farther, you will be able to bury better the phaco needle and gain a better purchase on the lens for the chopping maneuvers.

Chapter 7 Supracapsular quick-chop phaco: a capsule-free posterior chamber approach

William F Maloney

THE 30-YEAR EVOLUTION OF PHACO: 1967–97

Phacoemulsification (phaco) has more or less reinvented itself in each decade of its 30-year existence. If the following sequence of phaco's evolution continues, we are now on the verge of another new phaco approach:

- Anterior chamber phaco   1967–77
- Posterior chamber phaco   1977–87
- Endocapsular phaco   1987–97

I am still not sure that supracapsular will be the next generation of phaco, since I feel that it is still really in its formative phase. However, I can say that I believe my present supracapsular technique has surpassed my endocapsular technique and I continue to perform supracapsular phaco with increasing confidence and enthusiasm. My supracapsular experience has taught me that the location of maximum safety for both the capsule and the endothelium is still within the posterior chamber, but outside the relatively inhospitable environment of the capsular bag.

SURGICAL TECHNIQUE

Preparation, anesthesia and incision for supracapsular phaco are done according to the surgeon's preference, after which the following sequential steps are performed.

CAPSULORHEXIS

Viscoelastic of choice is instilled into the anterior chamber and supplemented as needed in sufficient amounts to maintain a flat anterior capsule throughout the creation of a 5–6-mm-diameter continuous circular capsulorhexis (CCC) utilizing either cystotome or forceps.

HYDRODISSECTION

A 26- or 27-gauge polished round cannula is used to perform hydrodissection. Up to 1.5 ml of balanced salt solution (BSS) (or xylocaine in topical/intracameral cases) is injected under the anterior capsular rim until a fluid wave is seen to pass beneath the entire width of the nucleus. Hydrodissection is gently continued until, in most cases, the opposite equator of the nucleus spontaneously 'tilts' out of the capsulorhexis at the conclusion of the maneuver. In the event that this spontaneous 'lens tilt' does not occur, nuclear rotation is performed.

NUCLEAR ROTATION (OPTIONAL)

The same hydrodissection cannula is used to gently rotate the nucleus first in one direction and then the other, ensuring that the nucleus is free of all cortical attachments. Hydrodissection is then repeated. If at this point the lens tilt again fails to occur, the supracapsular approach should be converted into any preferred endocapsular technique.

LENS TILT (FIG. 7.1)

With the larger CCC, hydrodissection normally results in a spontaneous 'lens tilt' which begins the sequential process of overturning the nucleus and, in so doing, removing it from the capsular bag. Again, if after the first three steps above this lens tilt does not occur, then the endocapsular approach should be utilized.

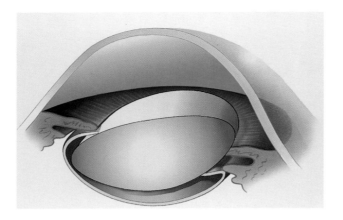

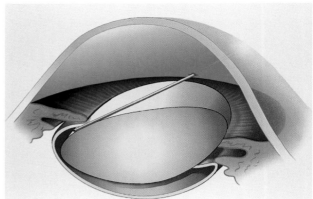

a

Figure 7.1. *Lens tilt. Hydrodissection lifts the nucleus through the CCC and begins lens transposition outside of the capsular bag.*

INITIAL TRANSPOSITION: POSTERIOR SWEEP (FIG. 7.2)

The hydrodissection cannula is used to gently further depress the posterior half of the tilted nucleus and then smoothly sweep the posterior equator of the nucleus across the posterior capsule (Fig. 7.2a,b) until the superior equator is just beyond the vertical midline (Fig. 7.2c). The hydrodissection cannula is removed.

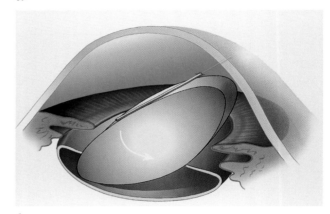

b

COMPLETE TRANSPOSITION: THE VISCO-INVERTED NUCLEUS (FIG. 7.3)

Viscoelastic is steadily instilled as needed while its cannula slowly continues the transposition of the nucleus until it is once again oriented horizontally, but now lies upside down.

FINAL REPOSITION IN POSTERIOR CHAMBER (FIG. 7.4)

The viscoelastic cannula adjusts the final position of the inverted nucleus into the supracapsular space; behind the iris but above and completely outside the collapsed capsular bag. Viscoelastic is supplemented as desired.

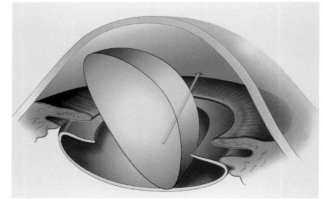

c

Figure 7.2. *(a-c) Initial lens transposition. The nucleus is partially inverted to a point just past the vertical midline.*

PHACO ON THE FLIP SIDE

All of the usual endocapsular techniques (both cracking and chopping), as well as single-piece, power-based

emulsification, can be used with the supracapsular approach. In my experience, all benefit from the increased efficiency which results from the enhanced followability of the 'misfit' upside-down nucleus

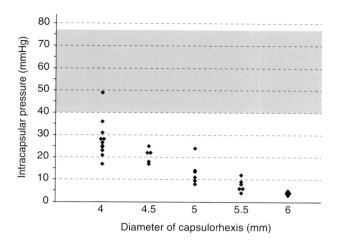

Figure 8.6. *Intracapsular fluid pressure measured during hydroexpression of the nucleus in 32 cadaver eyes. The fluid pressure correlated significantly with the diameter of the capsulorhexis opening. The shaded area shows the pressure range at which rupture of the posterior capsule was induced during hydroexpression of the nucleus in 16 cadaver eyes with a small capsulorhexis opening (<4 mm).[9] It appears that hydroexpression may be hazardous in cases with a small capsulorhexis opening as fluid pressure may reach the rupture point of the posterior capsule. Reprinted with permission.*

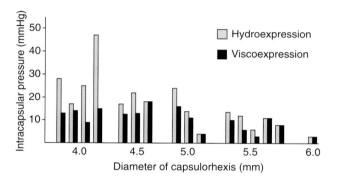

Figure 8.7. *Comparison of intracapsular fluid pressure. Intracapsular fluid pressure measured during hydroexpression and viscoexpression of the nucleus in pairs of cadaver eyes. Viscoexpression is carried out at a lower fluid pressure than hydroexpression – especially in eyes with a small capsulorhexis.[10] Reprinted with permission.*

technically difficult.[10] Even though it may be possible to tilt the nucleus by fluid pressure, the pressure decreases quickly, whereupon the capsulorhexis edge again tightens around the nucleus, thus resisting further expression. As a consequence, some manipulation will be needed to get the nucleus out of the capsular bag, and this may stress the zonular fibers.

In cases with a small capsulorhexis opening (<5.5 mm) or in otherwise difficult situations, the use of a viscoelastic to express the nucleus seems to be safer. Viscoelastic material disperses more slowly than BSS, acts more locally to lift the nucleus, and stays in the bag after the nucleus has been tilted. Experiments performed on human cadaver eyes have shown that the time of nucleus expression can be increased up to 25 s when the viscoexpression technique is used.[10] This means that the tension in the capsulorhexis edge has time to relax, reducing the forces needed to express the nucleus (Fig. 8.7). Accordingly, the risk of rupturing the posterior capsule will be reduced (Fig. 8.6).[9]

CONCLUSION

In extracapsular cataract extraction, hydroexpression of the nucleus can be recommended in cases with a relatively large capsulorhexis opening (diameter >5.5 mm). When the capsulorhexis opening is smaller or in otherwise difficult cases, viscoexpression of the nucleus should be preferred.

REFERENCES

1 Gimbel HV, Neuhann T. Development, advantages, and methods of the continuous circular capsulorhexis technique. *J Cataract Refract Surg* 1990; **16:** 31–7.

2 Thim K, Krag S, Corydon L. Stretching capacity of capsulorhexis and nucleus delivery. *J Cataract Refract Surg* 1991; **17:** 27–31.

3 Colvard DM, Dunn SA. Intraocular lens centration with continuous tear capsulotomy. *J Cataract Refract Surg* 1990; **16:** 312–14.

4 Thim K, Krag S, Corydon L. Capsulorhexis and nucleus expression. *Eur J Implant Refract Surg* 1990; **2:** 37–41.

5 Almallah OF. Capsulorhexis complications with planned extracapsular cataract extraction. *J Cataract Refract Surg* 1989; **15:** 232–3.

6 Maher JF. Nucleus expression after capsulorhexis. *J Cataract Refract Surg* 1988; **14:** 693.

7 Corydon L, Thim K. Continuous circular capsulorhexis and nucleus delivery in planned extracapsular cataract extraction. *J Cataract Refract Surg* 1991; **17:** 628–32.

8 Corydon L. Modified forceps for capsulorhexis. *J Cataract Refract Surg* 1991; **17:** 99.

9 Krag S, Thim K, Corydon L. Strength of the lens capsule during hydroexpression of the nucleus. *J Cataract Refract Surg* 1993; **19:** 205–8.

10 Thim K, Krag S, Corydon L. Hydroexpression and viscoexpression of the nucleus through a continuous circular capsulorhexis. *J Cataract Refract Surg* 1993; **19:** 209–12.

Chapter 9   **Phakosection—cataract surgery**

David J McIntyre

PATIENT SELECTION FACTORS

One of the features of the phakosection technique is its broad applicability to cataracts of all types and stages of maturity. Enhanced surgical safety is a benefit to very elderly patients with advanced dense cataract development as well as the younger working population with immature cataracts.

SURGICAL SAFETY

I believe that the safety of cataract surgery can be greatly enhanced by approaching the cataract as three separate tissue portions that typically have different hardness or viscosity:

1) The nucleus at the center of the cataract in adult patients has a very high viscosity which prevents simple aspiration.
2) The epinucleus which surrounds the nucleus has an intermediate level of viscosity which can be aspirated, although requiring high vacuum pressure.
3) The peripheral cortex which lies just under the capsule has the lowest viscosity and is easily aspirated.

It is my opinion that the most hazardous moment of cataract surgery is when the epinucleus is being aspirated. At that time, sudden clearing of the aspiration device will allow the adjacent cortex to be aspirated very rapidly and the peripheral and/or posterior capsule may then be impacted and torn by the aspirating force. In order to eliminate this risk, I have established a personal policy to never aspirate the epinucleus from its position within the capsular bag. Once the epinucleus is removed, then the peripheral cortex can be stripped from the periphery and aspirated with relative safety.

SURGICAL PREPARATIONS

PROPHYLACTIC ANTIBIOTICS

Preoperative prophylactic topical antibiotics are used for 2 days prior to the surgical procedure. While there is no clear proof that this affects the incidence of bacterial endophthalmitis, its use appears prudent.

PATIENT GENERAL MEDICATION

Patients are instructed to continue their normal general medical treatments and medications up to and following the time of surgery. Patients who are using aspirin or coumadin for prophylactic clotting control do not change their medication schedule. Patients who are being treated with general anesthesia and/or heavy sedation with consequent increased risk of aspiration are instructed to have clear liquids only for 12 h prior to surgery. Patients with diabetes who fall into this category also have their antidiabetic medications fractionated during the same preparatory period.

FOR EFFECTIVE CATARACT SURGERY, WIDE PUPILLARY DILATION IS A MAJOR BENEFIT

We dilate our patients' pupils with a combination of cyclopentolate, phenylephrine, and an antiprostaglandin. The antiprostaglandin is quite efficient at maintaining pupil dilation during the trauma of the surgical procedure. Drops are repeatedly instilled during the 30–40 min prior to surgery.

ANESTHESIA

While it is clearly established that some patients can satisfactorily undergo cataract surgery with only topical and/or intracameral anesthesia, we are concerned about the risks of injecting periocular anesthetics after the procedure has been initiated. Consequently, about 20% of our patients are being operated upon with a peribulbar anesthetic which is injected following an intravenous dose of methohexital.

Our injection routine is a mixture of 3/4% Marcain with 4% lidocaine and a small amount of hyaluronidase. The volume injected ranges from 6 to 10 ml total in a combined superior and inferior peribulbar injection.

OCULOPRESSION

This is applied for approximately 20 min following the peribulbar injection, when utilized to more rapidly dissipate the anesthetic fluids and reduce vitreous volume.

SKIN AND CONJUNCTIVA PREPARATION

Diluted Iodophor skin preparation solution is applied to the external surfaces of the lids and brow area throughout the period of oculopression and immediately prior to the surgical procedure.

SURGICAL APPROACH AND PREPARATIONS

For the past 6 years I have found that approaching the eye from the temporal limbus affords much more comfortable and facile access to the ocular contents. Operating from the temporal side, however, requires that most of the furniture and personnel within the operating room be repositioned. It has been very satisfactory, with the surgeon and surgical assistant facing one another across the surgical field, with the instrument table to the side of the surgical assistant.

The surgical field is draped in the usual fashion with a lash-line barrier drape held in position by the lid speculum.

The lid speculum must be of appropriate design, with its supporting structures lying over the nose rather than the lateral canthus.

I have found that traction sutures are completely unnecessary with the temporal approach to cataract surgery.

One of the major advances in recent cataract surgical technique is the self-sealing incision. As popularized by Singer,[1] a properly constructed 'frown' approach scleral tunnel results in a self-sealing incision with minimal astigmatic effects. Positioning of a self-sealing tunneled incision must be carefully planned in patients who have previously had intraocular surgery, as close proximity to a previous limbal incision can produce unexpected astigmatic results.

The self-sealing tunnel incision may be made in the peripheral clear cornea. However, it is my view that the additional safety that results from covering the incision site with conjunctiva is extremely important. Consequently, I begin the incision with a limbal peritomy and complete the closure with conjunctival coaptation to fully cover the scleral surface of the surgical wound.

An anterior chamber maintainer is utilized intermittently throughout the procedure to provide an inflow of irrigating solution. The infusion pressure is varied by raising and lowering the reservoir of balanced salt solution (BSS). The volume of flow at any particular time is determined by wound leakage and rate of aspiration. In order to adequately maintain the chamber volume and avoid so-called 'mini-collapses', a large-bore chamber maintainer is required. Mine has an inside diameter of 0.9 mm. The maintainer tip is threaded metal, which allows it to be screwed into a properly sized paracentesis, achieving excellent retention. It is my routine to turn the maintainer off during capsulorhexis when the anterior chamber is filled with air and also during cutting and extraction of the nuclear fragments when a viscoelastic agent is in use. During the remainder of the procedure, the maintainer is running with the bottle height adjusted for the needs of the moment.

INCISIONS

A paracentesis is made through the peripheral clear nasal cornea ½ cm³ of 1% non-preserved lidocaine is infused and the chamber maintainer is screwed into position (Fig. 9.1). The valve is then opened, inflating the anterior chamber.

A temporal peritomy is done and episcleral vessels are cauterized as required with a bipolar cautery (Fig. 9.2). The actual site for a frown incision is selected and marked with calipers set for 5.5 mm (Fig. 9.3). A frown incision is made with a diamond blade, seeking a depth of approximately one-half the scleral thickness (Fig. 9.4). With a double-beveled angled 'crescent' dissecting blade, the tunnel is dissected forward into the peripheral clear cornea at a depth of one-third to one-half the scleral thickness (Fig. 9.5). The anterior chamber is not entered.

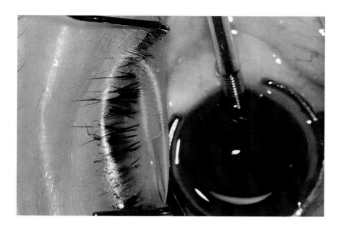

Figure 9.1. *The large-bore anterior chamber maintainer is screwed into the nasal cornea through an appropriate paracentesis to achieve firm retention.*

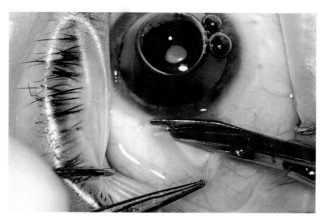

Figure 9.2. *A temporal peritomy sets the stage for closure of the conjunctiva over the tunnel incision at the end of the procedure.*

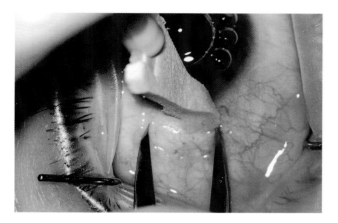

Figure 9.3. *The anticipated tunnel length of 5.5–6 mm is marked with a caliper.*

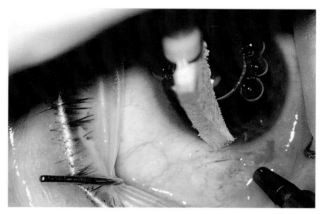

Figure 9.4. *With a diamond blade, the frown incision is made to a depth of one-third to one-half the scleral thickness.*

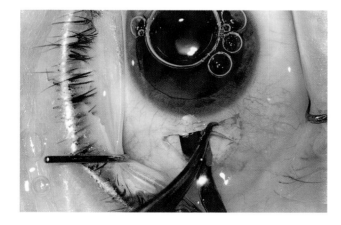

Figure 9.5. *The tunnel is dissected with a double-beveled angled crescent knife without entry into the anterior chamber.*

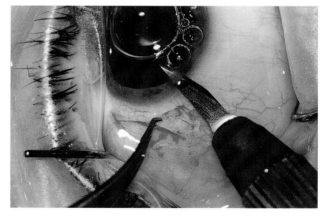

Figure 9.6. *A working paracentesis is made to the surgeon's 'strong side'.*

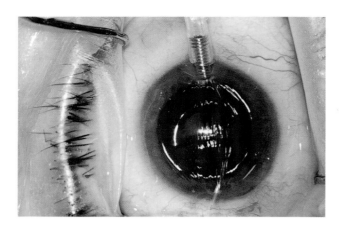

Figure 9.7. *Capsulorhexis is performed with a hooked cystotome under a large air bubble.*

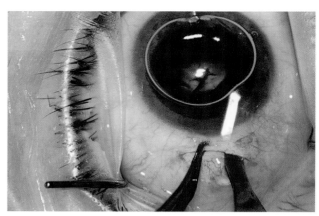

Figure 9.8. *The tunnel incision is fully opened with the double-beveled angled crescent blade, ensuring that the internal dimension is at least as great as the external frown.*

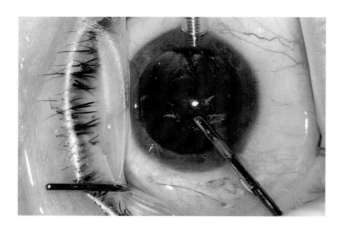

Figure 9.9. *Debulking aspiration removes the cortex and epinucleus overlying the compact central nucleus within the capsulorhexis space.*

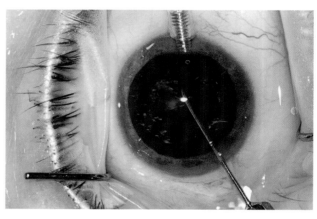

Figure 9.10. *Hydrodelineation and dissection of the compact nucleus is a combination of mechanical and hydraulic forces.*

A paracentesis is made to the right (for a right-handed surgeon) of the dissected tunnel through the peripheral clear cornea (Fig. 9.6). This paracentesis must be adequate for the unobstructed passage of the 21-gauge debulking cannula.

THE ANTERIOR CAPSULAR INCISION

As popularized by Neuhan,[2] I prefer to make a continuous-tear capsulorhexis in the anterior capsule. The capsulorhexis must be of sufficient size to allow dissection and tilting of the nucleus present in the

specific case—generally, 6–6.5 mm is sufficient. I make the capsulorhexis tear with a cystotome made from a 27-gauge ½-inch hypodermic needle. The tip is simply bent to a small sharp hook and the shaft angled 45°. It is also my preference to perform the capsulorhexis under a large air bubble. Three benefits are achieved with air:

1) Air is retained very well in the anterior chamber.
2) The progressing tear of the anterior capsule is clearly visible, as the highlights reflect from the bottom of the air bubble.

3) The absence of fluid in the anterior chamber eliminates the magnification effect of the corneal curvature—thus when the capsulorhexis appears to be 6 mm, it is in fact 6 mm.

With the anterior chamber maintainer valve shut off, the hooked cystotome is introduced through the tunnel incision, making its own perforation into the anterior chamber. The surgical assistant supplies an air bubble from an air-filled syringe through the sterile extension tube on which the cystotome is mounted. During the procedure, the assistant is able to inject additional air if needed. The capsulorhexis begins with a perforation in the center of the anterior lens capsule, and then spirals into a circular tear by engagement and rotation of the capsular flap (Fig. 9.7). This is a deliberate and controlled technique and can be achieved in the majority of cases.

If there is posterior vitreous pressure or if there is loss of anterior chamber volume, the forces on the capsule may cause the tear to extend into and be trapped by the fibers of the zonule. Occasionally, such a capsulorhexis can be retrieved by judicious use of the hooked cystotome or a capsule forceps. However, if this is not possible, completion of the anterior capsulectomy by multiple puncture can-opener technique is a satisfactory second choice.

There are cases where can-opener technique may be the only practical form of anterior capsulectomy. Such cases include those with very poor visualization resulting from corneal disturbances and those patients with a small and undilatable pupil.

COMPLETION OF THE TUNNEL INCISION

After completion of the capsulorhexis, the tunnel incision is then completed into the anterior chamber, usually perforating through its center area with the 15° super-sharp and completing the full opening of the tunnel with the double-beveled angled 'crescent' knife (Fig. 9.8).

PHAKOSECTION OF THE NUCLEUS

Following the philosophy of treating the three portions of the cataract as separate tissue entities, I first expose the anterior surface of the compact central nucleus. This is done by aspiration of the overlying cortex and epinucleus within the area of the capsulorhexis with a debulking cannula through the paracentesis (Fig. 9.9). The chamber maintainer is running at a relatively high bottle height and residual air bubbles are aspirated from the chamber. The debulking 21-gauge cannula is mounted on a 3-ml syringe filled with a small amount of BSS and its orifice is directed downward onto the face of the nucleus. With rapid, firm aspirating movements, small sections of the cortex and epinucleus are aspirated. As the cannula orifice meets the surface of the compact nucleus, it obstructs the orifice, thus preventing any further aspiration. The cortex and epinucleus are thus removed within the space of the capsulorhexis, which extends out to approximately the diameter of the nucleus. There has been no hydrodissection up to this stage.

The compact nucleus is then hydrodissected from its position within the epinucleus without disturbing the epinucleus itself; thus the epinucleus and surrounding cortex continue to lie within the capsular bag, providing a barrier between the surgeon and the posterior capsule. Dissection of the nucleus is done with a hydrodissecting 27-gauge cannula mounted on a 3-ml syringe filled with BSS. The technique is a combination of mechanical and hydraulic forces, starting by 'scratching' over the area of the anticipated equator of the nucleus and then combining small-volume brief injections of BSS (Fig. 9.10).

When the nucleus has been delineated and hydrodissected around two-thirds of its circumference, rotation of the hydrodissecting cannula will elevate one edge of the nucleus from the epinuclear bowl (Fig. 9.11). This is not an attempt to bring the nucleus entirely into the anterior chamber, but only to tilt it sufficiently to provide access to its equator. The chamber maintainer valve is then turned off and a small amount of high-viscosity hyaluronic acid is injected into the anterior chamber over the surface of the tilted nucleus (Fig. 9.12). The phakosection spatula and single cutter are then inserted, with the spatula passing under the center of the nucleus and the cutter over its surface. The cutter is gently but firmly pressed through the nucleus down to the surface of the spatula, dividing the nucleus (Fig. 9.13). Depending on the size of the nucleus, it may be divided into two, three or four fragments. The intent is to divide the nucleus into long, slender fragments which have a small cross-section for removal through the tunneled incision. After cutting of the nucleus, both the spatula and the cutter are removed from the anterior chamber. A small additional amount of viscoelastic is inserted and, with its cannula, the first fragment for extraction is

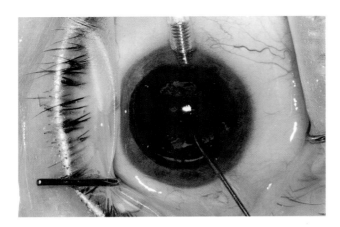

Figure 9.11. *The defined compact nucleus is tilted to expose an equatorial margin by rotating the hydrodissection cannula.*

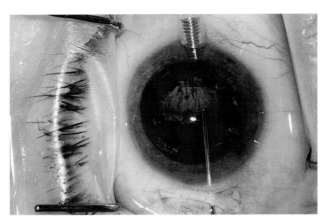

Figure 9.12. *Viscoelastic is injected to protect the corneal endothelium from the exposed nucleus.*

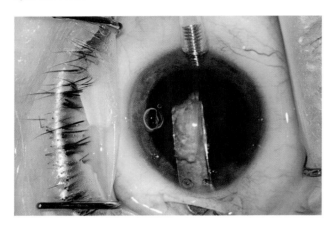

Figure 9.13. *With the nucleus spatula and single cutter, the nucleus is divided into two or more long, slender fragments.*

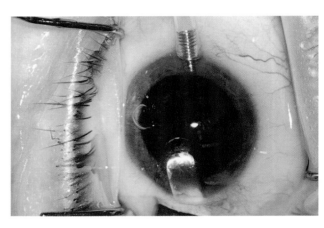

Figure 9.14. *With the nucleus spatula and extractor, the first half of the nucleus is extracted from the anterior chamber.*

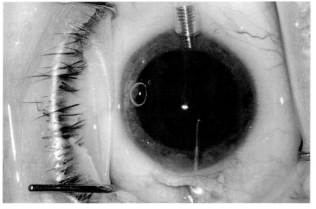

a

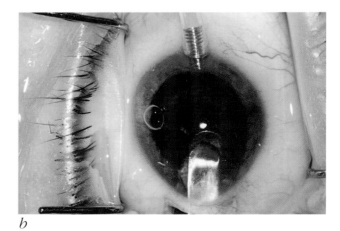

b

Figure 9.15. *(a) The remaining half of the nucleus is covered with additional viscoelastic and aligned toward the tunnel incision. (b) With the nucleus spatula and extractor, the second half of the nucleus is extracted from the anterior chamber.*

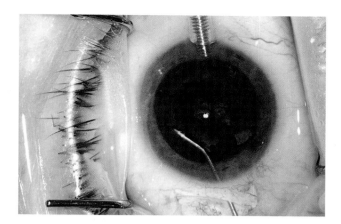

Figure 9.16. *The epinuclear bowl is hydrodissected and hydroexpressed from the capsular bag.*

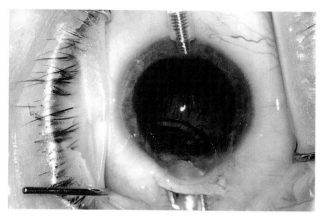

Figure 9.17. *The entire epinuclear bowl is hydroexpressed from the anterior chamber with the irrigating spoon.*

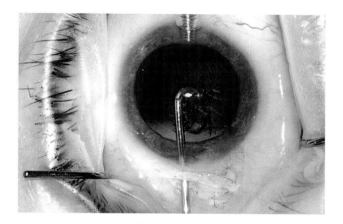

Figure 9.18. *Binkhorst-style curved cannulas are very effective for removing the peripheral cortex underlying the tunnel incision.*

positioned in alignment with the tunnel. The spatula is then reintroduced along with the extractor and, with the spatula below and the extractor above, the first fragment is gently extracted from the anterior chamber (Fig. 9.14). During this maneuver, the extractor blade remains parallel to the iris plane, while the tip of the spatula is elevated very slightly in order to ensure a grip on the fragment. For removal of each additional fragment, a small amount of viscoelastic is added, and the fragment is positioned and removed with the two instruments (Fig. 9.15a,b). For this stage of the procedure, I normally use between 0.1 and 0.2 ml of viscoelastic. It has been my experience that high-viscosity hyaluronic acid provides the greatest stability while requiring the smallest volume for the procedure.

EPINUCLEUS

After the nuclear fragments have been divided and removed, the anterior chamber maintainer is again turned on. The hydrodissection cannula, mounted on a 5-ml syringe filled with BSS, is inserted and, as it enters the tunnel, it allows escape of the viscoelastic material. A stream of BSS is then injected under the margin of the capsulorhexis, causing a hydrodissection of the entire epinucleus (Fig. 9.16). In some cases, a small amount of mechanical 'milking' is required to dislodge the epinucleus. Occasionally, there will be a spontaneous expulsion of the epinucleus. More frequently, an irrigating spoon mounted on a 3-ml syringe filled with a small amount of BSS is used to open the valve of the tunnel incision while providing additional BSS infusion to extrude the epinucleus (Fig. 9.17). With this technique, the epinucleus is removed by pressure rather than vacuum, thus minimizing risk to the posterior capsule.

THE RESIDUAL PERIPHERAL CORTEX

The peripheral cortex is then stripped from the periphery of the capsular bag and aspirated from the anterior chamber. The majority of the material is reached through the paracentesis with a straight side-ported aspirating cannula mounted on a 3-ml syringe filled with a small amount of BSS. Portions of cortex which lie under the incision are extracted with the right- and left-hand sharply curved Binkhorst-style side-ported cannulas (Fig. 9.18). The anterior

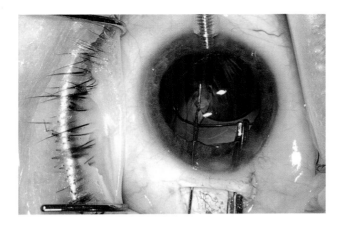

Figure 9.19. *The trailing haptic is placed directly into the capsular bag with the Dusek–McIntyre forceps.*

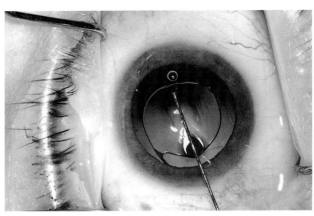

Figure 9.20. *Following removal of the chamber maintainer, hydration of the paracenteses, bipolar coaptation of the conjunctiva, and deepening of the anterior chamber with BSS, a touch of the cannula on the central cornea demonstrates that the intraocular lens is in a central position within the capsular bag and that all incisions are watertight.*

chamber maintainer supplies replacement volume while this aspiration is being completed.

The central posterior capsule may be polished or scrubbed with the aspirating cannula by turning its aspirating port downward and applying minimal digital aspirating force to the syringe.

LENS INSERTION

The implant, which in my current technique is a 5.5-mm round optic one-piece polymethylmethacrylate lens, is inserted directly into the capsular bag while the maintainer is running at a low pressure level. Insertion of the leading haptic is assisted by a 30-gauge cannula

filled with a small amount of BSS. The lens is held in position by a touch of this cannula while the introduction forceps are removed and the trailing haptic is placed into the capsular bag with the Dusek–McIntyre forceps (Fig. 9.19). It is my preference to rotate the haptics within the capsular bag to a horizontal position for maximum vertical stability.

The procedure is then terminated by removal of the chamber maintainer, coaptation closure of the conjunctival peritomy, hydration of the paracenteses, and deepening of the anterior chamber with a 30-gauge cannula mounted on a TB syringe filled with a small amount of BSS (Fig. 9.20). Atropine and topical antibiotics are instilled and, if desired, a protective dressing is applied. The patient is immediately ambulatory and discharged without restriction for examination in 24 h.

REFERENCES

1 Singer JA. Frown incision for minimizing induced astigmatism after small incision cataract surgery with rigid optic intraocular lens implantation. *J Cataract Refract Surg* 1991; **17** (suppl): 677–88.

2 Neuhann T. Theoric und Operationstechnik der kapsulorrhexis. *Klin Monatsbl Augenheilkd* 1987; **190**: 542–5.

Chapter 10 **Lasers in cataract surgery**

D Michael Colvard

INTRODUCTION

For decades, the use of a laser to remove cataracts has been a dream for ophthalmologists. In recent years, substantial progress has been made to bring this concept out of the realm of fantasy.

The lasers presently under clinical development for cataract surgery in the USA are all solid-state lasers. A solid-state laser is one in which a crystal, rather than a gas, holds the excitable element. This specific element, which is called the dopant, emits a specific wavelength which gives each laser its particular characteristics. By scientific convention, when referring to a laser the dopant is mentioned first, followed by the name of the crystal. In common parlance, however, this notation convention is ignored. The Nd:YAG is typically called by its crystal (the 'YAG laser'), and the Er:YAG is called by its dopant (the 'erbium laser'). The Nd:YAG, whose crystal is yttrium–lithium–fluoride, is generally referred to simply as the 'picosecond laser'.

All three of these solid-state lasers have undergone clinical evaluation in the USA. In this discussion, the companies sponsoring the research and the principal investigators for each of the lasers will be identified. An overview of the technology, instrumentation, surgical techniques, clinical experience and potential advantages over standard ultrasonic methods of cataract extraction will be provided.

Nd:YAG LASERS

At present, there are two groups actively involved in the development of Nd:YAG devices for cataract surgery, the ARC Laser Group, led by Dodick, and the Paradigm Medical Industries group, led by Eichenbaum.

ARC Nd:YAG LASER

Introduction

In 1991, Dodick in New York outlined a method of cataract removal using laser energy. He described the use of a pulsed Q-switched Nd:YAG laser similar to capsulotomy lasers to ignite a plasma on a titanium target plate. This creates an acoustic wave that may be used to disrupt a cataractous lens.[1]

Description of the technology

A standard Nd:YAG laser, which delivers near-infrared energy with a 1.064-μm wavelength, is used to generate a laser pulse with a width of 6 ns. This laser pulse is channeled into a 300-μm quartz fiber. The fiber is inserted into an irrigating and aspirating handpiece through the infusion channel. At the end of the infusion channel is a titanium target. The fiber terminates approximately 1.3 mm in front of the target. When the laser pulse strikes the titanium target, a plasma is ignited (Fig. 10.1). This results in

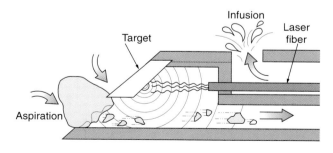

Figure 10.1. *In the Dodick Nd:YAG handpiece, laser energy strikes a titanium plate. A plasma is created, providing acoustic activity which results in nuclear disruption.*

a shockwave which is used to fragment nuclear material that has been drawn into the handpiece by aspiration and the flow of balanced salt solution (BSS).

Surgical technique

Two 1.6-mm clear corneal incisions are made with a paracentesis knife. Through one is inserted an infusion probe. Through the second is inserted an aspiration probe containing the laser fiber and titanium target. This is done after a standard 6-mm capsulorhexis is performed. The nucleus is ablated with repeated laser pulses at 1–6 H. Following the ablation of the nucleus, the cortex is aspirated with the same probe. The wound is enlarged for the insertion of a foldable lens.

Clinical experience

To date, 41 cases have been performed in the USA by Dodick under an IDE from the FDA. Additionally, 400 cases have been performed in Europe where the device has been approved for clinical use.

Potential advantages over existing technology

Dodick and his colleagues have cited a number of potential advantages of the Dodick device. The laser handpiece is smaller, making it possibly more ergonometric than the standard currently available ultrasonic handpieces.

The technology produces no clinically significant heat at the incision. This would seem to eliminate the possibility of incision burns. Moreover, since no substantial heat is produced at the incision, infusion can be separated from aspiration and the laser energy chamber. This makes it possible to perform the entire cataract procedure through two small, separate side-port incisions.

It is also possible, though not proven, that this laser energy system may be gentler with ocular structures than ultrasonic devices. Dodick has found that moderately dense nuclear material can be removed with 200–500 laser shots at 10 mJ. This results in a net input of energy into the eye of 2–5 J which is believed by Dodick and his colleagues to be 'considerably less than that used for an ultrasound phaco'. Furthermore, the Dodick instrument operates at

1–5 Hz compared to 20 000–40 000 Hz for a standard phacoemulsification device. It is conceivable that this could potentially help to reduce collateral trauma to tissues such as the corneal endothelium (Dodick J, Grabner G and Alzmer E, personal communication).

PARADIGM Nd:YAG LASER

Introduction

The 'Photon' Nd:YAG laser probe under development by Paradigm Medical Industries of Salt Lake City is designed to be part of a 'Photon Ocular Surgery Workstation'. This assembly of instruments includes standard ultrasonic components for cataract extraction, as well as a bipolar cautery device.

Description of technology

Like the Dodick system, the Paradigm laser probe delivers pulsed ND:YAG energy via a quartz fiber. The Nd:YAG energy is delivered in proximity to the coaxial aspiration and irrigation ports, where an acoustic wave results in lens tissue disruption. A coaxial HeNe beam facilitates visualization at the treatment site (Fig. 10.2)

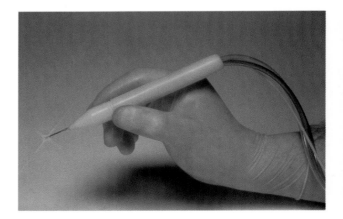

Figure 10.2. *In the Photon handpiece, a coaxial HeNe beam facilitates visualization at the treatment site.*

Surgical technique

The 'Photon' probe is used through a 2-mm incision and is used very much like standard phacoemulsification device for cataract removal.

Clinical experience

Phase 1 clinical trials were completed in 1997. These trials, conducted on cataracts of soft and moderate density, revealed surgical times roughly equivalent to that expected with standard ultrasonic devices. An absence of thermal rise at the incision or in the anterior chamber, and 'improved' chamber maintenance with reduced fluid exchange, are said to have been noted by investigators.

Potential advantages over existing technology

Paradigm has described a number of potential advantages of its laser probe over standard ultrasonic equipment. Like the Dodick group, it believes that the device provides a gentler mechanism for lens removal than may be found with phacoemulsification. It points out that the tip of the probe is smooth, and suggests that it is less likely to inadvertently injure structures such as the posterior capsule. The company also emphasizes the ability of the heat-free probe to allow for a tighter incision seal during lens removal. This, it believes, produces a more stable anterior chamber, reduces fluid flow through the chamber, and allows for higher vacuum settings (Millar RW, personal communication).

Er:YAG LASERS

Although a number of companies are investigating the Er:YAG laser for a variety of ophthalmic applications, at present only Premier Laser Systems of Irvine, California, led by Cozean, has performed clinical studies for cataract extraction in the USA.

Introduction

The erbium laser probe, designed for cataract extraction by Premier Laser Systems, is part of a multipurpose device for ophthalmic surgery. The laser system has been approved by the FDA for blephroplasty and skin resurfacing. It is in clinical trials for the treatment of glaucoma, and is in preclinical evaluation of photokeratectomy. The Premier erbium laser has been approved by the FDA for anterior capsulotomy and is entering phase 2 clinical trials for cataract extraction.

Description of technology

Energy from the Er:YAG laser with a wavelength of 2.94 µm had the highest absorption in water of any available laser. As a result of this high level of absorption, laser energy is confined and tissue penetration is less than 1 µm in tissues such as the human lens.[2] A cavitation effect caused by the collapse of a laser-induced bubble at the tip of the probe results in an acoustic wave. It is primarily this acoustic energy which brings about tissue disruption.[3,4] When the laser is used in cataract surgery, a zirconium–fluoride optical fiber and a silica tip are employed to bring the energy into the eye. The laser delivers a 300-µs pulse with multiple spikes in the nanosecond range. It has a power range from 5 to 290 mJ with a repetition rate from 5 to 30 Hz.

Surgical technique

For anterior capsulotomy, a silica tip, designed to deliver energy at a 90° angle to the axis of the fiber, is used. With the use of this tip, a circular capsulotomy can be fashioned by directing the laser energy at levels of 12–15 mJ at 10–15 Hz towards the capsule (Figs 10.3 and 10.4). Cataract removal is performed using a silica tip with an 800-µm bulb. This gives a focused spot size of approximately 0.5 mm. The energy levels of 20–75 mJ at 10–15 Hz are used to produce cataract disruption.[5] The procedure can be performed using side-port aspiration and with irrigation and the laser probe introduced through a second side-port, or, in a second iteration, the laser tip and the aspiration–irrigation lines are contained in a single handpiece.

Clinical experience

The laser, as noted above, has been fully approved for anterior capsulotomy and has been found effective in phase 1 clinical trials for cataract disruption.

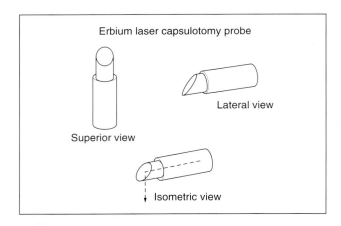

Figure 10.3. *A laser tip, designed specifically for anterior capsulotomy in the Premier laser system, directs Er:YAG energy at 90° to the axis of the optical fiber.*

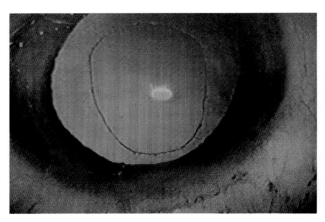

Figure 10.4. *A circular capsulotomy can be fashioned by simply drawing a circle on the anterior capsule with the Premier device.*

Potential advantages over existing technology

Like proponents of the Nd:YAG technology, advocates of the Er:YAG point to superior handpiece ergonomics, the smooth-tipped probe and a potentially more gentle cutting mechanism as advantages of this modality over phacoemulsification. A clear advantage of this device over standard ultrasonic instruments is its ability to perform a circular anterior capsulotomy.[6]

Nd:YLF LASERS

The Nd:YLF laser, manufactured by Intelligent Surgical Lasers, Inc. (ISL) of San Diego, California, represents the only laser modality in our discussion which has been used clinically without a fiber optic delivery system. This device utilizes a beam directed through the cornea and focused into the capsular bag. Although this laser is not under active clinical investigation at this time in the US, the technology is of sufficient interest that it is included in this discussion.

Introduction

The Intelligent Surgical Nd:YLF laser system was designed as a multipurpose device. It was developed primarily for its potential refractive surgical applications but was studied, under the direction of Schzanlin, for its usefulness in cataract surgery.

Description of technology

The crystal of the Nd:YLF laser, as noted previously, is yttrium–lithium–fluoride. This crystal allows for the generation of very fast pulses of energy (one trillionth of a second) which are focused to a very small spot size. A computer–assisted tracking system is included in the ISL device in an effort to localize and direct the bursts of laser energy within the capsular bag.

Surgical technique

Surgery with the ISL Nd:YLF 'picosecond' laser is a two-stage procedure. The patient is seated at a workstation (Fig. 10.5), and the laser energy is delivered through the cornea and into the nucleus of the cataract (Fig. 10.6). The intention is to soften the nuclear material so that only aspiration is needed. In the clinical study, the softened cataract was removed 18–24 h after the laser treatment.

Clinical experience

Approximately 100 patients were studied using this technique. In this initial group of patients, there were

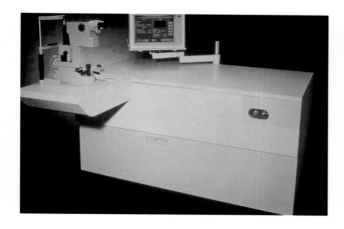

Figure 10.5. *The Intelligent Surgical Lasers Nd:YLF system utilizes a workstation. Patients are treated by this laser prior to the removal of cataract material.*

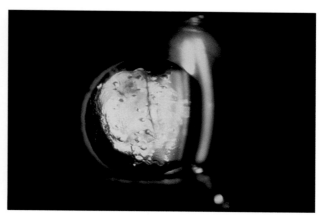

Figure 10.6. *The Nd:YLF laser softens the nucleus, facilitating cataract removal.*

no postoperative problems with increased pressure or anterior chamber inflammation. The surgeons found that while the laser did soften the nucleus and reduced average phacoemulsification time, it did not eliminate the need for ultrasonic energy altogether. ISL was encouraged by this initial work, but for a variety of reasons has not proceeded with additional investigation (Schzanlin D, personal communication).

Potential advantages over existing technology

The goal of the ISL Nd:YLF procedure is to make the second stage of the process solely an irrigation–aspiration maneuver. The realization of this goal could potentially simplify nucleus removal in cataract surgery.

SUMMARY

In summary, three very interesting laser modalities, representing the efforts of four laser companies, have been discussed. Each laser discussed is in a phase of developmental evolution, and each laser shows promise as a useful clinical device.

Many ophthalmologists believe that laser technology in some form holds the future of cataract surgery. The putative advantages of laser technology over standard ultrasonic methods for cataract extraction, however, remain largely unproven. Additional clinical research, coupled with technical development and clinical refinement, is needed if the dream of safer, gentler cataract surgery through laser technology is to be realized.

REFERENCES

1 Dodick JM, Christian J. Experimental studies on the development and propagation of shock waves created by the interaction of short Nd:YAG laser pulses with a titanium target: possible implications for Nd:YAG laser phacolysis of the cataractous human lens. *J Cataract Refract Surg* 1991; **17**: 794–7.

2 Lin CP, et al. High speed photograph of Er:YAG laser ablation in fluid. *Invest Ophthalmol Vis Sci* 1990; **32**: 2546–50.

3 Berger JW, D'Amico DJ. Modeling of Er:YAG laser mediated explosive photo vaporization: implications for vitro retinal surgery. *Ophthalmic Surg Lasers* 1997; **28**: 133–8.

4 Shi WQ, et al. Tissue interaction with mid-infrared lasers in saline. *Bull Am Phys Soc* 1991; **36**: 1991.

5 Stevens G, et al. Erbium-YAG assisted cataract surgery, work in progress.

6 Colvard DM, Kratz RP. Cataract surgery utilizing the erbium laser. In: Fine IH, ed. *Phacoemulsification: New Technology and Clinical Application* (Thorofare, NJ: Slack, 1996) 161–80.

Chapter 11 **The Catarex™ Technology**

Richard P Kratz, Soheila Mirhashemi, Michael Mittelstein and John T Sorensen

INTRODUCTION: THE TECHNOLOGY

Catarex™ is a fundamentally new and different technology that appears to represent a breakthrough in cataract surgery because of its potential advantages over extracapsular cataract extraction (ECCE), phacoemulsification (phaco) and other technologies under development.

DESCRIPTION OF TECHNOLOGY: THE SYSTEM

Several generations of progressively refined and improved functional prototypes of the system have been developed and tested. This system consists of a console, and a detachable handpiece with connecting catheter and fluid lines.

The latest-generation console is software driven and houses a high-speed motor, a fluidic pump system, a means for adjusting irrigation pressure and flow, an electrosurgical generator, a power supply, and associated electronics. A multifunctional foot pedal controls most of the console functions. Various operational parameters are set via a touch-activated video screen, which also functions to display various information to the user during operation.

The detachable handpiece incorporates a 1.5-mm-diameter impeller-tipped probe. The handpiece with associated connecting catheter and fluid lines are provided sterile for use and interconnect with the console. When attached to the console, the connecting catheter mechanically couples the motor in the console to the impeller located at the tip of the handpiece probe.

A specialized electrosurgical probe has also been developed for creating an entry site into the anterior lens capsule. This electrosurgical probe is provided sterile and also attaches to the console. When placed against the anterior lens capsule and activated, this specialized electrosurgical probe easily and reproducibly creates a round entry hole through the anterior lens capsule, which is properly sized for subsequent insertion of the Catarex™ probe.

SURGICAL TECHNIQUE

A 2.5-mm scleral, limbal or clear-cornea incision is made in the eye, sized for a tight fit of the probe. In contrast to Phaco and ECCE, the anterior lens capsule is not removed in this procedure. Instead, a 1.5-mm-diameter entry site is made in the lens capsule using a specially developed electrosurgical probe. Next, a small bolus of saline solution is injected into the lens capsule via a cannular sized such that it completely covers the capsular opening, effecting hydrodissection. The surgical probe is then inserted through the incision in the eye and through the lens capsule by stretching the entry site. Activation of the probe causes a small, partially shielded, high-speed impeller located at the tip of the probe to rotate. The impeller is designed such that its rotation induces vortex fluid flow within the lens capsular bag. This induced fluid flow draws lens and cortex material to the tip, where it is rapidly reduced upon contact with the rotating impeller. During removal of the lens material, the capsular bag is distended by the infused fluid, allowing the induced vortex to clear all of the contents of the bag without causing damage to the capsule. Keeping the bag expanded is essential to the success of the procedure. In contrast to phaco, which requires the surgeon to carve out the lens material through continuous manipulation and movement of the phaco probe, the Catarex™ probe can be held in a relatively stationary position within the lens capsule, while the induced fluid flow draws the cortex and lens material to the probe tip for reduction. In a manner similar to that in phaco, irrigation and aspiration flow provided via the probe is used to remove the reduced lens and cortex material from the lens capsule. At that point, the intraocular lens (IOL) is prepared for insertion.

Thus, the cataractous lens and cortex material are rapidly removed in a single step, through a 2.5-mm incision in the eye, leaving the lens capsule mostly intact. The clean lens capsule, having only a 1.5-mm opening, provides a highly desirable cataract removal outcome for future refilling with a liquid polymer injectable lens substitute. With Catarex™ it is anticipated that the surgical procedure time will be reduced relative to phaco.

PRECLINICAL AND CLINICAL EXPERIENCE—EXPERIMENTAL STUDIES

A set of various experimental studies has been performed to establish the proof-of-principle of the new technology. A number of the lenses examined in enucleated eyes had hard cataracts and were successfully removed with the Catarex™ technology. A brief description of these studies follows.

HUMAN CATARACT LENSES EMBEDDED IN GELATIN

The objective of these ex vivo studies was to demonstrate that human cataracts could effectively be reduced within the human lens capsule.

Fresh human cadaver cataract lenses contained within their intact lens capsules were embedded into gelatin. The probe was introduced into the lens capsule via a single puncture entry site. It was observed that human cataract lenses and associated cortex material were reduced and completely removed from the mostly intact lens capsule using Catarex™, typically within 2 min of probe activation.

EX VIVO STUDIES IN THE INTACT WHOLE PIG EYE

Numerous series of studies were conducted using the excised whole pig eye model. The objective of these ex vivo studies was to establish the appropriate operating parameters for this system and to determine

if the lens and cortex material of the intact whole pig eye could be removed without gross disruption of the lens capsule.

Fresh excised pig eyes were used for the experimental model. A standard slit blade (typically 2.65 mm) was used to make a clear corneal incision into the eye. As typically done during phaco, a viscoelastic was injected into the anterior chamber between the cornea and lens capsule to restore the volume of the anterior chamber of the eye. A specialized electrosurgical probe was then introduced through the incision and placed against the lens capsule. When activated, the electrosurgical probe created a small, circular entry hole about 1.5 mm in diameter through the anterior lens capsule. A small bolus of balanced salt solution (BSS) was injected into the lens capsule to cause a hydrodissection separation of the lens cortex from the lens capsule. A 1.5-mm probe was inserted into the lens capsule via the anterior entry site. The probe was activated, and the effectiveness of the lens and cortex reduction and removal was observed. In addition, gross postsurgical examination of the lens capsule was performed via the operating microscope to observe whether the posterior and anterior faces of the lens capsule remained mostly intact..

It was observed that the vortex formation of the system could effect rapid and reproducible reduction and removal of the lens and cortex material from the mostly intact lens capsule in a single step through a 1.5-mm anterior lens capsule entry site in the whole pig eye model.

The time of probe activation resulting in complete reduction and removal of the lens and cortex material was typically less than 3 min, and often within about 1 min. Gross postsurgical observation indicated successful removal of the lens and cortex material without disruption of the posterior or anterior lens capsule.

Some of the pig eyes from these studies were subsequently fixed in formalin and sent to an independent pathology laboratory for analysis. Results of the gross and microscopic examination of these eyes confirmed that the lens and cortex material were absent while the posterior and anterior lens capsules were intact except for the electrosurgically induced anterior lens capsule entry site.

EX VIVO STUDIES IN THE INTACT WHOLE PIG EYE USING MIYAKE PREPARATION

Additional ex vivo studies were performed in the excised pig eye model in the same manner as described above, except that the Miyake preparation of the eye was utilized. In the Miyake preparation, the whole eye is carefully sectioned such that the lower half of the eyeball containing the optic nerve is removed and the remaining upper half of the eyeball is mounted onto a clear glass slide. By the utilization of such an experimental preparation, the procedure could be observed from behind the lens capsule. From this perspective, the support of the lens capsule by the zonules (which are hidden from view by the iris when the procedure is conventionally viewed from above the lens capsule) can be directly observed during the procedure. Thus, any movement or stresses imposed on the zonules caused by the procedure can be experimentally observed. In addition, the posterior lens capsule can also be directly observed during the procedure using the Miyake preparation. The objective of these studies was to observe if the vortex fluid action would grossly disrupt or stress the zonules which support the lens capsule.

When the procedure was performed in the excised pig eye using the Miyake preparation, it was observed that very little movement of the posterior lens capsule and concomitant transmission of stresses to the zonule were induced during lens and cortex reduction and removal.

Interestingly, studies have been performed by other investigators using the Miyake preparation to observe zonule movement and stress during phaco procedures. In comparison, it would appear that the Catarex™ technology appeared to cause less gross capsule movement and stress to the zonule than that observed to occur during the phaco carving procedure.

IN VIVO STUDY IN THE LIVE SWINE MODEL

A study was performed to demonstrate the proof-of-principle of the Catarex™ lens removal technology in a live animal model. The objective of this study was to evaluate the ability of this system to remove the crystalline lens from the eye of a live pig.

An adult pig was selected for lens extraction. Atropine ophthalmic solution was instilled in both eyes. Intravenous mannitol was infused to control intraocular pressure. A clear corneal incision was made with a 2.65-mm keratome in one of the eyes. Viscoelastic was injected into the eye to maintain anterior chamber depth. The specialized electrosurgical probe was used to create a circular opening in the anterior lens capsule of about 1.5 mm diameter. BSS

was injected via a cannula through the lens capsule entry site to hydrodissect the lens cortex from the lens capsule bag. The probe was inserted into the lens through the anterior lens capsule entry site; the nucleus and cortex were reduced by the vortex action, and the fragments were removed by irrigation and aspiration flow. Viscoelastic was injected into the empty lens capsule to distend the capsular bag, which could then be examined for gross integrity under the surgical microscope. The corneal incision was closed with a single interrupted suture.

Postsurgical examination with the operating microscope indicated that the anterior and posterior faces of the lens capsule appeared intact. The crystalline lens appeared to be absent and only a small amount of cortex appeared to remain within the capsule sac. Upon gross pathologic examination, the capsule entry site was revealed, with absence of lens and lens cortical material. The posterior and anterior faces of the lens capsule were grossly intact. Upon microscopic evaluation, the zonules were present and only a small remnant of cortical material was noted in the equatorial region within the lens capsule.

POTENTIAL ADVANTAGES OVER EXISTING TECHNOLOGY (i.e. PHACOEMULSIFICATION)

Catarex™ may offer potential advantages over phaco and ECCE cataract removal. These potential advantages will be explored during our continuous investigation:

- The cataract lens and cortex materials are removed in a single step.
- The technology may be safer, since the probe is held in a relatively stationary position during lens reduction.
- The cataractous lens-reducing procedure is performed completely within the lens capsule, eliminating the potential risk of damage to the corneal endothelium lining.
- The handpiece is substantially smaller in size and weighs less than phaco handpieces, so surgeon control and comfort are enhanced.
- Delivery of the mechanical energy, which rotates the impeller, is very efficient, virtually eliminating concerns about heat build-up in the probe or heat-induced corneal burn.

One truly outstanding and exciting distinction that sets the Catarex™ procedure apart from other approaches is the fact that the lens capsule remains functionally intact after surgery. As discussed previously, implantation of most IOLs does not restore accommodation. In the future, it would be highly desirable to refill the lens capsule with a liquid polymer injectable lens substitute after the natural cataract lens has been surgically removed. In theory, refilling the lens capsule with such an elastomeric material would allow the eye to be able to change the shape of the substitute lens and thus function in a natural manner, restoring accommodation. Restoration of accommodation would represent the ultimate postsurgical endpoint for cataract treatment. A number of major ophthalmic companies are known to be working on the development of liquid polymer injectable lenses as substitutes for the human lens. This technology can achieve lens and cortex removal while leaving the lens capsule functionally intact; thus, Catarex™ represents the enabling technology for such future use of injectable lens substitutes.

Chapter 12 **PhacoTmesis**

Aziz Y Anis

HISTORICAL EVOLUTION

Prior to 1980–81 I had relied upon manual cataract removal. I had at that time developed and refined my dry intercapsular cataract extraction (DICE) technique, in which I used a similar method of anterior capsulotomy as the envelope technique used by Albert Galand. I did not use any irrigation to maintain the anterior chamber but I filled it with viscoelastic and I completed the whole procedure (sliding the nucleus out from the capsular bag and then aspirating the cortex strip by strip) without any irrigation; hence the name 'dry technique'.

I have to admit that at that time I was still very critical of phacoemulsification; the criticism was mainly of the techniques used then rather than of the technology itself. Since then, both technology and techniques have been improved and refined to provide a highly controlled and precise method for small-incision cataract extraction.

During my work with the DICE technique, I used to separate the anterior capsule from the anterior cortex by gently lifting the anterior capsule with a cyclo-dialysis spatula and sweeping it from side to side. In one instance I was handed a 30-gauge cannula instead of the cyclo-dialysis spatula, and the syringe contained some balanced salt solution (BSS), some of which was accidentally injected during the maneuver. I observed the fluid quickly cleave between capsule and cortex all around the equator separating the posterior capsule from the posterior cortex and nucleus. I started intentionally repeating this process in surgery after that, and even though I did not meet any major complications, I returned to using the cyclo-dialysis spatula for fear of rupturing the posterior capsule with fluid pressure that could be trapped posteriorly. I mentioned this observation a couple of times and eventually it developed into what we now know as hydrodissection. This led me

to the thought of injecting deeper into the substance of the lens, expecting to fragment segments of the cortical and nuclear periphery and eventually wash the fragments out of the anterior chamber through a small incision. I planned to rotate the lens and continue this fragmenting process by water wedging until the whole nucleus and cortex were extracted. Another option that I thought of was that, after creating many fragmenting cracks in the nucleus, I would introduce a wide-bored cannula and manually aspirate the fragments. When I started experimenting with these concepts I found that instead of the segmental fracturing that I expected, the fluid cleaved between the outer lamella of the nucleus and created concentric cleavage circles as seen through the microscope. I called this process hydrodelineation. Even though hydrodissection and hydrodelineation were widely adopted by standard phacoemulsification surgeons to facilitate their techniques of standard phacoemulsification, my objectives were quite different. I was hoping to develop a non-ultrasound small-incision technique. This was actually achievable in relatively soft nuclei, where a 30-gauge cannula or needle is able to penetrate the nucleus almost to its center; however, it was not possible to penetrate 2+ or harder nuclei.

Therefore, I decided to provide the cannula with more aggressive penetrating power by propelling it with ultrasound. Alcon worked with me to realize this objective, and together we developed hydrosonics. Hydrosonics combines an ultrasonic handpiece with a specially configured 29-gauge cannula that is ultrasonically driven and which contains a pump mechanism that automatically injects small increments of BSS. Also I described another handpiece with a rotating tip that could easily bore into the now softened and fragmented nucleus and simply aspirate it and the cortex, possibly again in a dry manner. However, the aspirating rotating-tip handpiece was never developed in conjunction with hydrosonics.

After hydrosonics was formally introduced by Alcon on the Master 10,000 series and later on the Legacy 20,000 in 1988–89, I started using it in a modified phacoemulsification method which I called hydrosonic phacoemulsification, in which I simply used the phacoemulsification tip as a means of aspirating the hydrosonically fragmented and mashed nuclear and cortical matter, with my foot in position 2 on the foot control most of the time. I only pressed onto position 3 to provide ultrasonic power when I met a slightly larger fragment that occluded the tip and would not aspirate.

I was still not completely satisfied that I had fulfilled my objectives. I also realized that there was a reluctance on the part of surgeons to use two handpieces to extract the nucleus while more refined and controlled techniques like divide and conquer and phaco chop and others were introduced which facilitated phacoemulsification dramatically and increased the number of phacoemulsification surgeons in leaps and bounds.

It was obvious to me, however, that in all these techniques the burden of precision and safety in the procedure, particularly in protecting the posterior capsule, lay on the surgeon's shoulders. There was no inherent feature in the instrument itself to protect the posterior capsule.

During a coffee chat late in 1988 with Mark Steen, I sketched an idea roughly on a napkin. It was a concept for a surface discriminating instrument. It was simply a small 1.5-mm-diameter band ring at the tip of an aspirating rotating cannula (Fig. 12.1). I thought that if this cannula rotated at a very high speed it would scrape off slivers of the nucleus within the sphere formed by the rotating ring, and these would pass through the cannula to be eliminated. I thought that if the advancing edge of the band was relatively sharp and the receding edge was relatively thick (Figure 12.2), the sharp edge would cut efficiently and the cavitation behind the receding edge would further facilitate the process. I visualized that this cutting and cavitation would only occur in the complex fibrillar, lamellar structure of the nucleus and cortex, but to the capsule smoothly stretched by the appropriate intracameral pressure regulated by the bottle height, the instrument would be no more than a smooth-surfaced polishing sphere.

Using a prototype unit I wrapped a bar of hand soap with Saran Wrap and I was delighted to see the tip sink into the soap like a hot nail in butter but stop dead as soon as it hit the Saran Wrap. I could not cut into it while still rotating at full speed. Later, a simple pump mechanism and passive irrigation were added.

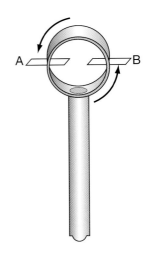

Figure 12.1. *Initial concept of rotating ring on aspirating cannula.*

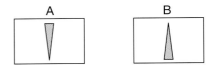

Figure 12.2. *Proceeding edge of ring – sharp (A); receding edge of ring – blunt (B)*

We tested it on pigs' eyes, using a dental drill to provide a very high speed of rotation that reached almost 400 000 rev/min. The pigs' lenticular matter disappeared in no more than a couple of seconds, while the capsule remained intact in spite of touching it with the tip. With that crude model, however, the very high speed caused considerable chattering. The same rapid elimination of lenticular matter happened with cadaver eyes that had very soft lenses.

I elected to work with Chiron on this project and I insisted having Mark Steen to conduct the research and development on the instrument. At first I called the device the 'phacomole', because it bore into the lens and ate it from the inside out. However, I thought it sounded unscientific, and chose the Greek term for cutting, 'tmesis'. In my first presentation of this technology in the ASCRS meeting in 1989, I introduced the term. PhacoTmesis received immediate acceptance and recognition.

I signed an exclusive agreement with Chiron in 1990 with the great promise of prompt development. Unfortunately, progress was very slow. However, during that time we found that the rotating-ring concept, even though extremely safe for the posterior capsule, was not practical in removing a regular 3 or 3+ cataract. The procedure took a longer time and the rotating ring provided less access to the aspirating cannula. We therefore modified the tip by creating a short longitudinal slit at the end of a zero-degree cannula and offset the two halves slightly as in Fig. 12.3. This provided very much the same mechanism as the rotating ring in cutting and cavitation, and it provided a terminal access port for the lenticular matter to be aspirated. However, this configuration reduced or eliminated the surface discrimination provided by the ring, and the slits on either side slowed the aspiration because of the difficulty in occlusion. At this time I decided to add ultrasound to the rotation, hoping that the combined energies would produce a greater cutting and aspirating effect than ultrasound alone.

This provided an engineering challenge for Mark Steen, but he successfully designed a handpiece that included both a motor and an ultrasonic transducer to produce both movements simultaneously at the tip. It cut through hard nuclei with apparently no resistance. Nuclear tissue appeared to break down ahead of the tip.

In March 1993 we performed the first phacoTmesis procedures and in 1994 premarket approval was obtained.

An interface unit called the Synergist, which contains the ultrasound driver and an interface board to utilize the fluidics of any existing phacoemulsification machine was developed.

I continued to use the Synergist unit fitted on my Alcon Legacy phacoemulsification machine and was able to explore its unique features and develop the optimum technique that utilizes these features. In August 1997, by mutual agreement I withdrew the license from Chiron and I continued to use Tmesis as my only method for small-incision cataract surgery until the present date. In March 1998 I signed a global license for Alcon to include the Tmesis technology in its cataract machines.

CURRENT TMESIS INSTRUMENT

The Tmesis equipment that I presently use and which other surgeons such as Brint, Rheinhardt Koch, Budo and others use, comprises the following.

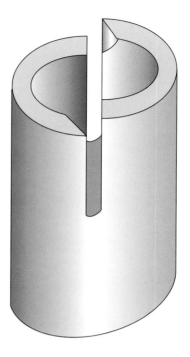

Figure 12.3. *Original concept of rotating ultrasonic fragmenting cannula with split at the tip and offset halves.*

SYNERGIST UNIT (FIG. 12.4)

The Synergist unit is the power unit for the Tmesis handpiece and contains the ultrasonic driver and the interface board. It is about 12 in long by 12 in wide by 2 in high. On the back is the power cord and the port for the special cable that connects it to the ultrasonic port on the host machine. The end of the cable that plugs into the host machine carries the port for the handpiece cable. Also on the back of the Synergist unit is a control button for the balance between rotation and ultrasound (Fig. 12.5).

When the arrow is at 12 o'clock, both rotation and ultrasound start simultaneously when the foot control reaches position 3. From there on further depression of the foot control increases ultrasonic power linearly. Rotation is standard at 4000 rev/min. An ultrasonic power ceiling is set on the host machine. If the control button is turned to the left, ultrasound starts first and rotation begins with further depression of the foot control. If the button is turned to the right, rotation will start first, and will be followed by ultrasound.

Synergist* Interface

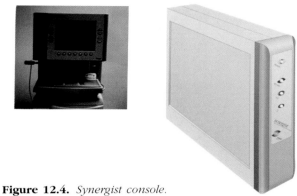

Figure 12.4. *Synergist console.*

Normal

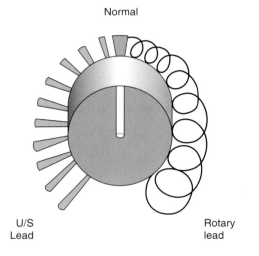

U/S
Lead

Rotary
lead

Figure 12.5. *Control button on back of synergist. In the normal position ultrasound. Turn dial to the left for ultrasound first followed by rotation. Turn dial to the right for rotation first followed by ultrasound.*

CONNECTING CABLE

Each host machine requires a special cable configured to fit its specifics.

TMESIS HANDPIECE (FIG. 12.6)

The Tmesis handpiece is an intricately engineered, precise, high-technology instrument. It is almost the

same size as a standard phaco handpiece, or slightly larger. It contains a high-technology mini-motor to provide high-speed rotation and a composite crystal to provide ultrasonic linear oscillation simultaneously.

As mentioned before, we have experimented with different rotation speeds, reaching as high as 40 000 rev/min, and came to the conclusion that the optimum rotation speed combined with ultrasonics was somewhere between 3000 and 5000 rev/min.

TMESIS TIPS

The optimum tip size and configuration, which was found by trial and observation over an expanse of thousands of cases, was 0.6 mm with a zero-degree blunt and smoothly polished tip edge. The placement of the tip should be done very carefully by a well-trained surgical technician using a special wrench. Extra care should be exercised not to bend the tip at the hub during installation or by leaning the handpiece in any way that would cause pressure on the side of the tip. A special silicone irrigating sleeve is provided with the tip (Fig. 12.7).

HIGH-MAGNIFICATION OBSERVATION OF THE EFFECT OF TMESIS ON THE NUCLEAR TISSUE

Since 1994 I have been using Tmesis routinely as my only instrument for cataract surgery. So far I have performed approximately 3000 Tmesis procedures. Some very clearly defined observations have been made by the other surgeons who have used Tmesis in a large number of cases.

These observations are:

*   The cutting performance of Tmesis, such as in creating a groove in the nucleus, is characteristically resistance-free, no matter how hard the nucleus is.
*   The anterior chamber remains absolutely stable without the slightest hint of any vacuum surge. Prolonged occlusion and vacuum build-up never happens, no matter what vacuum level is used.
*   No wound burn has ever been observed, no matter how long the ultrasonic time.
*   Even in the obvious presence of a posterior capsular tear before complete elimination of the nucleus,

Rotary-Ultrasonics
Handpiece Cut-Away

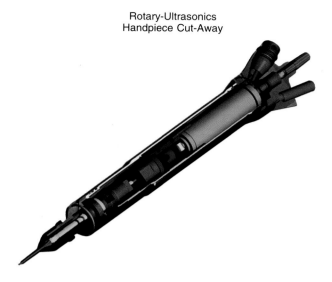

Figure 12.6. *Tmesis handpiece cut-away.*

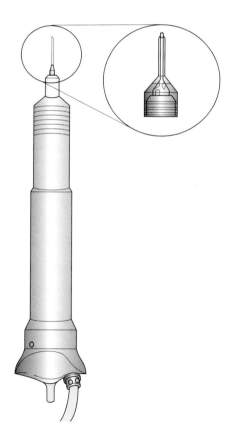

Figure 12.7. *Tmesis handpiece with silicone irrigating sleeve.*

vitreous entanglement does not appear to happen and the capsular tear does not appear to enlarge.

Since the observations are quite different from the experience with standard phacoemulsification, I tried to find logical explanations for these observations. In January 1998, I solicited the assistance of the Engineering School at the University of Nebraska. Professor Alexander devised a method to observe and analyse what happens at the Tmesis tip under high magnification (Fig. 12.8).

The method of analysis comprised of:

- Television camera coupled with optical magnification system.
- N_2 Laser$_m$ = 337 mm with pulse length = 10 ms.
- Trigger signals from television camera synchronized with N_2 laser firing.

The laser was placed at one end of a 12-foot table and the television camera was lined up with it at the other end. A holding chamber filled with BSS and containing a human cadaver nucleus was placed midway, intercepting the direct line between the laser and the camera. The resulting image is more or less a silhouette.

The Tmesis handpiece was fixed vertically above, with the tip immersed in the BSS solution above the nucleus. Directional controls could move the handpiece up, down, sideways, forwards and backwards under ×500 magnification.

The following observations were made:

In fluid above the nucleus:

- Ultrasound alone: at 70% power, showed no significant cavitation bubbles.
- Rotation alone: at 4000 rev/min, showed no discernible effect.
- Combined rotation and ultrasound produced a marked formation of well-formed, sizeable cavitation bubbles. The significant observation was that the bubbles did not disperse but rather crowded together to form a convex cushion covering the cross-sectional area of the tip opening and extending a significant distance beyond the tip (Fig. 12.9).

When the tip was advanced towards the nucleus:

- With ultrasound alone, the advancement of the tip would produce no effect until the tip touched the nucleus, and it then would grab it.

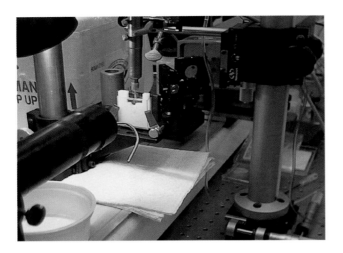

Figure 12.8. *Set-up for high-magnification analysis of effect at Tmesis tip.*

Figure 12.9. *Cavitation bubble cushion limited to tip aperture without dispersing.*

- With rotation only, small vortices would extend from the tip to the nucleus, producing no significant effect until the tip grabbed the nucleus.
- With combined ultrasound and rotation, as the tip approaches the nucleus the cavitation bubble cushion touches it first and disintegrates the nuclear tissue ahead of the tip so that the tip is practically unable to make direct contact with the tissue as long as it is active (Fig. 12.10). I labeled this effect macroablation. This macroablation is sufficient to explain many of the observations mentioned above.
- There is no resistance in cutting, because macroablation disintegrates the nuclear tissue ahead of the tip and therefore, since the end of the tip never actually touches the tissue, there is no sensation of any resistance.
- The anterior chamber depth is characteristically stable, since the nuclear tissue is finely disintegrated by macroablation. There are no nuclear fragments large enough to occlude the Tmesis tip for a length of time sufficient to cause build-up of significant negative pressure and subsequent surge.
- Wound burn does not happen, since there are no occasions of prolonged occlusion to cause increased heat accumulation. Unlike the standard phaco tip, where the surface of the cannula remains in the same position in relation to the incisional tissues while oscillating linearly at ultrasonic speed, thus permitting heat to accumulate on the areas of maximum friction which lie

against the anterior and posterior lips of the incision, the constant rotation of the Tmesis tip prevents any heat accumulation on any particular area of the surface. This area is constantly cooled by the irrigating fluid on either side of the tip formed by the vertical compression of the irrigating sleeve caused by the incision.
- Vitrectomy is possible because macroablation has the same disintegrating effect on the vitreous as it has on the lenticular tissue, and thus tmesis acts as an extremely efficient vitrectomy instrument.

TECHNIQUE

The basic general principles that differentiate Tmesis techniques from standard phacoemulsification techniques are based upon Tmesis' unique capabilities.

For example, the macroablation feature is capable of creating a nuclear groove deep enough to fracture the nucleus with two or three passes. Macroablation can create a very short, deep groove which is particularly helpful in small pupils. This is in contrast to creating a groove with standard phacoemulsification, where shallow strips are sculpted using numerous passes to prevent occlusion and transfixation of the nucleus. The macroablation feature is capable of removing most of the bulk of the nucleus by simply hovering over the

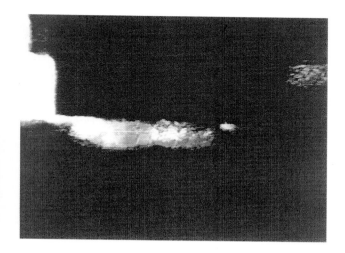

Figure 12.10. *No-touch disintegration of nuclear tissue by cavitation bubble cushion ahead of tip (macroablation).*

tissue at a very short distance without actually making contact, and so it is preferable not to divide the nucleus into small pieces.

In contrast with standard phacoemulsification, the nucleus has to be divided into small fragments by fracturing or chopping and feeding the small fragments to the phaco tip to aspirate them wth high vacuum levels, which is never needed in Tmesis.

The smooth, blunt, zero-degree tip is used to remove any residual cortex, and with the proper fluidic parameters it is used to scrub and remove any thin cortical filaments or cells off the posterior capsule and the equator, in contrast to standard phacoemulsification, where another handpiece is needed.

CRACK, DEBULK AND TUMBLE TECHNIQUE

I have developed this technique.

INCISION

A 2.5-mm incision is made with a diamond keratome. A vertical incision about half the thickness of the peripheral cornea is made just outside the clear cornea. The keratome is then introduced obliquely through the vertical incision to enter the anterior chamber, forming an internal corneal valve.

CAPSULORHEXIS

A 7–8-mm-diameter capsulorhexis is performed.

HYDRODISSECTION

Using the original hydrosonic cannula on a syringe, careful cortical cleavage hydrodissection is performed manually. When done carefully, this maneuver permits the cortex to be separated clearly with the nucleus from the capsular bag at the same time.

HYDRODELINEATION

Using the cannula, hydrodelineation is performed.

FRACTURING GROOVE

The fluidic parameters for the fracturing groove are as follows:

- Ultrasonic power ceiling: 70%
- Vacuum: zero
- Aspiration flow rate: 30 ml/min

Two or three passes are enough to form a deep groove along the diameter of the nucleus. Vacuum is reduced to zero in this phase, in order not to grab onto the nucleus. The nucleus is now fractured into two halves with cracking forceps or manually.

DEBULKING

Using the same parameters as above, the tmesis tip is moved back and forth over each half of the nucleus to macroablate as much of the central core as possible.

ASPIRATION

The nucleus is now rotated so that the dividing crack is 90° to the tip. The distal nuclear half is now tumbled so that the equator presents in the pupillary area and the posterior surface of the nuclear equator. The vacuum is increased to 200 mmHg. Tumbling of the half-nuclear shell can be accomplished by applying the Tmesis tip to its anterior lip and establishing occlusion by aspiration only and towards the pupillary center. Tumbling can also be done with a careful scooping maneuver with the silent tip or with a nuclear manipulator. Once the half-nuclear shell is tumbled, the Tmesis tip is applied directly against the smooth surface of the equator and aspiration is started only to achieve firm occlusion; Tmesis power is then started, to revise a chunk of the nuclear shell. This process is repeated until the nuclear half is aspirated. The same tactic is used to aspirate the remaining half. If the hydrodissection was done carefully and well, there is usually no remaining cortex. If there is any residual cortex, the Tmesis tip is used in the aspiration/irrigation mode to remove it.

To remove any thin cortical filaments and epithelial cells, the vacuum is reduced to zero, the aspiration flow rate is reduced to 5 ml/min, and the Tmesis tip is applied directly to the posterior capsule and the equator to scub it clear. (Careful inspection of the edge of the tip should have been done prior to surgery to ensure its perfect smoothness and the absence of any sharp imperfection.)

VITRECTOMY

If an accidental tear in the posterior capsule occurs or if an intentional anterior vitrectomy is required, for example to remove asteroid hyalosis after a posterior capsulorhexis is performed, the Tmesis tip is used with the following fluidic parameters:

- Ultrasonic power: 70%
- Vacuum: 200 mmHg
- Flow rate: 30 ml/min

During all phases of the operation, the irrigation fluid bottle is kept at a height of 80 cm.

Chapter 13 Cataract rehabilitation in Asia: the role of extracapsular cataract extraction

Arthur SM Lim and Ronald LS Yeoh

THE CATARACT PROBLEM

Cataract is the leading cause of blindness in the world today and is responsible for 50% of all blindness.[1] In developed nations, cataract patients have ready access to the latest, safest and best techniques in cataract surgery. Currently, this usually means some form of small-incision cataract surgery with a posterior chamber lens implant done under local or topical anaesthesia. In developing countries, however, access to an acceptable level of cataract surgery is more difficult (Fig. 13.1). There are a number of reasons for this, and these will be touched on later. There is thus a great divide between the 'haves' and the 'have-nots'; on the one hand, patients having 6/6 (20/20) vision after surgery, and on the other, patients remaining blind and miserable, indefinitely. There is therefore the problem of mass cataract blindness which arises because patients have no choice but to become blind; a modern tragedy in the twentieth century (Fig. 13.2). Cataract blindness adds to existing economic difficulty because a blind person becomes an added burden to both the family and the state.

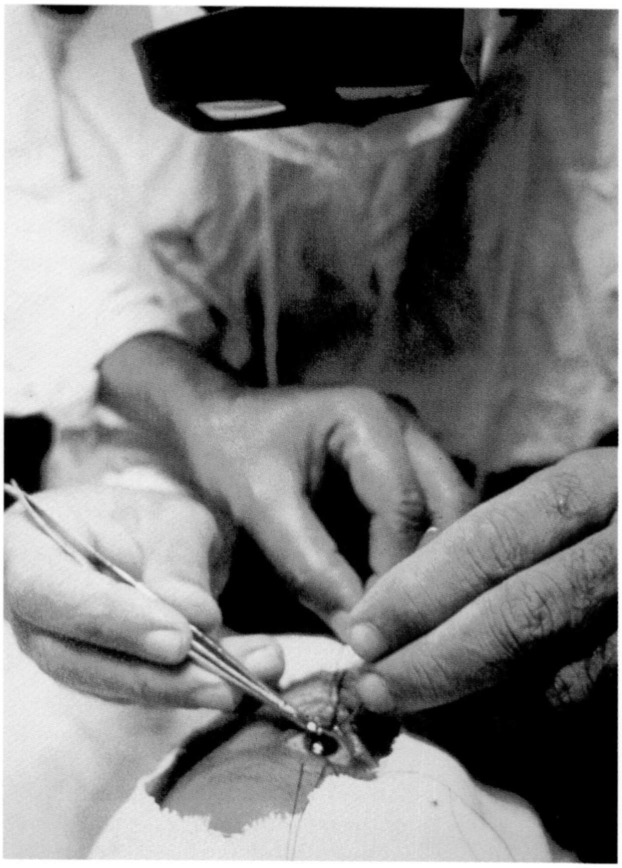

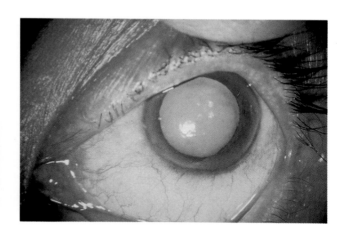

Figure 13.1. *Cataract surgery under difficult conditions.*

Figure 13.2. *Mature, blinding cataract.*

The Indian sociologist Rajendra T. Vyas made a touching statement in 1990:

> In developing countries, there are inadequate or absolutely no old age pensions or disability allowance schemes. Thus when a person becomes blind, he would be unemployed and have no means of supporting himself and his family. This often results in starvation and early death. The family then becomes destitute ... While blindness from cataract is easily reversible, colossal numbers exist in the rural communities of the developing countries. The rural people wait helplessly for the day of deliverance from their miserable existence. We have to ask ourselves whether we are going to allow them to pass their days in darkness and destitution?

In this chapter, we present the current situation in Asia, a diverse continent which encompasses developing, developed and newly industrialized countries. We discuss the current techniques used to approach mass cataract blindness and the problems associated with prevention of cataract blindness, and state our vision for the future. The comments we make may be applicable to other countries in the world.

MASS CATARACT BLINDNESS VERSUS SOCIAL VISUAL DISABILITY

How bad is the cataract problem? In the wealthier Asian countries, cataract is not a significant cause of blindness; diabetic eye disease is. Indeed, in most developed countries, cataracts are frequently operated on at a relatively early stage. In the poorer developing countries, however, cataract blindness is foremost. These numbers are increasing annually as healthcare workers battle the tide of an aging population. Many poor people cannot access cataract surgery; Taylor, in 1995,[2] indicated that only one out of six cataract patients has access to surgery.

An estimate by the WHO in 1990 of 20 million blind from cataract and increasing by 2 million every year[1] is probably conservative today. By extrapolation, cataract-blind people in India number 6–8 million, in China 4–6 million, etc. This relentless increase is worsened by the failure of existing cataract programmes to make an impact on case numbers.

Table 13.1
Per capita income and GNP for some Asia Pacific countries.

Country	Per capita income (1985)	Per capita GNP (1993)
Japan	US$8,316.00	US$31 490
Hong Kong	US$6,311.00	US$18 060
Singapore	US$5,847.00	US$19 850
Taiwan	US$3,142.00	US$10 852
South Korea	US$1,954.00	US$7 660
Malaysia	US$1,574.00	US$3 140
Thailand	US$579.41	US$2 110
India	US$220.00	US$300
Nepal	US$139.00	US$190
Bangladesh	US$128.61	US$220
China	–	US$490
Australia	–	US$17 500
New Zealand	–	US$12 600

Source: Far East Economic Review Asia 1987 Yearbook and Far East Economic Review Asia 1996 Yearbook. (Hong Kong: Review Publishing Co)

WHY HAVE WE FAILED IN ASIA?

That the cataract problem is worsening year by year is not in question; we have to question why. There are many reasons, some within and some outside our control.

It has to be remembered that Asia is a diverse continent of countries and economies with great differences (Table 13.1). The wealthier nations have few problems; it is the less wealthy developing countries that have the biggest problems with mass cataract blindness.

DEMOGRAPHY

As the global population ages, we are becoming victims of medical science's success in increasing lifespan. Cataract is well known as a condition of the elderly.[3] The population numbers vary tremendously; China has a billion people, and India not many fewer, whilst Singapore only has 3 million. The peoples of Asia are also diverse, with differing needs and perceptions.

GEOGRAPHY

Many poor people are scattered far and wide in rural and difficult-to-reach communities in vast countries like India and China. Delivering meaningful health care to them is a major logistic exercise. Hospitals, equipment and expertise tend to be concentrated in city centres, far from rural communities.

RESOURCES

Japan is one of the richest countries in the world, and yet Asia also has countries with very low per capita incomes (Table 13.1). Resources may be made available through organizations like the WHO, IAPB, the World Bank, etc., but a critical evaluation shows that the mass cataract blindness situation is not improving.

TRAINED SURGEONS

For many developing nations, in the rural communities, there is a shortage of eye surgeons trained in modern cataract surgery, i.e. extracapsular cataract extraction (ECCE) and intraocular lens (IOL) implantation. In locations where there may be adequate numbers of eye surgeons, they may be concentrated in the city centres.

THE ICCE VERSUS ECCE CONTROVERSY

The current surgical technique practised in most mass cataract blindness programmes (up to two-thirds) is intracapsular cataract extraction (ICCE) with aphakic glasses, a 30-year-old technique.[4] Many reports indicate that the majority do not benefit from this operation.[5] ICCE done in eye camps without microscopes and sometimes with poor facilities has led to criticism because of poor visual results and high complication rates[6] (Fig. 13.3). An estimated 40–80% of people who have had ICCE do not have aphakic glasses when re-examined.[7–9] Indeed, uncorrected aphakia is an important cause of blindness. It is well established that ECCE with a posterior chamber IOL is the operation of choice for most cataracts.

It is not surprising that ICCE for the masses has not really worked; the visual result is suboptimal, the complication rate is high and there is little incentive for young doctors to perform this operation.

Why, then, is this outdated surgical technique still practised for the masses blinded by cataract? Why is

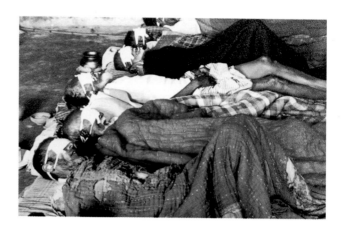

Figure 13.3. *Eye camp.*

this technique recommended when we would not choose to have it used on ourselves? The powers that be deem this technique to be expedient and cheap. The question that needs to be asked is whether expedience justifies an inferior operation.

Some of the arguments against the wider use of ECCE + IOL involve the relative lack of trained microsurgeons, microscopes and implants. Posterior capsule opacification can also pose a problem. None of these problems are insurmountable with proper organization and distribution of resources.

LOW-COST ECCE AND IMPLANT TECHNIQUES

There have been numerous queries on how to proceed with quality ECCE and posterior chamber implant (PCI) without high cost.

One reason is that the numerous options advocated are confusing for many ophthalmologists. Some important basic considerations for achieving good results should therefore be stressed. It is emphasized that many of the recent 'advances' are more for fine-tuning surgical techniques and should be considered to be alternatives and not advances.

Cost need not be high if instruments are kept simple. The main cost is the proper training of the surgeon. One must also invest in a good operating microscope with coaxial light, because good

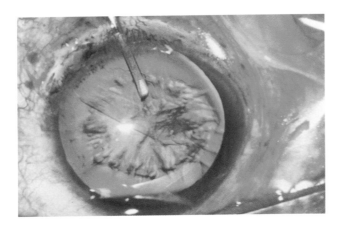

Figure 13.4. *Can-opener capsulotomy.*

visualization is important. The other costs include: cost of the implants, which will decrease in the near future; cost of viscoelastic material, a useful but not essential item; cost of infusion fluid, which can be made much cheaper; and the cost of other equipment, such as diamond knives and automated infusion/aspiration machines, which are not essential, but convenient to have.

It is important to remember the factors important for the success of ECCE and PCI surgery:

- Good microsurgeon.
- Good operating microscope with coaxial light.
- Soft eye by compression for at least 10 min.
- Well-dilated pupil; infusion fluid with 1 : 1 000 000 adrenaline to keep pupil dilated.
- Anterior capsulectomy (can-opener technique) with bent tip of disposable needle (Fig. 13.4).
- Nucleus expressed gently.
- Cortex removal by Simcoe or similar system. The technique of aspirating cortex is important.
- Understanding of important reflexes—ring reflex, radiating lines.

It is just as important to know that many innovations are useful but not essential:

- Viscoelastic material.
- Balanced salt solution (BSS) or special BSS.
- Mechanical aspiration.
- In-the-bag insertion of implant.
- Diamond knife.

OPERATING MICROSCOPE

It can never be overemphasized that an operating microscope with good coaxial light is essential for successful ECCE.

RED REFLEX

The red reflex shows up many important structures which are otherwise not seen.

IMPORTANT SILHOUETTES

Most important is the appearance of the posterior capsule when it is caught in the aspirating port. It appears as radiating black lines converging towards the aspirating port. It is an extremely important physical sign because, when it is present, the instrument must not be moved, as any movement may tear the posterior capsule. Careful infusion of fluid will push the posterior capsule away from the port.

RING REFLEX

This is an important reflex and is due to indentation of the posterior capsule by the aspirating cannula. It indicates that the posterior capsule is intact and bulging against the cannula.

BASIC MICROSURGERY

COMMON ERROR: HIGH MAGNIFICATION

A common error is to use high magnification when suturing. It is important not to use high magnification when suturing, because the needle, needle-holder and forceps will be out of view of the microscope. This makes suturing extremely difficult.

Magnification of ×5 or ×6 is adequate for most purposes. Magnification of higher than ×10 is usually unnecessary. During precise dissection, such as dissecting the scleral flap, some surgeons use higher magnification.

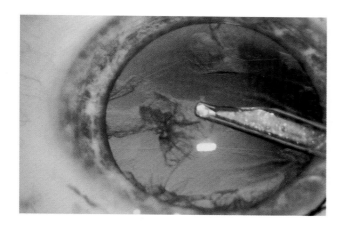

Figure 13.5. *Low-cost Simcoe cannula.*

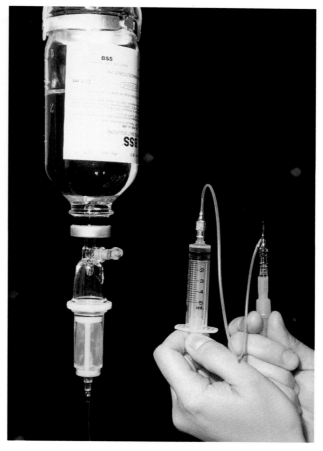

Figure 13.6. *Manual irrigation/aspiration.*

INFUSION/ASPIRATION SYSTEM

There are several useful infusion/aspiration systems used to remove the cortex. The most popular system is the Simcoe cannula (Fig. 13.5).

The Simcoe cannula has advantages over the McIntyre and other systems. Because it is flat, it opens the wound less than a circular cannula would. Accordingly, less fluid leaks out of the wound and the anterior chamber is maintained more effectively.

There is increasing acknowledgement by implant surgeons who have performed thousands of ECCEs, that the Simcoe manual technique to aspirate the cortex is not only the most economical but also provides the best control. The aspiration can be completed in less than 3 min with less than 5 ml of fluid.

The curve of the cannula avoids the prominent frontal bone and the nose and therefore does not interfere with intraocular manipulation of the cannula. This also simplifies aspiration of the cortex at 12 o'clock.

This system can be worked with one hand holding the probe and with the other hand doing the aspiration. It is preferable to use a 5-ml syringe for better control, instead of a 20-ml syringe as was originally suggested. It is important to avoid having air in the syringe, as this would interfere with control. The infusion of fluid is better through a drip with the bottles set at 60 cm above the eye, adjusted if desired, rather than a bulb (Fig. 13.6).

INSTRUMENTS

A small number of instruments is required and they are:

- microforceps
- micro needle-holder
- blade-holder for razor blade
- corneal scissors (right/left)
- Kelman–McPherson angled forceps
- Sinskey hook.

THE IMPLANT—CHOICE AND POWER

There are several hundred types of lens implant, and the choice can be difficult. It should be emphasized

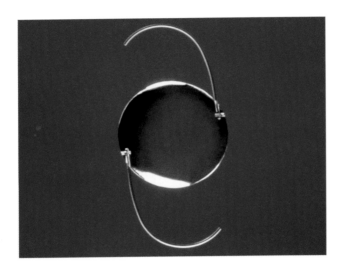

Figure 13.7. *Sinskey-style implant.*

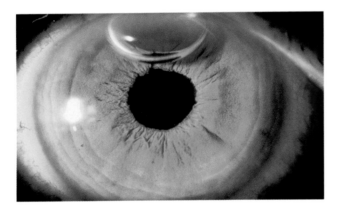

Figure 13.8. *Successful ECCE +IOL.*

that good results are achieved because of good surgery. Most modern implants from reputable implant companies of good standing will produce high-quality implants. It is best to avoid cheap implants from new, unfamiliar manufacturers.

The Sinskey implant is a good implant to use (Fig. 13.7). Modification includes angulation.

Most surgeons today will calculate intraocular implant power with corneal curvature measured with the keratometer and axial length of eye measured with ultrasonography.

Planned microscopic ECCE with posterior chamber implant can be done safely, producing excellent results, by trained eye surgeons using low-cost techniques (Fig. 13.8).

WHAT PRICE PHACOEMULSIFICATION?

Small-incision cataract surgery with foldable implants is currently widely practised in developed countries. It is also widely practised in the more developed Asian economies, but only in the major Asian cities, where an estimated 50–80% of cataract procedures are done using phacoemulsification (phaco) techniques. The increased capital and recurring costs of phaco have restricted its use in rural communities.

Nevertheless, even while there is debate on the ECCE versus ICCE issue for mass cataract blindness, there is an ever-increasing body of ophthalmologists who are advocating the somewhat controversial use of phaco in eye camps. Mehta has carried out successful eye camps in rural areas using phaco.[10] Maloney also feels that phaco has much to offer in the treatment of mass cataract blindness (Maloney WF, personal communication).

The justification advanced is that phaco with use of a 5-mm IOL may be done without suturing and with rapid visual rehabilitation. The cost of the phaco machine is reduced with volume surgery and there are cost savings resulting from fewer sutures being used.

In trained hands, phaco clearly offers excellent results. However, we have to bear in mind the difficulties in training enough phaco surgeons in this high-technology operation. The phaco learning curve has potentially serious complications. Phaco machines also need maintenance.

Clearly, the debate still rightly centres on ICCE or ECCE + IOL as the procedure of choice for mass cataract blindness. To even consider phaco as a valid alternative requires a paradigm shift as far as mass cataract blindness is concerned. Although this sounds far-fetched, it is not beyond the realms of possibility, and in years to come phaco for the masses, in appropriate situations, may yet come to pass.

CATARACT TECHNIQUES IN ASIA IN THE YEAR 2000

By the year 2000, quality cataract surgery will spread throughout Asia. The demand for quality eye care, in particular quality cataract surgery and phaco, will increase.

It is likely that less than 10% of cataract surgery in Asia will be done by phaco at the turn of the millenium. This is largely related to cost. While phaco is in the ascendancy in many Asian cities, quality ECCE and posterior chamber IOL implant surgery will still be the mainstay of cataract care. Most skilled surgeons with appropriate training will achieve 6/12 or 20/40 vision in 98% of their patients.

THE WAY FORWARD

Success in the visual rehabilitation of the millions of cataract-blind patients hinges on the premise that these unfortunate patients should not undergo a procedure with poor results. If an operation is not good enough for us, it should not be good enough for the mass cataract blind. The challenge therefore is to deliver high-quality ECCE and IOL to the masses. The directions we should take are as follows:

1) Getting a consensus among prevention of blindness workers, non-governmental organizations, the WHO, IAPB and ophthalmologists that ICCE is an obsolete, irrelevant technique that does more harm than good in the long run. We strongly hold the view that ICCE is obsolete. It is wrong to recommend it.
2) Getting a consensus that ECCE + IOL is the way to go.
3) Unity in action among all the above groups to raise and suitably allocate resources from the World Bank, WHO etc. These resources can then be allocated to fund microscopes, IOL development and YAG lasers. Low-cost, locally manufactured IOLs of excellent quality are already available in many parts of Asia. Ideally, the allocation of these funds should be tied to the use of ECCE + IOL.
4) Train adequate surgeons: we have long recognized that the way forward in delivering high-quality cataract surgery to the masses is not simply to do eye camp after eye camp but to run regular surgical training courses for rural ophthalmologists who may have no experience whatsoever of ECCE techniques. In China, we have helped to set up several implant training centres over the past 10 years starting in Tianjin and then in Xiamen and Jinan. The Tianjin International Intraocular Implant Training Centre (Fig. 13.9) was set up in 1989 and has since trained 1500 ophthalmologists from all over China[11] (Fig. 13.10). These surgeons have been performing more and more ECCE + IOL operations in China.

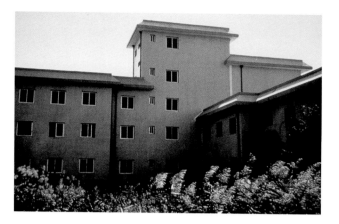

Figure 13.9. *Tianjin International Intraocular Implant Training Centre.*

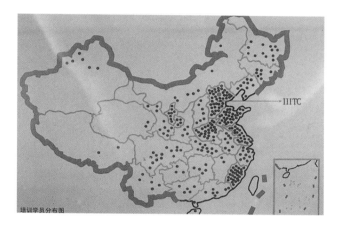

Figure 13.10. *Trained ECCE surgeons in China.*

Ophthalmologists from Singapore, the USA, Europe, Australia and Japan have all visited the Tianjin Centre and conducted numerous teaching courses and live surgery demonstrations. This centre in Tianjin can serve as a model for other developing countries.

VISION FOR THE FUTURE

As the 21st century beckons, eye surgeons of the world, together with the WHO and non-governmental organizations, should work hand in hand to eradicate the modern tragedy of cataract blindness. This should take the form of a concerted effort to train adequate numbers of ECCE surgeons, distribute resources appropriately to support ECCE and ensure accurate data collection for audit purposes.

International leaders frequently mention human rights. Can it not be said that the restoration of normal vision to the blind of the world can be considered as the most important human right? Are leaders of ophthalmic organizations guilty of failure to take adequate action? Are we, as eye surgeons, guilty of omission, for failing to help and react strongly? Tianjin has succeeded; should the rest of the world not follow?

When the human misery of millions of blind cataract victims continues to increase in the poor areas of the world, at a time when normal vision can be restored at low cost to all, we must press for action.

REFERENCES

1 World Health Organization. *Cataract* (Geneva: WHO Publications, 1990).

2 Taylor HR. Public health perspective for cataract surgery. Delivered at the 2nd International Ophthalmological Conference in Beijing, China, 4–8 July 1995.

3 Taylor HR, West SK, Rosenthal FS, et al. Effect of ultraviolet radiation on cataract formation. *N Engl J Med* 1988; **319:** 1429–33.

4 Lim Arthur SM. *The Human Right to Normal Vision* (Singapore: World Scientific Publishing, 1997) 30.

5 Sommer A. Obstacles and opportunities. New frontiers in ophthalmology. In: *Proceedings of the XXVI ICO*, 18–24 March 1990 (Amsterdam: Elsevier Science, 1991) 3–6.

6 Khan MD, Rahman A, Khan MA, et al. New trends in eye camp surgery. *Asia Pacific J Ophthalmol* 1991; **3**: 57–9.

7 Brilliant GE, Brilliant LB. Using social epidemiology to understand who stays blind and who gets operated on for cataract in a rural setting. *Soc Sci Med* 1985; **21:** 553–8.

8 Tabarra KF, Ross-Degnan D. Blindness in Saudi Arabia. *JAMA* 1986; **255:** 3378–84.

9 Faal H, Minassian D, Sowa S, Foster A. National survey of blindness and low vision in the Gambia. *Br J Ophthalmol* 1989; **73:** 82–7.

10 Mehta K. Phacoemulsification: the ideal technique for eye camps in India: an in-depth analysis. Presented at the 10th International Meeting on Cataract, Implant, Microsurgical and Refractive Keratoplasty, New Delhi, India, September 1997.

11 Chee C, Yeoh R. The International Intraocular Implant Training Centre—Tianjin, China (IIITC). *Asia Pacific J Ophthalmol* 1996; **8**: 14–16.

Chapter 14 Cataract surgery in emerging nations: role of phacoemulsification

Surendra Basti

Phacoemulsifcation (phaco), with its well-recognized benefits such as early visual rehabilitation, freedom from sutures and ability to permit controlled nuclear removal and in-the-bag intraocular lens (IOL) fixation, is currently the most frequently utilized technique of cataract removal in the developed world.[1] In the developing (used in this chapter synonymously with 'emerging') world, while this is not so, it certainly has caught the imagination of ophthalmologists and is possibly the most debated ophthalmic surgical procedure. This difference between the developing and the developed world in terms of adaptation to and utilization of phaco exists for several reasons. Intracapsular cataract (ICCE) is still the predominantly used technique. Also, since a large cataract backlog (the untreated cataract-blind population) exists in these economically less privileged countries,[2] the immediate need is probably to decrease/eradicate this backlog using cataract-removal techniques that are inexpensive. Thus phaco, which is a technique dependent on the utilization of expensive and sophisticated technology, is less widely used in the developing world at the present time. However, even in these countries in urban areas, the technique has been used for nearly a decade[3] and this use is increasing. The fact that some innovations pertaining to phaco are being published in the recent peer-reviewed literature from this part of the world bears testimony to this.[4,5]

The intent of this chapter is to present the current status of phaco in developing nations and to put in perspective the role that this procedure might have in this region in the coming decade. It must be mentioned that the author's views are largely based on extensive teaching and surgical experience in India, China and Thailand and close interaction with other surgeons in developing nations in Asia and in developing countries in Africa, Europe, and South and Central America. In a sense, therefore, this chapter is likely to provide an Asian perspective of phaco in the developing world.

CURRENT STATUS OF PHACO IN THE DEVELOPING WORLD

As might be expected, even within the developing world there is no uniform picture with regard to the degree of proficiency attained by surgeons performing phaco and the percentage of surgeons performing phaco. It appears that the amount of phaco being performed closely mirrors the degree of economic wellbeing of a given country. There clearly are several countries, such as Burma, Ethiopia, Cuba and Sudan, where there is almost no phaco being performed. As might be obvious, all of these countries are economically backward at the present time. In other countries whose economies are more healthy such as Malaysia, China India, Taiwan, El Salvador and Barbados, phaco is being used quite extensively, especially in urban areas. If one were to look closely at the scenario in India as reflecting that in the latter group of countries, the following pertinent facts might be interesting to note. There are approximately 9000 ophthalmologists in India for a population of 950 million. The WHO[2] estimated that there are 4.5 million people blind because of cataract in India. It might be surprising to note that phaco is actively being performed by less than 5% of ophthalmologists at the present time. A detailed account of the situation follows and might help understand what are the limitations at the present time, and what might serve as a predictor of trends for the near future.

Table 14.1.
Models of phaco machines presently available in India. The last three machines are locally manufactured.

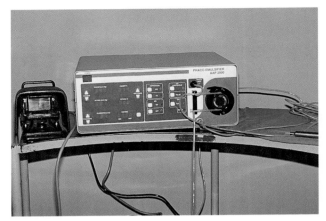

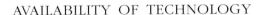

AMO Opsys
AMO Opsys MMP
AMO Diplomat
Alcon Universal–I
Alcon Universal–II
Alcon Legacy
Optikon Quasar
Optikon Pulsar—2000
Nidek CV—12000
Nidek CV—6000
Oertli Quinto
Provision Quantum
DORC
US—15000
Mentor
Performa 20/10
Universal—2000
IMD
APPA–2000
Ascon
Surgicon Synthesis

AVAILABILITY OF TECHNOLOGY

Almost every manufacturer of phaco machines, IOLs and viscoelastics operating on a global scale has a distributor network in India. Thus there are 19 models of phaco machines available (Table 14.1). Except for the Alcon Legacy and the AMO Diplomax, which may be considered higher-end machines and cost between US$60 000–70 000, most of the others cost between US$10 000–20 000. There are also three Indian manufacturers of phaco machines, and these machines cost between US$7000–10 000. The most popular of these is shown in Fig. 14.1. This machine has most of the features of imported phaco machines in the same category. It is estimated that approximately 650 phaco machines have been sold in India as of October 1997. Of these, only 10–20 belong to the higher-end group. Of the remaining machines sold, the market share of the Indian manufacturers is about 20%.

A similar situation exists for viscoelastic materials. There are several manufacturers of 2% methylcellulose in India (Fig. 14.2). The cost of a 2-ml vial is in the range of US$3–5. Sodium hyaluronate is available from international manufacturers and costs approximately US$45 for 0.4 ml. There are no Indian

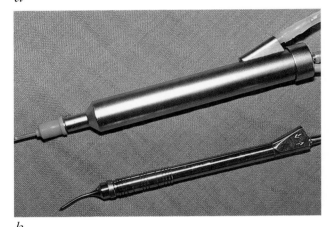

a

b

Figure 14.1. *Phaco unit (a) and handpiece (b) manufactured in India. This unit compares favourably with imported international brands that are more expensive.*

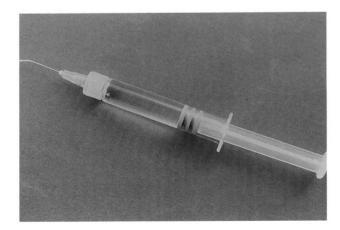

Figure 14.2. *Two per cent methylcellulose dispensed in a preloaded syringe.*

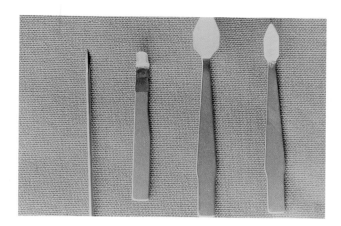

Figure 14.3. *Reusable blades for phaco wound construction. The cost of one set of blades for phaco is approximately US$4.*

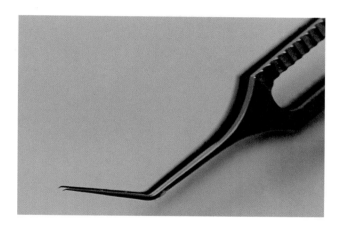

Figure 14.4. *Utrata forceps made of titanium. The cost is a tenth of the cost of similar forceps marketed in the USA.*

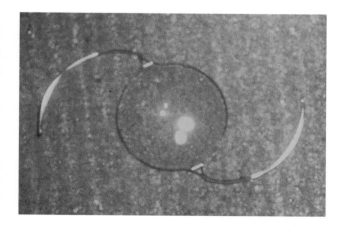

Figure 14.5. *Single-piece, all-PMMA, tumble-polished IOL with capsular C-haptics suitable for in-the-bag placement.*

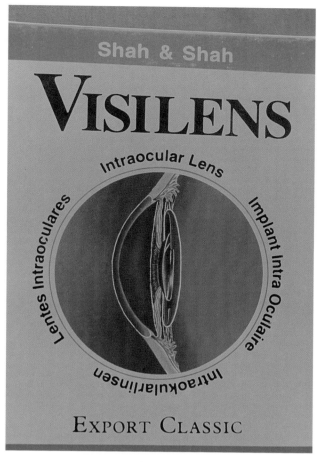

Shah & Shah

VISILENS

Intraocular Lens

Lentes Intraoculares

Implant Intra Oculaire

Intraokularlinsen

EXPORT CLASSIC

Figure 14.6. *Three-piece silicone foldable IOL manufactured in India.*

manufacturers of sodium hyaluronate preparations at the present time.

Instrumentation for sutureless wound construction (Fig. 14.3) is also made locally in India. These blades are reusable and each blade costs between US$2–4. Microsurgical instruments made of steel or titanium are available. The Utrata forceps shown in Fig. 14.4 is made of titanium and costs US$50.

Almost every international manufacturer has made its IOLs available in India. While an imported all-polymethylmethacrylate (PMMA) IOL costs US$30–50, a similar IOL manufactured in India (Fig. 14.5) costs US$7–10. With regard to foldable IOLs, most imported silicone IOLs cost US$60–70, while a local manufacturer (Fig. 14.6) charges approximately half that. Acrylic IOLs are available from Alcon and cost about US$100. There are no local manufacturers of IOLs of this material.

It is clear from the above that access to technology is clearly not a deterrent to widespread use of phaco in India. The availability of phaco machines, microsurgical instruments, viscoelastics and IOLs from Indian manufacturers has also made the cost of performing phaco significantly less than in the developed world.

ACCESS TO PHACO TEACHING PROGRAMMES

There are four training programmes providing hands-on training to practising ophthalmologists available at the present time. These programmes can systematically teach between 30 and 45 ophthalmologists in a year. Residency programmes are just beginning to include teaching phaco,[6] although at the present time these number less than five. Over a hundred workshops and wet labs on phaco have been conducted in the last 2 years.

Access to a proper initiation programme is a limitation at the present time, and several hands-on training programmes are necessary for proper teaching of phaco techniques to neophyte surgeons.

PROFICIENCY WITH EXTRACAPSULAR CATARACT EXTRACTION AND IOL IMPLANTATION (ECCE + IOL)

An important reason why phaco is performed by only few surgeons at present is that ECCE + IOL using modern microsurgical techniques is routinely performed by only 20.3% of ophthalmologists, as noted in a recent survey.[7] In the last few years, however, due to an initiative taken by the World Bank[8] and non-governmental organizations (NGOs) such as Sight Savers, several microsurgery training programmes have become functional.

It is likely that proficiency with ECCE + IOL will be attained by a large majority of surgeons in the coming few years. This might be the first step towards more widespread use of phaco.

SUMMARY OF THE CURRENT STATUS OF PHACO IN INDIA AND ITS SIMILARITY TO THAT IN OTHER COUNTRIES WITH A SIMILAR ECONOMIC BACKGROUND

As indicated above, factors that are responsible for phaco being performed by a minority of surgeons

are: few surgeons with proficiency with ECCE + IOL; few training programmes in phaco; and cost considerations. For the reasons discussed above, it is likely that the percentage of surgeons performing phaco will steadily increase in the years ahead. The scenario is very similar in other countries with similar economic backgrounds (Gangopadhyay N, MD personal communication).

ROLE OF PHACO IN DEVELOPING NATIONS: PUTTING THINGS IN PERSPECTIVE

This could be discussed along two lines: the role of phaco in today's medical and socio-economic scenario, and the role of phaco in the coming decade.

COST VERSUS BENEFIT OF PHACO IN DEVELOPING NATIONS TODAY

In the developing world, the average annual income at the present time is between $100 and $200. Because of poverty, ignorance and the unavailability of access to medical care without spending a disproportionately large (based on their income) amount of money, a considerable number of patients in rural areas consider decreasing vision caused by age-related cataract to be the 'beginning of the end' and leave it untreated. Against this background, if one were to prioritize goals of alleviating cataract blindness in the developing world, providing the benefits of early visual rehabilitation by utilizing techniques that are novel to practising ophthalmologists and at costs that cannot be passed on to the patient would probably receive least priority. Hence, all major public health efforts are being directed towards extending medical care to all parts of these countries. Until recently, ICCE was literally the only surgical technique utilized, especially in rural areas. However, with epidemiological studies[9] bringing to light the loss of man-hours resulting from patients losing or breaking their aphakic spectacles, initiatives are being taken to familiarize more and more surgeons with IOL techniques. Studies are underway to determine which type of IOL technique[10] would be best suited for these countries.

In urban areas, phaco is increasingly utilized because more surgeons are already familiar with

ECCE + IOL and are hence in a position to make the transition to phaco. Also, patients in these areas are wiling to share the increased costs of phaco, understand the benefits of the procedure and opt for it. Because of this, it is almost mandatory for surgeons to perform the procedure to stay competitive in the services they offer to their patients.

COST VERSUS BENEFIT OF PHACO IN DEVELOPING NATIONS IN THE NEW MILLENNIUM

As mentioned in the earlier part of this chapter, widespread availability of advanced medical care is inevitable with enhanced economic growth. There are signs that several developing countries, such as China, India, Korea, Taiwan and Malaysia, are now on the threshold of a great improvement in their economies. The various training programmes for IOL surgery that are presently underway, and the patient preference for IOLs over aphakic spectacles, are likely to result in a quantum leap in the number of surgeons performing ECCE + IOL. Attempts at achieving better uncorrected visual acuity are a natural step forward, and phaco makes this possible to a large extent. It is thus likely that surgeons performing ECCE + IOL will increasingly make the transition to phaco in the years ahead. What of cost considerations? Greater local manufacture of instrumentation and surgical materials necessary for phaco is likely to further decrease the cost of performing the procedure. Economic growth in these countries in the near future will also translate to a better paying capacity of patients. Are the benefits of phaco meaningful to patients belonging to lower socio-economic strata? I believe that they are. Earlier visual rehabilitation will mean less time away from work and hence less financial loss. In fact, the benefits of phaco are probably more meaningful to patients from these strata than they are to more affluent patients, who are in a position to absorb some financial stress. It is very likely that phaco will be the predominant technique of cataract extraction in developing countries in the early part of the 21st century.

REFERENCES

1 Leaming DV. Practice styles and preferences of ASCRS members—1996 survey. *J Cataract Refract Surg* 1997; **23:** 527–35.

2 Thylefors B, Negral AD, Pararajasegaram R, Dadzie KY. Global data on blindness. *WHO Bull* 1995; **73:** 115–21.

3 Mehta KR. Phakoemulsification cataract extraction with foldable IOLs—first 50 cases. *Ind J Ophthalmol* 1989; **37**(2): 80–3.

4 Vasavada AR, Desai JP. Stop, chop, chop and stuff. *J Cataract Refract Surg* 1996; **22**(5): 526–9.

5 Basti S. Different faces of the white cataract: a phaco surgeon's perspective. *Aust NZ J Ophthalmol* 1999; in press.

6 Thomas R, Naveen S, Jacob A, Braganza A. Visual outcome and complications of residents learning phacoemulsification. *Ind J Ophthalmol* 1997; **45**(4): 215–19.

7 Gupta AK, Ellwein LB. The pattern of cataract surgery in India: 1992. *Ind J Ophthalmol* 1995; **43:** 3–8.

8 Jose R, Bachani D. World Bank-assisted cataract blindness control project. *Ind J Ophthalmol* 1995; **43:** 35–43.

9 Murthy GVS, Gupta SK, Talwar D. Assessment of cataract surgery in rural India. *Acta Ophthalmol Scand* 1996; **74:** 60–3.

10 Snellingen T, Gupta S, Huq F, et al. The South Asia cataract management study. I. The first 662 cataract surgeries: a preliminary report. *Br J Ophthalmol* 1995; **79:** 1029–35.

Topical anesthesia resurfaced in this decade as a useful tool after Fichman's suggestion regarding the use of tetracaine 0.5% applied to the eye as the only anesthetic for cataract surgery.[7] Other agents, such as bupivicaine and lidocaine, have been popularized because of a reduced tendency to cause corneal epitheliopathy and a longer period of action as compared with tetracaine. However, patients are not universally comfortable with topical anesthesia as the only agent. Many surgeons employ small amounts of intravenous, oral or sublingual sedation as an adjunct. However, in 1995 Gills suggested the routine use of intracameral non-preserved lidocaine in addition to topical anesthesia with or without systemic sedation,[8] although the concept had been mentioned earlier by Fichman, who considered intraocular tetracaine for use in difficult case situations. The safety and efficacy of intracameral lidocaine has been further established by Koch[9] and Masket with Gokmen in separate studies.[10] In the latter investigation, approximately 40% of more than 300 patients receiving only topical anesthesia required intraoperative conversion to a deeper level of local anesthesia, whereas fewer than 1% of 300 cases receiving intracameral lidocaine had need for an additional local anesthetic method. In the same study, safety was measured by comparing the degree of corneal edema on the first postoperative day between the two groups; a reduced likelihood for corneal edema was associated with the use of intracameral non-preserved lidocaine hydrochloride 1%, but this finding may be related to the use of chop-style phacoemulsification for the latter group. Nevertheless, based upon the early postoperative appearance of the cornea, non-preserved lidocaine is seemingly non-toxic, although Koch reports reduced contrast sensitivity and visual acuity in the first few hours after surgery.

Other methods to provide ocular anesthesia for cataract surgery without the risks of blind pass, sharp-needle orbital injection have evolved along with topical anesthesia. Posterior sub-Tenon's infiltration employs a blunt cannula (Fig. 15.1) to place local anesthesia directly in the retrobulbar space. A conjunctival button-hole incision, performed under topical anesthesia, is necessary for the cannula to gain direct access to the sub-Tenon's space. This method was suggested as an alternative to sharp-needle orbital injection,[11] and has been further popularized by Greenbaum as a primary method for cataract anesthesia; he coined the term 'parabulbar' anesthesia to describe the concept.[12] Additionally, the method may be used for surgeons in transition to

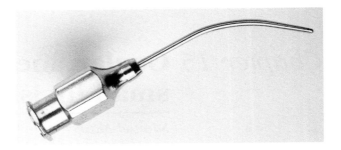

Figure 15.1. *Blunted reusable cannula for sub-Tenon's (parabulbar) anesthesia. (Courtesy Rhein Medical, Tampa, Florida.)*

topical/intracameral anesthesia and is very useful to convert from topical methods in cases where complications occur, surgery is prolonged, or the patient is otherwise in need of a deeper level of anesthesia. As long as the cataract incision is self-sealing, the parabulbar infiltration may be given at any time during the surgery. Depending on the nature of the agent used for infiltration, parabulbar anesthesia may provide complete ocular akinesia and amaurosis. Other alternatives include anterior subconjunctival injection given diffusely or only focally in the region of the incision, so called 'pin-point' anesthesia.[13]

It is evident that traditional ocular anesthesia for cataract surgery, utilizing sharp needles passed blindly through the skin of the lids or the conjunctiva, engenders risks (Table 15.1) that are avoidable with topical/intracameral or other recently developed means for applying local anesthesia. However, in addition to the greater safety associated with newer anesthetic systems, topical and topical/intracameral methods avoid the need for patching and allow the patient the use of the eye immediately following surgery in the overwhelming majority of cases. Advantages, therefore, include safety, improved cosmetic effect, ability to use the eye immediately following surgery, and the ability to move and fixate the eye during surgery in response to the surgeon as an aid to the procedure (Table 15.2).

Depending on the experience of the surgeon, certain conditions may contraindicate the use of topical/intracameral anesthesia (Table 15.3). Given the ability to move the eye, the patient can aid the surgery or create significant obstacles; cataract surgery under topical/intracameral anesthesia is, by necessity, interactive. Poor patient cooperation is a

Table 15.1

Risks of injection anesthesia

Damage to optic nerve
Retrobulbar hemorrhage
Ocular penetration/perforation
Central nervous system anesthesia
Apnea
Unintended bilateral ocular anesthesia
Damage to extraocular muscles/diplopia
Aesthetic blemish

Table 15.2

Advantages of topical/intracameral anesthesia

Avoids pain, blemish and risk of injection anesthesia
Allows immediate useful vision after surgery
Eliminates the need for patch after surgery
Reduces anxiety and/or heavy sedation associated with
    injection anesthesia
Compatible for patients on anticoagulants
Patients can aid surgeon by moving eye for favorable
    exposure

Table 15.3

Contraindications to topical/intracameral anesthesia

Relative
    Language barrier
    Anticipated difficult surgery
    Poorly cooperative patient
Absolute
    Total deafness
    Coarse nystagmus

relative contraindication, as is the inability of the surgeon and patient to adequately communicate in the same language. Often, an interpreter or bilingual family member can be present in the operating theater in order to facilitate surgery without the need for injection anesthesia. However, absolute congenital deafness with speaking difficulty is an absolute contraindication, since the patient may become disoriented under the surgical drapes and cannot be expected to communicate by the usual means of lip-reading or sign language; patients of this nature often require general anesthesia. Ocular conditions may

also act as relative or absolute contraindications: cataracts too dense to allow fixation on the microscope light, potentially complicated surgery (preoperative zonulysis, etc.) and nystagmus are common examples. Nevertheless, the huge majority of patients may safely experience small-incision cataract surgery under topical/intracameral anesthetic with very limited sedation.

METHODS

I prefer the use of lidocaine HCl 4.0% non-preserved for topical anesthetic. It is long-acting and non-mucogenic. (Previous experience with 0.75% bupivicaine HCl suggests that it causes undesired mucus production.) Intracameral anesthesia is achieved with unpreserved lidocaine HCl 1.0%. Some surgeons advocate diluting the intracameral agent with balanced salt solution (BSS) in order to raise the pH and reduce the mild discomfort associated with anterior chamber instillation.

1) Administer topical proparacaine HCl 0.4% to initiate anesthesia with little sting. Administer dilating agents (cyclopentylate or tropicamide and phenylephrine 2.5%), topical antibiotics, a topical non-steroidal anti-inflammatory drug (NSAID), and lidocaine HCl 4.0% four times at 5-min intervals prior to surgery.

2) After the patient is brought into the theater, several drops of the 4.0% lidocaine are administered prior to the sterile 'prep'. The latter begins with instillation of two drops of half-strength Betadine solution (not Betadine scrub) directly to the operative eye. At this time, very small amounts of intravenous sedation may be given, depending upon the mental and medical status of the patient, the anxiety of the surgeon, and the observations of the anesthetist or equivalent. I generally ask that 0.5–1.0 mg of midazolam HCl be administered intravenously.

3) During the draping process, communicate with the patient about the operative process. Tell them that they will feel slight pressure from the lid speculum and that they will need to fixate on the light of the microscope. Tell them that requests to look up, down, etc. should be achieved by moving the eye and not the head. Reassure them that they will feel no pain.

4) Begin surgery with the microscope light at low levels of illumination, sufficient only to perform a paracentesis. Place 0.2 ml of non-preserved lidocaine HCl in the anterior chamber and follow that with the viscoelastic of choice. The anesthetic will be washed out as the viscoagent fills the chamber if the lip of the side-port is depressed as the viscoelastic is injected. Slowly increase the microscope light and perform the clear corneal incision. Continue with routine surgical procedure.

5) Generally, no further anesthesia is necessary. However, in situations with prolonged surgery or very sensitive patients, additional intracameral anesthetic may be administered for complaints of 'pressure' or intraocular pain. For surface discomfort the conjunctiva may be swabbed with a pledget of any sterile topical anesthetic, but care should be taken to avoid placing the agent near or in the incision if it contains preservatives. Additionally, small increments of intravenous sedation can be added as may be (rarely) necessary.

6) In the very unlikely case that the patient cannot tolerate the microscope light even at low illumination and continues to squeeze the lids against the speculum, additional doses of intravenous medicine can be given until the intracameral anesthetic is administered. In my observations, once the eye has received the intracameral agent, all lid squeezing and signs of anxiety or discomfort abate rapidly. However, in extreme situations or should an operative complication occur that will significantly prolong surgery, one can stop surgery, given a self-sealing incision, pressurize the eye to normal, and administer deep sub-Tenon's local anesthetic with a blunt cannula (Fig. 15.1) through a conjunctival button-hole entry in the superior or inferior nasal quadrant.

Prior to incising the conjunctiva, a pledget of local anesthesia may be placed on the area for a few moments. The cannula should reach the retrobulbar space with ease if the button-hole opening includes Tenon's capsule. Only 2.0 ml of local agent is necessary, given direct access to the muscle cone. Relative amaurosis will be achieved in a matter of seconds, and, with strong local agents, akinesia can be established in a few minutes.

REFERENCES

1 Leaming DV. Practice styles and preferences of ASCRS members—1996 survey. *J Cataract Refract Surg* 1997; **23**: 527–35.

2 Cionni R, Osher R. Retrobulbar hemorrhage. *Ophthalmology* 1991; **98**: 1153–5.

3 Duker JS, Belmont, JB, Benson WE, et al. Inadvertent globe perforation during retrobulbar and peribulbar anesthesia. *Ophthalmology* 1997; **98**: 519–26.

4 Hay A, Flynn Jr HW, Hoffman JI, Rivera AH. Needle penetration of the globe during retrobulbar and peribulbar injections. *Ophthalmology* 1991; **98**: 1017–24.

5 Grizzard WS, Kirk NM, Pavan PR, et al. Perforating ocular injuries caused by anesthesia personnel. *Ophthalmology* 1991; **98**: 1011–16.

6 Masket S, Tennen DG. Astigmatic stabilization of 3.0 mm temporal clear corneal cataract incisions. *J Cataract Refract Surg* **22** (10): 1451–5.

7 Fine IH, Fichman RA, Grabow HR. *Clear-corneal Cataract Surgery and Topical Anesthesia.* (Thorofare, NJ: Slack, Inc.,1993.)

8 Gills JP, Cherchio M, Raanan MG. Unpreserved lidocaine to control discomfort during cataract surgery using topical anesthesia. *J Cataract Refract Surg* 1997; **23**: 545–50.

9 Koch PS. Anterior chamber irrigation with unpreserved lidocaine 1% for anesthesia during cataract surgery. *J Cataract Refract Surg* 1997; **23**: 551–4.

10 Masket S, Gokmen F. Efficacy and apparent safety of intracameral lidocaine as a supplement to topical anesthesia. *J Cataract Refract Surg* 1998; **24** (7): 956–60.

11 Stevens JD. A new local anaesthesia technique for cataract extraction by one quadrant sub-Tenon's infiltration. *Br J Ophthalmol* 1992; **76**: 670.

12 Greenbaum S. Anesthesia in Cataract Surgery. In: Greenbaum S, ed. *Ocular Anesthesia* (WB Saunders, 1997) 1–55.

13 Fukasaku H, Marron JA. Pinpoint anesthesia: a new approach to local ocular anesthesia. *J Cataract Refract Surg* 1994; **20**: 468.

Chapter 16 Free-hand clear corneal incision with Legacy 20,000 aspiration bypass system

James A Davison

INTRODUCTION

In 1992 I was inspired by Fine to adopt clear corneal temporal incisions for cataract surgery. Fine's pioneering work and his scientific presentations convinced me that clear corneal temporal incisions would be superior to the corneoscleral incisions from the superior approach that I was making at the time. I adopted Fine's keratome technique, but in 1993 I adopted a refinement that I learned from David Brown (Fort Myers, Florida). Brown employed a free-hand technique using a diamond blade made by Diamatrix, Inc. (BUCK knife, Brown Universal Cataract Knife). Having one blade that could accomplish everything was very appealing, especially in our setting of operating in multiple hospitals and multiple cities and towns in urban and rural Iowa. Hospitals, of course, were reluctant to purchase seemingly expensive diamond blades, since steel blades had got the job done. To them, even though disposable steel could be proved to be cumulatively expensive, at least the cost per case was predictable and seemed small relative to the high expense of a single diamond blade. Since the BUCK knife was a universal diamond blade, I initially purchased three (two for use and one for backup) and took them to the various locations where I operated, where they were rented by the hospitals from me. I was soon able to convince each hospital to purchase their own, as we were providing a superior technique more efficiently (faster and with ultimately less total expense). Because of the availability of the knives, many of my partners also adopted the technique, so that multiple surgeons were able to accomplish clear corneal temporal incisions at multiple locations using the same diamond blades without the extraordinary expense and unnecessary redundancy associated with various types and sizes of keratome-style diamond knives.

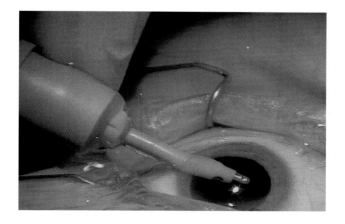

Figure 16.1. *Easy access is obtained for the irrigation/aspiration (I/A) tip through the temporal palpebral fissure. The surgeon has an opportunity to use his left index finger as a fulcrum to create finer control of the I/A tip.*

The advantage of clear corneal temporal surgery is that it not only creates the cleanest, most precise incision furthest way from the visual axis, but also allows safer access to the intraocular contents (Fig. 16.1). No longer did I have to struggle to get over the brow and endure the substantial corneal distortion and compromised visibility that accompanied superior corneoscleral incisions. The temporal pathway provided me with safer access and has improved my cataract surgery substantially.

My average induced keratometric astigmatism with clear corneal temporal incision free-hand technique is 0.2 diopters of flattening at 6–8 weeks. Because of this small amount, I perform all cases, regardless of preoperative astigmatism, with a clear corneal temporal technique. I feel that this location gives me the best chance to perform my best cataract surgery for each patient, regardless of their anatomy. I have been able to routinely prescribe a spectacle lens change at 2 weeks after the surgery. Because of the incision's safety and stability, I see my patients about 40 min after surgery. I find that their wounds are secure, their intraocular lenses (IOLs) are in place, their chambers are formed, and I can discharge them with drops (antibiotic and prednisolone acetate 1% four times a day for 2 weeks, then prednisolone acetate 1% twice a day for 2 weeks) and an instruction package, and just recheck them in 2 weeks for their final lens prescription. When possible, we have checked intraocular pressures (IOPs) several hours after surgery, and have found that, in patients without preoperative glaucoma, IOP ranges from 10 to 35 mmHg, with most in the normal range and only some in the mid-30s. Higher pressures may be found in glaucoma patients, whose topical non-miotic medication we restart on the day of surgery. I have found that it is not necessary to check them on the day after surgery. Again, with our relatively rural environment this reduces the risks, hazards and expense of travel for our patients and their families, and they have been uniformly very enthusiastic about this follow-up plan.

I have performed approximately 9000 clear corneal temporal incision cataract operations and have had only six wound leaks. Two were in patients in whom I considered placing a suture (I suture about 1% because of poor wound sealing). In one patient, I actually had the 10–O nylon open at surgery, but ultimately convinced myself that it was not going to be necessary to suture at the time. I ended up suturing both wounds later the same day because the patients demonstrated slightly shallow chambers and low IOPs. Two were very nervous, squeezing, eye-rubbing men who precipitated an iris prolapse 2 days and 3 days, respectively, after surgery. One was a man who struck his face, including his lid, against a kitchen counter during a fall. The sixth was a patient who was in a car crash and had an air bag explode in her face, prolapsing her iris (but leaving the IOL capsular bag, etc. intact) 2 weeks after surgery. In all of these cases, single or multiple 10–O nylon sutures were placed. Some loss of iris substance occurred during the repositioning process of the major traumatic cases. In no cases were the capsular bag, IOL or vitreous involved. I have had no cases of endophthalmitis.

In the earlier years of using this incision, I created a groove that was between 150 and 300 µm deep, depending on the blade stop calibration, and then completed the incision through the groove. Later, again at Fine's suggestion, I abandoned the groove

but continued to make the incision free-hand. The epithelial entry of the diamond is almost invisible 1 day after surgery, whereas the groove continues to be obvious indefinitely. Less foreign body sensation has been reported by my patients since I abandoned the initial groove. The non-groove technique actually makes the incision process a bit easier, rather than more difficult, since more tissue resistance is available without the weakening effect that the groove creates by disrupting the peripheral countertraction which is available with an intact cornea without the groove.

TECHNIQUE

All patients receive an antibiotic drop four times a day, starting 3 days prior to surgery. The patient is prepared and draped in the usual fashion, including placing dilute povodine iodine in the conjunctiva, which is rinsed with balanced salt solution (BSS), and an open wire speculum is put in place, curling the edges of the Visitec adhesive drape underneath the lash margin, and draping the lashes away from the operative field. A caliper is set at 2.8 mm (Fig. 16.2), and an indentation created on the corneal surface (Fig. 16.3). If desired, a 150–300-µm-deep groove can be created for a length of approximately 3.2 mm (the length that we will need for IOL insertion) (Fig. 16.4). In our current technique, however, the initial step is to create a paracentesis opening (Fig. 16.5), and this is followed by incision creation without a groove. The blade is placed against the cornea at the corneal limbus and driven into the stroma in a uniplanar fashion, not ever being parallel to the corneal surface. The Descemet's target entry point is 1.75 mm from epithelial penetration. The entry of the blade is ultimately accomplished with an oblique, right-to-left motion, rather than a direct straight-in penetration. This is done because the diamonds are sometimes a little dull or the cornea seems a little tougher, and straight-in penetration generates a 'pop' as the resistance gives way when the blade enters the anterior chamber, which can result in touching of the iris or lens, or generate an actual patient-movement reaction. If an oblique entry is utilized, there is more of a gradual entry, slowly slicing into stroma and arriving at Descemet's level more slowly so that this sudden loss of resistance can be avoided. The initiation point is slightly to the right. If the blade is slightly dull, a compression of tissue can be seen, especially in grooved cases, prior to entry (Fig. 16.6). It is more obvious in the grooved example because corneal

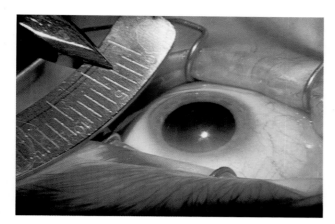

Figure 16.2. *The caliper is set at 2.8 mm.*

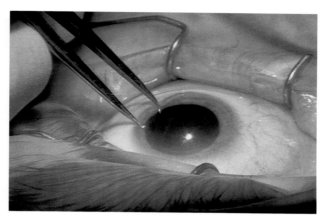

Figure 16.3. *A light indentation on the peripheral corneal surface is created with the pointed ends of the caliper.*

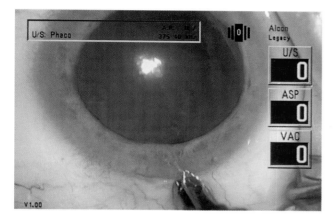

Figure 16.4. *A 150–300-μm-depth groove is created (older technique).*

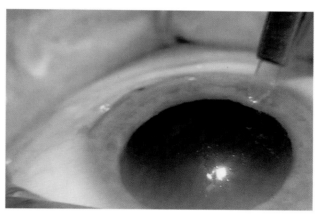

Figure 16.5. *A paracentesis incision is created with the diamond blade fully extended.*

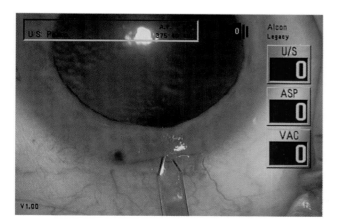

Figure 16.6. *An oblique entry is created as the blade not only is driven through the corneal stroma to Descemet's level, but also slices to the surgeon's left. Notice the compression of tissue being created because of the relatively dull blade, and the groove being used in this case.*

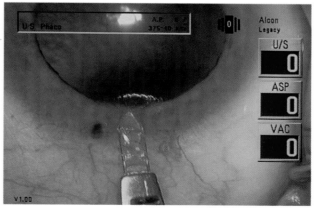

Figure 16.7. *Descemet's level is entered 1.75 mm from the epithelial level as the blade is swept to the left.*

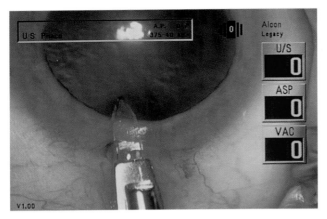

Figure 16.8. *The blade is swept to the left so that its lateral aspect is just underneath the indentation created by the caliper.*

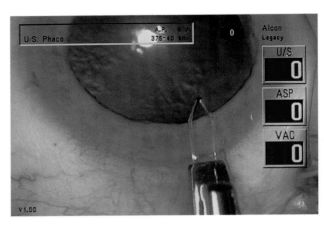

Figure 16.9. *The blade is swept to the right so that its lateral aspect is underneath the right indentation.*

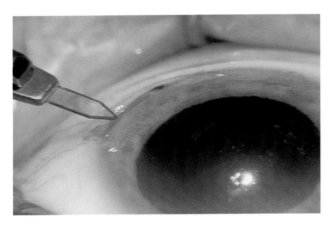

Figure 16.10. *The initiation of the incision is created at the epithelial level of the corneal portion of the limbus. The starting point is just to the right of center.*

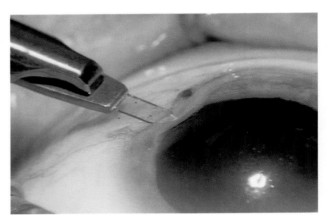

Figure 16.11. *Side view. A slight compressed indentation has been created before Descemet's membrane is penetrated.*

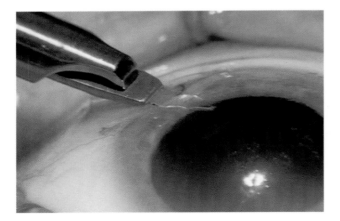

Figure 16.12. *Side view. The blade sweeps to the left.*

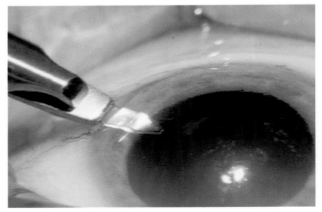

Figure 16.13. *Side view. The blade sweeps to the right. Note that the angle of the blade has not changed from the epithelial entry in Fig. 16.10.*

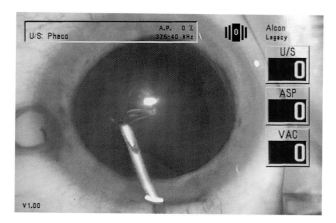

Figure 16.14. *The capsulorhexis is initiated centrally and swept to the left.*

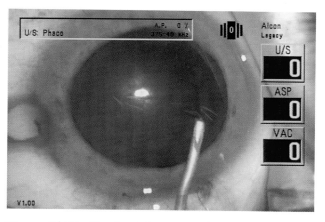

Figure 16.15. *The rhexis has spiraled to an approximate 2.5-mm radius.*

tissue tends to pile up in a distorted accumulation because of loss of peripheral corneal countertraction as the diamond blade pushes centrally. This is one of the reasons why grooving should be avoided, i.e. the accuracy of wound width creation is more consistent and the sudden release of compressed central stroma is less with non-grooved, uniplanar incisions. At approximately 1.75 mm into the cornea Descemet's membrane is encountered (Fig. 16.7). The blade is then simply swept to the left (Fig. 16.8), to the spot underlying the dimple that has been created with the caliper, and then to the right (Fig. 16.9). After the incision is created, the blade is carefully withdrawn, retracted and placed in its case. If a slightly dull diamond blade is employed, a slight sawing motion is necessary. This sawing motion should be of very low amplitude and not much force, while the blade is alternatively driven in and withdrawn. If too much of a cut is made while the blade is being driven in, the incision tends to extend centrally into the cornea making a longer than necessary corneal tunnel. If the incision is extended as the blade is being withdrawn, the length of the tunnel becomes shorter and the incision seems to extend peripherally, making a narrow flap. Interestingly, sometimes the exact opposite may seem to occur, therefore, if a sawing motion is needed, small movement, i.e. almost a micro oscillation created by finger motion, are necessary.

Seen from a side view, the blade enters the cornea at the limbal junction (Fig. 16.10); a slight dimpling can be seen just prior to Descemet's entry (Fig. 16.11). This is followed by a sweeping motion to the left (Fig. 16.12), and then a sweeping motion to the right (Fig. 16.13).

All subsequent steps in surgery are made with an attempt to keep the incision tunnel intact and not to disturb the corneal tissue. Stretching, tearing or cooking corneal tissue may compromise the ability of the incision to self-seal at the end of the case. However, the most common cause of the wound not sealing is a tendency for the tunnel shelf to be 1.5–1.25 mm rather than the critically necessary 1.75 mm needed for consistent self-sealing. Lengths greater than 2.00 mm may lead to oar-locking and an unsatisfactory cosmetic result. It is important for the incision not to be made more peripheral than the cornea; actually, a totally clear corneal incision without limbal bleeding is preferable. If it is more peripheral, conjunctival ballooning or subconjunctival hemorrhage may make the operation more difficult and generate patient complaints.

Preservative-free lidocaine 1% is irrigated over the corneal surface and the incisions and gently and somewhat slowly into the anterior chamber. This gentle instillation keeps the patient from feeling a stinging sensation. A total of 1.5 ml is usually used, divided somewhat equally over the surface and within the eye. Lidocaine instillation prior to viscoelastic placement allows the anesthetic to readily reach the ocular tissue. A capsulorhexis opening is created with a cystotome, starting centrally and sweeping to the left (Fig. 16.14). The rhexis continues towards the surgeon and by the time it sweeps past the third clock hour, the correct radius will have been achieved (Fig. 16.15). It is nice to have this transition towards the surgeon, as the important part of the intact capsular bag during the phacoemulsification and lens implantation process is the portion that is away from the

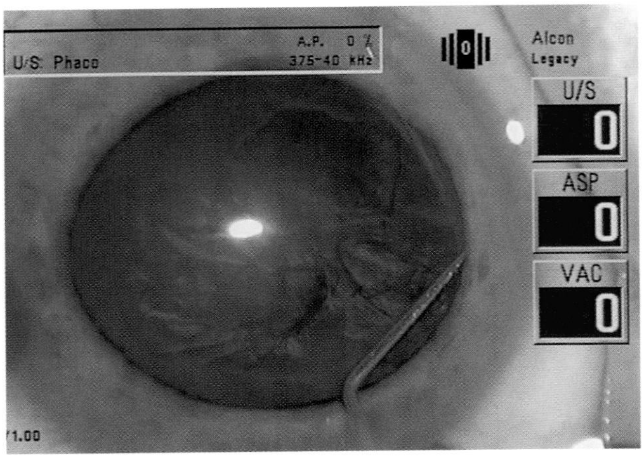

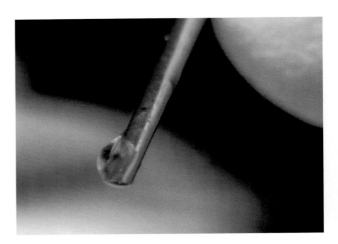

Figure 16.16. *A 30-gauge cannula is placed underneath the anterior capsule and a fluid wave was progressed almost all the way across the posterior cortical interface.*

Figure 16.17. *A 175-μm hole has been drilled into the shaft of the ABS phacoemulsification tip approximately 3 mm from the end.*

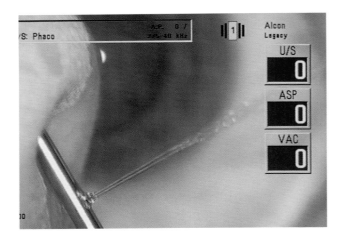

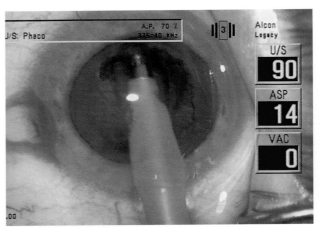

Figure 16.18. *My finger is occluding the phaco-emulsification tip aperture and the machine is in the reflux mode. Note the stream of BSS exiting the ABS aperture.*

Figure 16.19. *Deep grooves are easier to create because of the good visualization in front of and beside the 0.9-mm, 45° phacoemulsification tip.*

surgeon, i.e. the capsular bag that receives all the driving forces of phacoemulsification and lens implantation is 180° away from the incision.

Hydrodissection is accomplished with a 30-gauge cannula (Fig. 16.16). A 30-gauge cannula gives a fine directional quality to the dissecting fluid, resulting in a safe, low-volume and well-controlled process. Make sure to provide an incisional egress for BSS and/or viscoelastic.

PHACOEMULSIFICATION

I prefer the Alcon Legacy 20,000 phacoemulsification machine and the 0.9-mm micro tip with aspiration bypass system (ABS) opening in the shaft (Figs 16.17 and 16.18). In all cases, this smaller tip helps me to better appreciate my location within the three-dimensional canyon of the nucleus as it is being grooved.

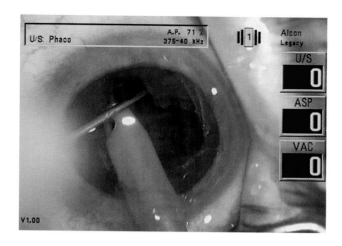

Figure 16.20. *Cross-handed posterior nuclear plate-tearing technique is employed.*

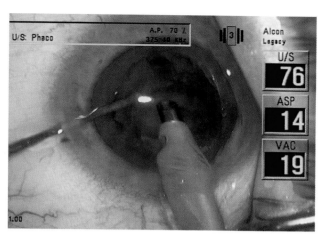

Figure 16.21. *Note the striae in the superficial layer of the corneal wound from distortion due to the phacoemulsification tip pushing against the right-hand side of the wound. Notice the tip position within the sleeve.*

It is especially good for small eyes, small pupils, and patients with pseudoexfoliation and loose zonular elements. A 175-μm hole has been placed in the shaft of the ABS phacoemulsification tip approximately 3 mm from the end. During quadrant removal, as complete aperture occlusion is accomplished, the ABS will permit a substantial amount of fluid to be withdrawn into the phacoemulsification tip from the ABS hole. I use settings of vacuum 500 mmHg, aspiration flow rate 30 ml/min in the normal quadrant removal phase, and with complete tip occlusion 11 ml/min can still be withdrawn through the ABS opening. Occlusion break does not cause anterior segment anatomy movement because complete occlusion and zero flow are not achievable. The entire process is mor fluid and dynamic rather than abrupt and choppy.

PHACOEMULSIFICATION—NON-OCCLUDED PHASE

Phacoemulsification is accomplished in Memory 1 (ultrasound 90% maximum, maximum vacuum potential 50 mmHg aspiration flow rate 14 ml/min). A divide and conquer method variation is used, employing a combination of capsular bag phacoemulsification and iris plane phacoemulsifica-

tion of nuclear fragments. Deep grooves are possible because of the good visualization around and in front of the smaller tip and also the 45° configuration of the tip itself (Fig. 16.19). Using a specially modified, 0.35-mm cyclodialysis spatula, a cross-handed cracking technique is used to tear the posterior nuclear plate from the periphery centrally (Fig. 16.20).

As phacoemulsification proceeds, the tip is allowed to go deeper and grooves are made. There is a tendency to 'see' just the tips of the phacoemulsification unit and assisting cyclodialysis spatula, but careful attention needs to be paid so that the instruments, especially the phacoemulsification tip, stay well centered loosely within the very center of the incision, both from left and right, and top to bottom. When the phacoemulsification tip is involved in creating a deeper pass, the tip is observed to be in an appropriate position. But because of the shallower depth of focus and narrower field associated with higher magnification during this process, the surgeon may not see that the cornea is distorted because the shaft of the phacoemulsification tip may be pushing against one of the wound tunnel walls (right, left, top or bottom) (Fig. 16.21). The friction generated can cause immediate heat absorption by any component of the elliptical corneal tunnel where contact has been made. Thermal absorption results in chemical collagen changes and ultimately wound shrinkage and poor wound sealing. Constant

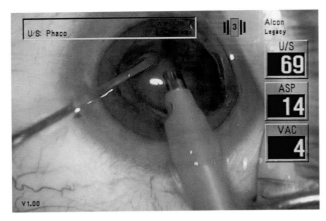

Figure 16.22. *The shaft of the phacoemulsification tip is now appropriately in the center of the elliptical wound tunnel. No corneal distortion is seen.*

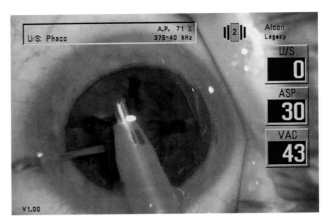

Figure 16.23. *The 45° tip aperture is applied to the wall of nuclear fragment and vacuum is allowed to build.*

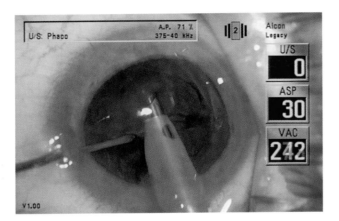

Figure 16.24. *As vacuum is building, the fragment is drawn central but also rotated so that the peripheral portion will become the superficial portion and the deeper, firmer portion will be removed last.*

awareness of shaft centration within the elliptical tunnel helps prevent this problem (Fig. 16.22). Focal heat absorption seems to be more frequent with the 0.9 mm tip, probably because of its smaller, more focally concentrated wound contact area and the necessary increased phacoemulsification time and intensity. The firmer the cataract, the more exaggerated the effect. After phacoemulsification is completed, the overlying cornea should be clear. Any overlying whitish change indicates thermal damage. Subtle thermal changes from this heat absorption are probably much more common than we realize with both the 0.9 mm and 1.1 mm tips.

PHACOEMULSIFICATION—OCCLUDED PHASE

The phacoemulsification machine is now switched to Memory 3 for most normal quadrant removals (phacoemulsification maximum energy 70%, vacuum 500 mmHg, aspiration flow rate 30 ml/min); if very soft lenses are being aspirated, an intermediate setting (Memory 2) is used to control speed and tissue access rates and basically to slow down the operation (phacoemulsification maximum energy 50%, vacuum 300 mmHg, aspiration flow rate 25 ml/min).

The flat aperture of the 45° tip is placed sideways against the flat wall of the separated nuclear quadrant. Vacuum is allowed to build, with very little ultrasonic energy applied so that the tip can bore into but still adhere to the quadrant (Fig. 16.23). As vacuum builds, the nuclear fragment is held even more securely on the phacoemulsification tip aperture. The tip is drawn centrally and rolled over so that the fragment is rolled centrally and vertically in a simultaneous unlocking motion (Fig. 16.24). The tip is rotated 90° so that the previously side-facing aperture faces upwards. The nuclear fragment is rotated so that it is basically within the upper capsular bag or lower iris plane, well away from the posterior capsule and corneal endothelium, with the tip aperture facing the corneal endothelium. The initial part of the nuclear fragment is aspirated with ultrasonic assistance while the rollover occurs. Vacuum is assisted by low levels of ultrasonic energy as needed, so that the rest of the quadrant can be aspirated while it is in that location (Fig. 16.25). A little more ultrasonic energy may be needed in the later phases

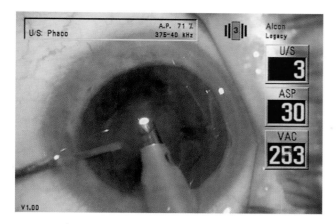

Figure 16.25. *The nuclear fragment is being removed. The phacoemulsification tip is facing the corneal endothelial surface. The softer peripheral nuclear material is now the most central and drawn in easiest.*

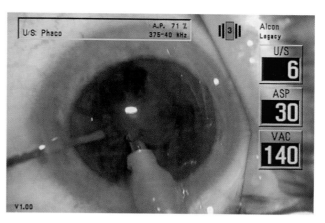

Figure 16.26. *The firmer nuclear material is being aspirated with low levels of phacoemulsification energy.*

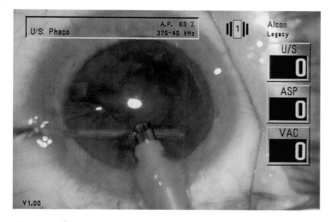

Figure 16.27. *The cyclodialysis spatula is protecting the posterior capsule and preventing additional peripheral nuclear pieces from being withdrawn.*

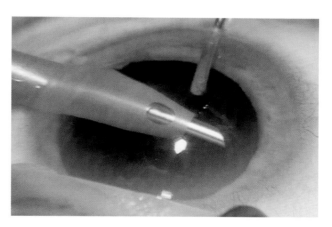

Figure 16.28. *Side view. The aperture of the 45° tip has been applied to the wall of the nuclear fragment and vacuum is allowed to build.*

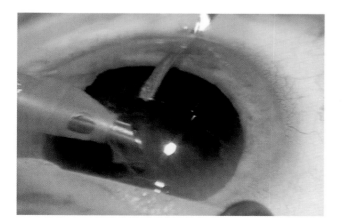

Figure 16.29. *Side view. The nuclear fragment is drawn centrally while simultaneously rolling it over 90°.*

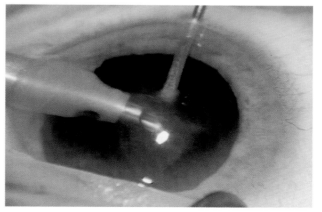

Figure 16.30. *The phacoemulsification tip is facing the endothelium and the nuclear fragment is being withdrawn.*

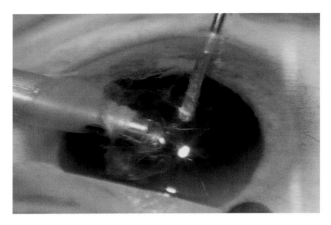

Figure 16.31. *The cyclodialysis spatula aids in positioning of the nuclear fragment.*

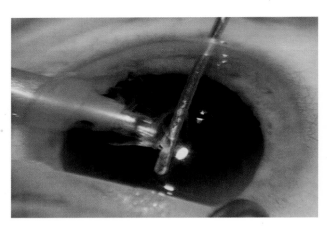

Figure 16.32. *The cyclodialysis spatula protects the posterior capsule against inadvertent aspiration.*

of nucleus removal, as the firmer portion of the deeper nucleus is ultimately the last to be acquired (Fig. 16.26). As the very last of the firm nuclear fragments are removed, the cyclodialysis spatula is placed immediately underneath the phacoemulsification tip to prevent aspiration of capsule or involuntary presentation of the next nuclear quadrant (Fig. 16.27). With this system, total occlusion is never achieved. The alternate flow through the ABS tip prevents it. This reduces any presumed dependence on machine software to prevent rebound after an occlusion break, because the break never happens.

From the side view, the nuclear wall is engaged with the face of the 45° tip. The quadrant is withdrawn and the tip rotated 90° so it faces superior (Figs 16.28, 16.29 and 16.30). The nuclear fragment is within the deeper iris plane and aspirated, with the cyclodialysis spatula assisting in procurement and manipulation of nuclear material while protecting the posterior capsule from inadvertent aspiration (Figs 16.31 and 16.32).

CORTEX REMOVAL

Cortex is removed with a 0.3-mm I/A tip with the machine in surgeon control of aspiration with setting limits of 50 ml/min and 500 mmHg maximum vacuum. The 0.2-mm tip can be used for small strings of cortex or in loose zonule situations in which I desire to engage less cortex with each withdrawal.

CAPSULAR VACUUMING

The 0.2-mm I/A tip is used to vacuum as much material as possible, with machine maximum presets of 11 ml/min and 11 mmHg.

INCISION ENLARGEMENT

When vacuuming of the posterior capsule is completed, viscoelastic is placed in the anterior chamber. The diamond blade is extended fully and the incision lengthened from 2.8 mm to approximately 3.2 mm to accommodate IOL insertion (Fig. 16.33).

INTRAOCULAR LENS IMPLANTATION

I feel that the following implantation technique is the most gentle on the incision tunnel tissue and also creates the least acute distortion of the acrylic IOL polymethylmethacrylate (PMMA) haptics. I currently prefer to implant acrylic IOLs. The AMO Array multifocal lens may be implanted in similar fashion with instruments appropriate for silicone IOLs. A 3.2-mm incision is generally needed for this, although 3.0 mm incisions may be used with a cartridge injector.

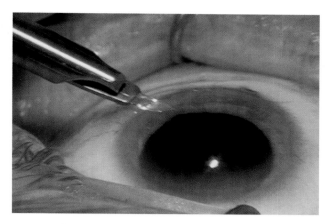

Figure 16.33. *The incision is enlarged from 2.8 to 3.2 mm with the diamond blade.*

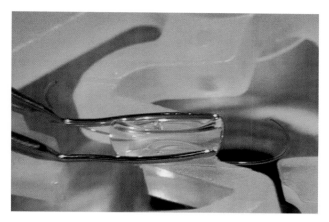

Figure 16.34. *The acrylic lens optic is grasped with implantation forceps.*

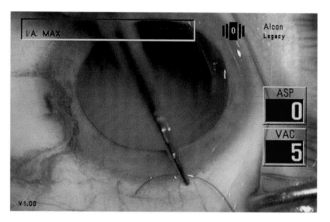

Figure 16.35. *The leading haptic is in a position to be straightened as the optic is pulled slightly away from the 0.12 forceps.*

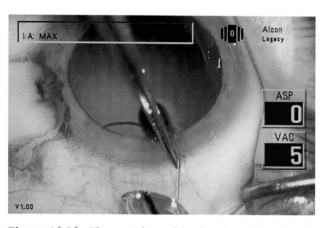

Figure 16.36. *The straightened leading haptic is placed in the anterior chamber.*

The folded lens is removed from the modified Acrypak compression device with insertion forceps (Fig. 16.34). The surface of the forceps' paddles are cleaned with an instrument wipe so that they do not harbor any foreign material that might be impressed on the optic surface. The leading haptic is extended with counterpressure by straightening, so that it can go through the incision (Figs 16.35 and 16.36). The superficial portion of the incision is lifted gently so that the optic can slide between the superficial portion and the deeper tunnel walls. Care is taken not to mar the lens with the 0.12 forceps. Care is also taken not to disturb the stroma or epithelium which makes up the surface of the

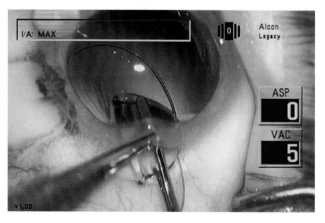

Figure 16.37. *The superficial portion of the wound is lifted with 0.12 forceps so that optic entry can be initiated.*

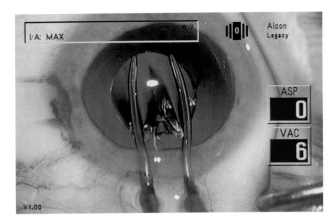

Figure 16.38. *The IOL is unfolded, being careful of the corneal endothelium.*

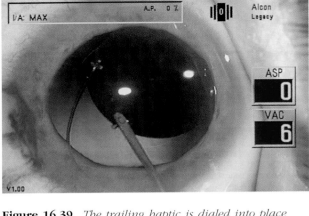

Figure 16.39. *The trailing haptic is dialed into place within the capsule bag.*

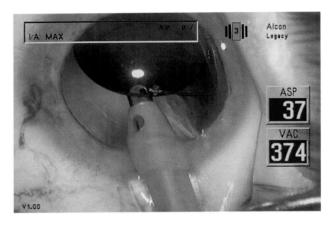

Figure 16.40. *Viscoelastic is removed with a 0.3 tip first in a retrolental position, later in the anterior chamber.*

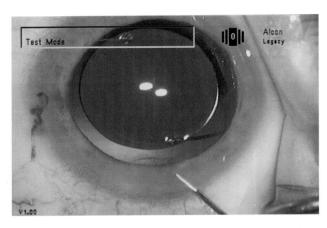

Figure 16.41. *Stromal hydration is accomplished with a 30-gauge cannula.*

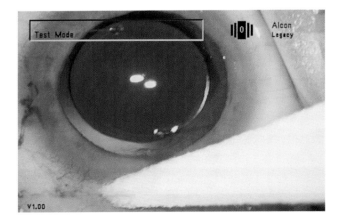

Figure 16.42. *IOP is adjusted to normal by wound compression with a Weck-cel sponge.*

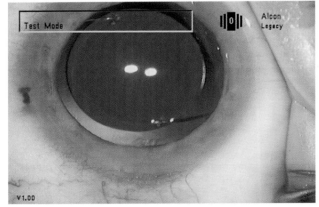

Figure 16.43. *The procedure is complete. Inspection of incision, paracentesis, anterior chamber, iris, rhexis, capsule, and IOL.*

superficial tunnel flap (if the wound is tight it should be extended). Globe stabilization through countertraction can be accomplished by placing a cyclodialysis spatula in the side-port incision. No substantial traction should be attempted with the 0.12 forceps on the wound edge, as disruption of the epithelium or stroma or both may occur. The 0.12 forceps should be used only to lift slightly (Fig. 16.37). The lens is allowed to unfold, again being careful of the endothelial surface of the cornea, not only centrally, but peripherally near the wound (Fig. 16.38). The lens is dialed into position with a Lester manipulator (Fig. 16.39). Viscoelastic is removed with the 0.3 I/A tip. Aspiration is not engaged until the tip has been placed under the IOL optic. If the tip is under the optic, the posterior capsule will not be encountered and all viscoelastic will be removed from the space between the posterior capsule and the optic of the IOL (Fig. 16.40). The tip can then be brought into the anterior chamber to finish thorough viscoelastic removal.

WOUND CLOSURE

The side-port incision is irrigated with a 30-gauge cannula, not only to close the side-port incision with stromal hydration, but also to make sure that there are no nuclear fragments are hiding there. The stroma is then hydrated with brief and minimal pressure from the 3-ml syringe through a 30-gauge cannula. Hydration of the stroma should be accomplished with the tip at mid-stroma, well away from the epithelial and the endothelial edges (Fig. 16.41). The eye is overinflated so that the tunnel interfaces become opposed. If the eye is left overinflated, the wound will seal but the IOP will be too high and the patient will be almost immediately uncomfortable. Normal pressure is obtained by expressing some of the fluid from the incision with gentle pressure using a Weck-cel sponge. If the wound is too well sealed and fluid will not express with this technique, it can be let out passively by placing the 30-gauge cannula within the side-port incision, but the appropriate pressure of the eye must be still be assessed by tactile sensation with the Weck-cel sponge over the incision. Pressure in the eye at the conclusion of this tamponade should be normal, i.e. not hard or soft (Fig. 16.42). When the IOP is normal to low normal, a final inspection is made. The external wound, internal wound, paracentesis, anterior chamber, capsulorhexis border, IOL and iris are all inspected to make sure that they are secure and their positions are appropriate and that no foreign bodies are present (Fig. 16.43). The wound edges may moisten a bit, but no frank gross leakage should be apparent. The speculum is then carefully withdrawn while the patient is asked to keep their eyes open. The adhesive drape can then be slowly removed, while again asking the patient to keep their eyes open. The patient is then asked to just close their eyes gently, but not to squeeze. Any remaining fluid is gently dried with a towel so that the patient does not feel like they have to reach up and wipe their eye. The patient is instructed to keep their eye closed for approximately 1 min. They may then open it, but they are shown where the incision is and instructed not to rub their eye. Antibiotic drops and prednisolone acetate 1% are started four times a day on the day after surgery. The antibiotic (which was started 3 days prior to surgery) runs out in a few days. After 2 weeks, the steroid is reduced to twice daily for 2 more weeks.

Chapter 17 **Clear-cornea cataract incision: astigmatic consequences**

Kimiya Shimizu

INTRODUCTION

Clear-cornea cataract surgery has a long history, and as the operative wounds become smaller, its effectiveness increases. Postoperative astigmatism and endophthalmitis used to be two major complications of clear-cornea incision; however, these problems have been almost solved by making the wound as small as 3.2 mm or less at the temporal site (and by using irrigation containing antibiotics). The author mainly performs cataract surgery through a temporal clear corneal incision under topical anesthesia, which has been made possible by corneal incision. A single-plane incision is made with 2.8 mm keratome and seals without suture. This method increases the indications for cataract surgery, simplifies the operation and reduces postoperative inflammation, such as cystoid macular edema (CME). This paper describes the surgical technique, advantages and disadvantages of this method. In addition, it outlines the future incision size for astigmatic neutral which leads to the effects of toric IOL and multifocal IOL in full range. Finally, the development of disposable tools to decrease the surgical cost and increase safety, which has arisen as a result of this technique, is discussed.

HISTORY

Clear-cornea cataract surgery was done by Albrecht von Graefe from about 1750, and has been used in extracapsular extraction for a long time. After the 1960s, due to the appearance of microscopy and delicate suture thread, the incision site of cataract surgery was transferred from the cornea to the limbus. On the other hand, Galand and Delmelle had conducted planned extracapsular cataract extraction (ECCE) by clear-cornea incision.[1] From the latter half

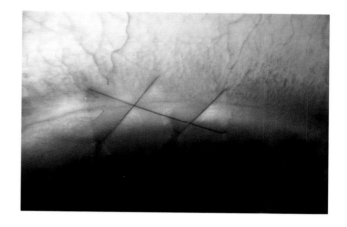

Figure 17.1. *Five-millimeter corneal incision with suture.*

of the 1980s, the indications for intraocular lens (IOL) were extended gradually, and the operation in patients with diabetes[2] and glaucoma[3] became commonplace. In these complicated eyes, scleral incision with a long tunnel or limbal incision caused synechiae or complicated surgery, and clear corneal incision showed better results in many cases. I therefore increased the indications for phacoemulsification (PE) with corneal incision, and found ease of operation, less postoperative inflammation, and broad indications for corneal incision. We reported PE through a clear corneal incision,[4] but as the incision in cataract surgery was 4 mm in foldable IOL and 5.5 mm in polymethylmethacrylate (PMMA) lenses with suture at that time (Fig. 17.1), postoperative astigmatism was a problem, and postoperative infection sometimes occurred. Noting the results of the secondary implantation of anterior chamber lenses by Masket,[5] we began to perform temporal corneal incision to reduce induced against-the-rule astigmatism. By this method, postoperative against-the-rule astigmatism was reduced, and the ease of operation was enhanced. In 1991, McFarland made the wound more scleral and introduced PE through a scleral pocket incision without suture.[6] With the development of foldable IOLs, the incision size could be reduced to 3.5 mm or less. From 1993, the appearance of disposable injections made it possible to reduce the incision size to 3.2 mm, and, from that time, sutureless surgery by temporal clear corneal incision became routine, and topical anesthesia also came to be employed in all cases. In 1994, with improvement of the disposable injector, the incision size became reduced to 2.8 mm,[7] and the knife used for incision was changed from a diamond keratome to a stainless disposable one, and the incision method was changed to single-plane incision. At the same time, the operation kit was changed to a disposable kit, which means that surgery is performed with a disposable kit only. For postoperative infection, we use irrigation solution with antibiotics, which was introduced by Gills.[8] With this irrigation, together with disposable kit, the complication of postoperative inflammation has been controlled at present. In addition, we obtained other advantages, such as reduction of postoperative inflammation and operation time.

ADVANTAGES OF CLEAR CORNEAL INCISION

SIMPLE AND FAST

In corneal surgery, only one single-plane incision is done with the disposable keratome, and no conjunctival incision, no scleral tunnel and no diathermy are necessary. It requires only one incision with the keratome, and marking the incision and enlargement of the wound is unnecessary. Therefore, uniform incision can always be obtained. As all operative procedures are performed through one wound, the operation time can be shortened.

CORNEAL INCISION FACILITATES TOPICAL ANESTHESIA

From 1985, I had performed cataract surgery under topical anesthesia with 4% cocaine,[9] but due to scleral incision, occasional pain occurred in diathermy and conjunctival incision. Therefore, topical anesthesia was not employed routinely at that

time. In 1990, we began to perform small corneal incision surgery, which made routine topical anesthesia possible, as neither coagulation nor suturing was required.[10] Since 1996, we have been using Gills' intracameral injection[11] of 0.5% lidocaine together with topical instillation in some cases.

TEMPORAL APPROACH SUITS CORNEAL INCISION

In limbal or scleral incision, postoperative redness becomes remarkable when the temporal approach is employed. However, temporal corneal incision hardly causes injection or bleeding. (Therefore, temporal incision is suitable for corneal incision.)

Temporal incision has four advantages. First, the approach to the anterior chamber is easier, especially in patients with a narrow palpebral fissure (Fig. 17.2). Furthermore, as inferior duction of the eyeball is not required with the temporal approach, the iris plane is always kept at right angles to the microscope to provide good visibility. The second advantage is that no pain may be caused, as patients are not forced to see downwards, and the palpebral fissure does not have to be forced to expand. The third advantage is that the cornea is oval and the optical center of the cornea deviates to the nasal area from the anatomic center. Therefore, in temporal incision, the distance is about 1 mm more from the optical center as compared with superior incision (Fig. 17.3). Thus, the operative invasion to the corneal center is minimal in

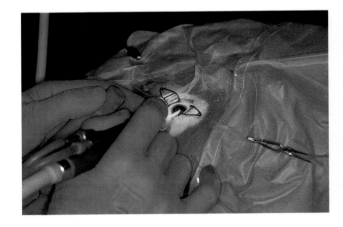

Figure 17.2. *The temporal approach is easier for cases with a narrow palpebral fissure.*

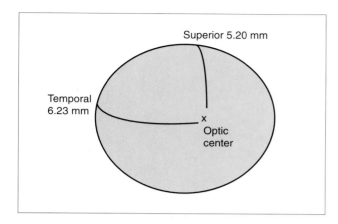

Figure 17.3. *Schema showing the distance from the corneal optical center to the corneal temporal and superior sites measured in 103 cases.*

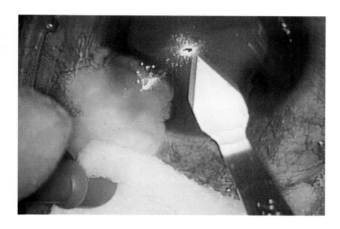

Figure 17.4. *Clear corneal incision in eyes with filtering bleb.*

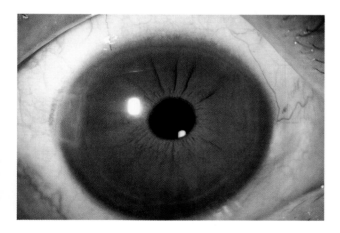

Figure 17.5. *The patient on the day after surgery. Almost no injection can be seen.*

temporal incision. As a result, surgically induced astigmatism is small and recovery of visual acuity is fast. The fourth advantage is that the wound will not separate when blinking, and temporal incision provides good adaptation of the wound.

LESS OPERATIVE INVASION

As no conjunctival incision or scleral dissection is done, clear corneal incision is advantageous in cases of glaucoma with filtering bleb (Fig. 17.4). In addition, as there is almost no postoperative injection (Fig. 17.5), an unnecessary worry of patients and families is avoided. As no bleeding occurs, a post-operative eye patch becomes unnecessary, and this is helpful for a one-eyed patient. Furthermore, as the distance between wound and iris is larger in corneal incision than in scleral incision, corneal incision causes less iris damage and iris invasion. To prove this, when the rate of CME was examined retrospectively with the same lens implantation, the rate was significantly less in the corneal incision group than in the scleral incision group[12] (Table 17.1).

FEWER TOOLS

In scleral incision, many tools are necessary, such as conjunctival scissors, diathermy, a knife for scleral half-layer incision, a blade for scleral dissection, and a keratome. In contrast, only one keratome is required in corneal incision. As the incision becomes smaller, I routinely use only one disposable keratome, and this makes the maintenance and management of tools easy. This method is also

Table 17.1
Incidence of CME.

	Corneal incision	*Limbal incision*
N (F/M)	132 (86/46)	334 (216/115)
Age	69.1 ± 12.4	69.8 ± 10.7
Operation time (min)	16.8 ± 6.4	21.0 ± 6.7
CME	0/132	13/334 (3.9%)*

* ($p < 0.05$, chi-square).

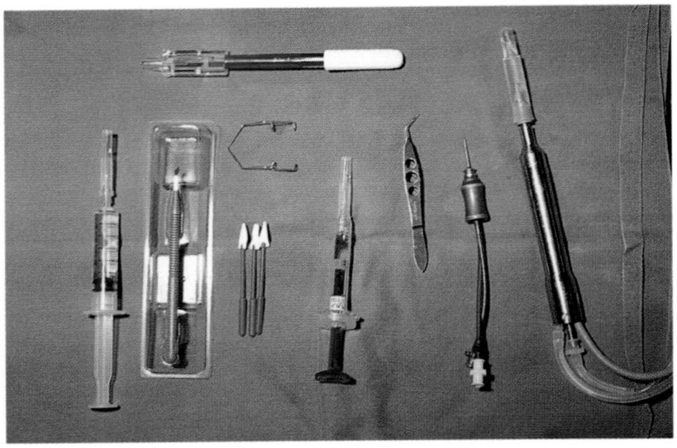

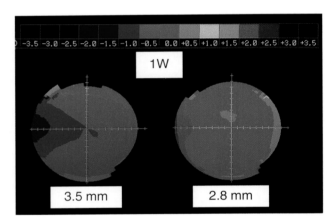

Figure 17.6. *Instrumentation of corneal incision. A few tools are necessary.*

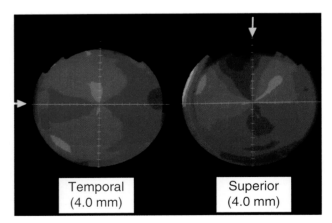

Figure 17.7. *Differential topography before and after surgery. The induced astigmatism is smaller in the 2.8-mm incision.*

Figure 17.8. *Differential topography before and after surgery. The induced astigmatism is about two-thirds in temporal incisions.*

advantageous for prevention of infection and for reducing the cost (Fig. 17.6).

DISADVANTAGES OF CLEAR CORNEAL INCISION

INFECTION

Infection is related to the wound size. Of the cases in our study, endophthalmitis occurred only in those with incisions of 4 mm or over. In temporal small incisions of 3.2 mm or less, with the use of an antibiotic in the infusion and with a total disposable kit, we have never experienced infection among more than 6000 cases.[13]

ENDOTHELIAL DAMAGE

As long as PE is performed in situ, endothelial damage rarely becomes a problem. Furthermore, low molecular weight hyaluronic acid has a strong protective effect on endothelial cells.[14] With the use of it prior to PE, endothelial cell loss is $4.4 \pm 9.1\%$ in my cases, which is the same as that with corneal or limbal incision.

ASTIGMATISM

With the same incision size, the induced astigmatism of corneal incision is larger than that of scleral incision. However, the surgically induced astigmatism decreases as the incision size decreases (Fig. 17.7), and the surgically induced astigmatism of temporal incision is about two-thirds of that of superior incision (Fig. 17.8). Thus when the temporal corneal wound is 2.64 mm, it is calculated to become zero. In today's corneal incision of 2.8 mm, induced astigmatism is 0.04 ± 0.55 D, which is larger than that in scleral incision.

SURGICAL PROCEDURE

TOPICAL ANESTHESIA

A first drop of 1% lidocaine is instilled just before sterilization of an eye. Just before the incision, an additional 2–3 drops are instilled on the conjunctiva to prevent the corneal epithelial damage. Occasionally, some sedation is introduced before surgery, but no akinesia is induced, and no further instillation is required. When complicated surgery is expected, intracameral anesthesia with 0.5% lidocaine is added by the technique introduced by Gills. Potential disadvantages of topical anesthesia are that the effect is less strong and the duration is slightly shorter (about 15–20 min).

NO SOFT EYE OR BRIDLE SUTURE IS REQUIRED

In principle, it is not necessary to obtain a soft eye by compression or massage. No bridle suture is required in any cases. Under topical anesthesia, the patient obeying the operator's instruction with regard to eye movement may provide a good operative field.

OPERATOR'S POSITION

When the operator is right-handed and the operative eye is the right eye, sit at a position of 10:30. When the operative eye is the left eye, sit at 4:00 (Fig. 17.9).

SINGLE-PLANE CORNEAL INCISION OF 2.8 MM

Basically, a single-plane incision is made. The incision site is better as far peripheral as possible within the cornea. If the incision is posterior to that, chemosis can decrease the visibility. In a two-plane incision, chemosis occurs less frequently, but the operation becomes complicated. A two-plane incision makes the surface area of the wound larger, and makes the hinge which allows the wound to gap. This is clearly seen by fluorescent staining of the wound postoperatively (Fig. 17.10). The length

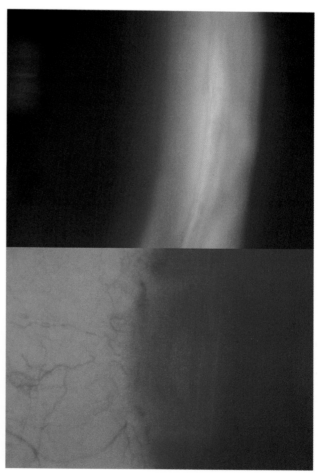

Figure 17.10. *Fluorescent staining. Single plane and double.*

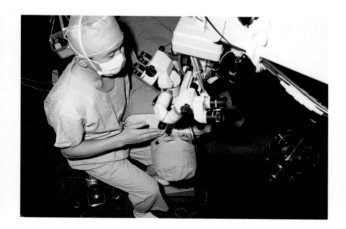

Figure 17.9. *The surgeon's position. In the case of the right eye, the surgeon sits at 10:30, and in the case of the left eye, the surgeon sits at 4:30.*

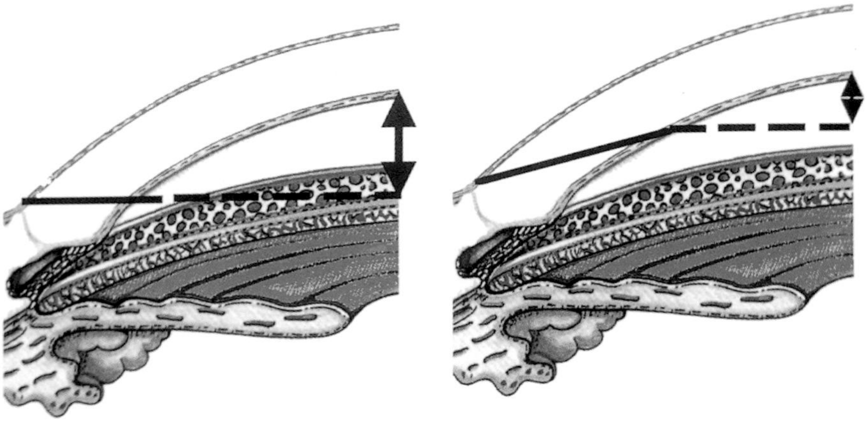

Short tunnel

Long tunnel

Figure 17.11. *When the tunnel is longer, the distance between tip and endothelium becomes closer, causing endothelial damage.*

of the corneal tunnel is ideally about 1.5 mm. A shorter tunnel decreases the self-sealing rate, while the visibility becomes better. A too long tunnel increases the self-sealing, but corneal folds sometimes disturb the visibility. Corneal endothelial damage also becomes greater (Fig. 17.11) as the distance between the phaco tip and corneal endothelium becomes shorter. Thus, when the operator performs corneal incision for the first time, it is recommended to make a rather shorter tunnel and to place 11-0 nylon single knot without being concerned with self-sealing. When you incise the cornea, do not fixate the eyeball at the temporal side, as an eyeball rotates slightly and the wound is sometimes twisted. As a result, the wound configuration becomes asymmetric. Instead, I compress the eye lightly at the nasal side using mercerol sponge, and this method makes it easier to incise the cornea. With the use of mercerol sponge rather than forceps, bleeding can be prevented (Fig. 17.12). The proper placement of the incision is important. If it is too anterior, the corneal tunnel becomes shorter, and the self-sealing effect is decreased. In contrast, if it is too posterior, conjunctival bleeding and/or chemosis sometimes occur.

So, before incising the cornea, dry the incision site and place the keratome just anterior to the terminal conjunctival vessels (Fig. 17.13). Then, advance the keratome straight about 1.5 mm into the corneal stroma. Next, direct the keratome slightly downwards to perforate Decesmet's membrane (Fig. 17.14). When the tip of the keratome appears in the anterior chamber, remove the mercerol sponge and

release the counterpressure. After that, advance the keratome, swinging it to both right and left sides. By doing this, the incision may be conducted safely without causing the collapse of the anterior chamber (Fig. 17.15). The length of the corneal tunnel is usually 1.5 mm, but if it is a complicated or hard nucleus case, it should be shorter. On the other hand, when the case has good mydriasis or a shallow anterior chamber, the incision site should be a little anterior, and the corneal tunnel should be longer to prevent iris damage and/or iris prolapse.

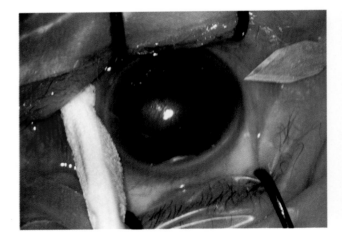

Figure 17.12. *Apply the counterpressure by mercerol sponge to fix the eye.*

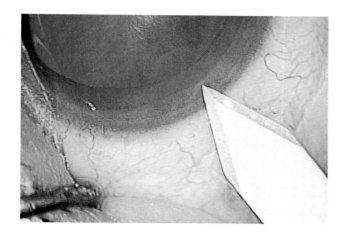

Figure 17.13. *Start the point of corneal incision.*

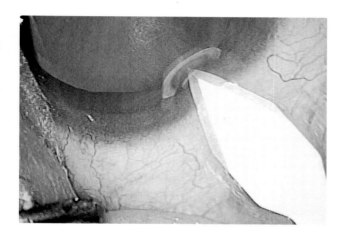

Figure 17.14. *Perforation of Decesmet's membrane.*

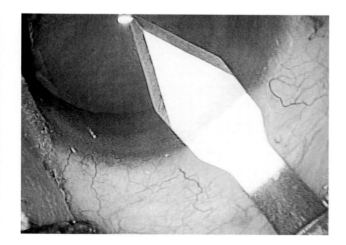

Figure 17.15. *Complete perforation.*

ANTERIOR CAPSULORHEXIS

Sodium hyaluronate is injected into the anterior chamber, and capsulorhexis is performed with the capsule forceps or a needle. When the incision is at the temporal site, the wound is not easily separated, and the capsulotomy can be manipulated much more easily.

HYDRODISSECTION

A 5-ml syringe with a blunt 27-gauge needle is used. Inject the balanced salt solution (BSS) in several directions, and confirm that the nucleus is completely separated from cortex.

PHACOEMULSIFICATION

Just before insertion of the ultrasound tip, low molecular weight sodium hyaluronate is injected. It has a stronger protective effect on the corneal endothelium during PE and aspiration.

To insert through an incision of 2.8 mm or less, a small US-tip[15] with an outer diameter of 0.9 mm is used (Fig. 17.16). With the use of a small US-tip, wound injury becomes less and the self-sealing rate can be increased. For safe and effective PE, it is important to adjust the flow rate and vacuum pressure at each phase of PE (multi-modulation

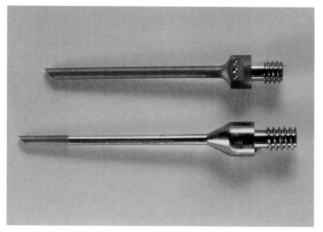

Figure 17.16. *Small US-tip and regular one. For 2.8-mm incisions, the small tip is preferable.*

phaco: MMP).[16] Use of the proper sleeve for the tip is also critical.

INTRAOCULAR LENS IMPLANTATION

After PE, high molecular weight sodium hyaluronate is injected into the anterior chamber before cortical aspiration. By use of a 2.8-mm disposable injector, a 5.5-mm three-piece silicone IOL (Fig. 17.17) is implanted. At that time, eyeball fixation is not necessary. Instruct the patient to look to the temporal side, and insert the injector utilizing the eye movement (Fig. 17.18).

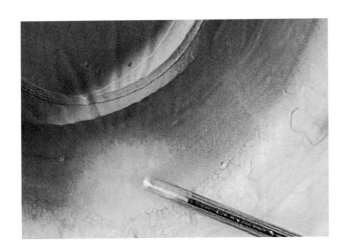

Figure 17.19. *Hydration.*

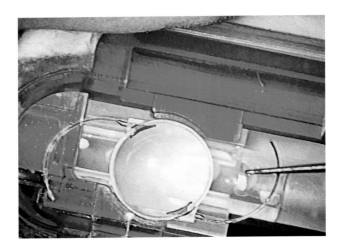

Figure 17.17. *Silicone lens placed in a cartridge.*

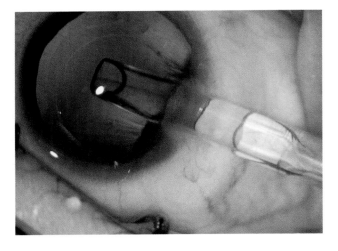

Figure 17.18 *A silicone lens is inserted through a 2.8-mm incision.*

HYDRATION AND INFUSION/ASPIRATION

The wound is deformed somewhat by surgery, so anterior collapse or IOL deviation may be caused by leakage after viscoelastics are aspirated with the I/A tip. To prevent this, hydration is performed before I/A tip insertion. After this, with use of a smaller inner diameter I/A tip rather than the normal one, cortex and sodium hyaluronate are aspirated at the same time. I sometimes perform cortical aspiration following IOL implantation. This is because, after IOL implantation, tension is always added to the lens capsule. So, even when the posterior capsule is aspirated, there is less chance of rupture. That is, as the space between the anterior and posterior capsules is wide, it is not easy to aspirate the capsule. To obtain the self-sealing wound, hydration is tried again. The method is to inject BSS containing an antibiotic into the corneal stroma of both left and right cut ends of the incision (Fig. 17.19). I use a 10-μg/ml solution of imipenem/cyrastatin. After hydration, the posterior lip of the wound is pressed with mercerol sponge to confirm that there is no leakage. The cornea becomes transiently opaque, but will become transparent by the next day.

After the eye speculum is removed, a disposable contact lens soaked in dichlorofenac sodium solution is put in place, and the operation is completed. By application of the contact lens, the wound can be protected, and postoperative foreign body sensation is reduced. As the use of a contact lens makes the eye patch unnecessary, it is helpful for one-eyed patients, and for those with astigmatic keratotomy

(AK), as a contact lens is useful to protect the wound. This contact lens is removed before the physical examination on the next day.

ASTIGMATISM CONTROL

NO INDUCED ASTIGMATISM

Based on our study, the wound size is determined to be 2.6 mm, which causes no astigmatism and which enables 100% self-sealing.

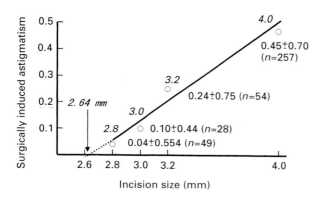

Figure 17.20. *Incision size and induced astigmatism in temporal corneal incision. When the incision is 2.64 mm, induced astigmatism is calculated to be zero.*

To determine the relationship between wound size and induced astigmatism, surgically induced astigmatism was examined in temporal corneal incisions of 4.0, 3.2, 3.0 and 2.8 mm, at 1 month after surgery. Calculating from the regression line, the surgically induced astigmatism became almost zero at an incision size of 2.64 mm[17] (Fig. 17.20), and this size is considered to be the target of small incision for the time being. The self-sealing rate was calculated similarly, and 100% self-sealing was obtained when the wound was 2.59 mm[18] (Fig. 17.21), which is almost the same as the astigmatic neutral wound size.

CONTROL OF PRE-EXISTING ASTIGMATISM

When a 2.6-mm incision is conducted no astigmatism is induced by surgery but it becomes impossible to control the preoperative astigmatism by cataract incision only. In other words, it is impossible to correct pre-existing astigmatism by small-incision cataract surgery. Especially in those with with-the-rule astigmatism, it becomes difficult to correct astigmatism by temporal incision. In cases with severe preoperative astigmatism, AK or foldable toric IOL becomes necessary.

When the patient has with-the-rule (WTR) astigmatism, I employ superior corneal incision. However, the superior approach causes more complications in shallow anterior chamber cases, a low self-sealing rate and late visual recovery. Thus, temporal corneal approach is superior except for correction of WTR astigmatism. Today, in cases with astigmatism over 1 D, I use the toric IOL[19] (Fig. 17.22) or astigmatic

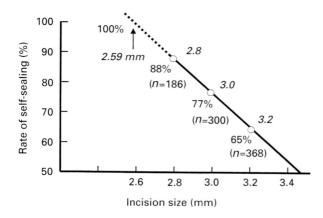

Figure 17.21. *Incision size and sealing rate. When the incision is 2.59 mm, the self-sealing rate is calculated to be 100%.*

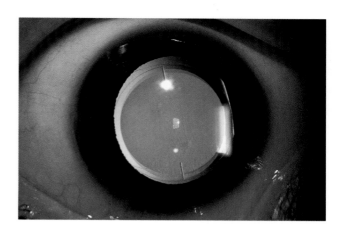

Figure 17.22. *Single-piece toric IOL with the line indicating the toric axis.*

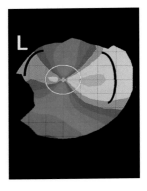

	Nas.	Temp.
OZ	6.0	6.0
Length	1.5	3.5
Degree	170°	0°
Depth	545	545

Figure 17.23. *Surgical plan of TOAK.*

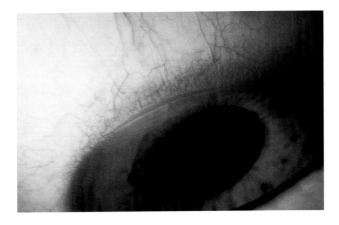

Figure 17.24. *Gills' limbal-relaxing incision.*

keratotomy combined with 2.8-mm temporal clear-cornea cataract surgery. As a result, two-thirds of all my cataract cases have less than 0.5 D astigmatism after surgery.

When the eye has preoperative symmetric astigmatism by videokeratoscopy, a toric IOL is implanted. When it is asymmetric, AK is the choice. A toric IOL is superior to AK in that it is non-invasive to the cornea, so it does not decrease the optical performance. Furthermore, additional tools and times are not required for toric IOLs. However, axis rotation sometimes occurs, decreasing the effects of cylinder correction. In such situations, repositioning is necessary.

In contrast, AK is useful for correction of asymmetric astigmatism, as it can adjust the depth and length of the incision with reference to videokeratoscopy (topography-oriented astigmatic keratotomy: TOAK)[20] (Fig. 17.23). In TOAK the corneal optical performance decreases when the optical zone is less than 6 mm, and/or overcorrection is caused. Therefore, I use the modified Gills' technique,[21] in which a limbal-relaxing incision is performed with a depth of 500 μm (Fig. 17.24). In this technique, the effects of correcting astigmatism are less strong, but no irregular astigmatism is caused and optical performance is not decreased.

When astigmatic control becomes possible, the effect of a multifocal IOL increases.[22]

Basically, it is desirable that the surgery is simple and causes minimal invasion. Before a non-invasive operative method by laser is developed, small-incision keratotomy under topical anesthesia will be the operative method which satisfies these requirements most.

REFERENCES

1 Galand A, Delmelle M. Preliminary report on the rigid disc lens. *J Cataract Refract Surg* 1986; **12:** 394–7.

2 Iwase H, Miyata K, Kohara M, Sshimizu K. Intraocular lens implantation in diabetic patients. *Act Soc Ophthalmol Jpn* 1988; **92:** 499–506.

3 Amano S, Shimizu K. IOL implantation in glaucomatous eyes. *Jpn J Ophthalmol Surg* 1990; **3:** 157–63.

4 Shimizu K. Small incision cataract surgery. *Ocul Surg News* 1991; **9**(Suppl): 2–15.

5 Masket S. Temporal incision for astigmatic control in secondary implantation. *J Cataract Refract Surg* 1986; **12:** 179–81.

6 McFarland SM. The clinical history of sutureless surgery. In: Gills JP, ed. *Sutureless Cataract Surgery* (New Jersey: Slack, 1992) 3–4.

7 Shimizu K, Komatsu M, Nakajima T. Development of a novel silicone IOL for small incision. *Jpn J Clin Ophthalmol* 1994; **48:** 1103–7.

8 Gills JP. Filters and antibiotics in irrigating solution for cataract surgery. *J Cataract Refract Surg* 1994; **17:** 385.

9 Murao T, Kinoshita Y, Shimizu K. Silicone lens implantation. *Jpn Rev Clin Ophthalmol* 1986; **80:** 2194–7.

10 Maruo T, Komatsu M, Shimizu K. Cataract surgery under topical anesthesia. *Jpn Rev Clin Ophthalmol* 1995; **89:** 450–2.

11 Gills JP, Cherchio M, Raanan MG. Unpreserved lidocaine to control discomfort during cataract surgery using topical anesthesia. *J Cataract Refract Surg* 1997; **23:** 545–50.

12 Kaburaki T, Shimizu K. The incidence of pseudophakic cystoid macular edema: clear corneal incision vs. limbal incision. *J Cataract Refract Surg* 1994; **20:** 43–5.

13 Shimizu N, Shimizu K. Incidence and prevention of endophthalmitis following cataract surgery. *Jpn J Clin Ophthalmol* 1997; **51:** 211–14.

14 Nagahara Y, Shoji N, Shimizu K, et al. Protection of corneal endothelium in phacoemulsification. *Jpn J Ophthalmol Surg* 1993; **6:** 459–63.

15 Shimizu K. S-tip phaco. *Jpn J Ophthalmol Surg* 1990; **3:** 399–402.

16 Shimizu K, Sugita G, Taniguchi S. Multi-modulated phaco-emulsification (MMP). *Jpn J Cataract Refract Surg* 1990; **7:** 86–94.

17 Shimizu K. Temporal clear corneal incision cataract surgery. *Jpn J Ophthalmol* 1995; **37:** 323–30.

18 Shimizu N, Shimizu K. Self-sealing wounds in temporal clear-corneal incision cataract surgery. *Jpn J Ophthalmol Surg* 1996; **9:** 397–401.

19 Shimizu K, Misawa A, Suzuki Y. Toric intraocular lenses: correcting astigmatism while controlling axis shift. *J Cataract Refract Surg* 1994; **20:** 523–6.

20 Furusawa N, Tanaka S, Shimizu K. Topography-oriented astigmatic keratotomy. *J Cataract Refract Surg* 1995; **21**(Suppl): 1–5.

21 Gill JP. The efficient cataract surgery: 8 steps to streamlining your procedures. *Rev Ophthalmol* 1997; **4:** 76–82.

22 Shoji N, Shimizu K. Clinical evaluation of a 5.5 mm three-zone refractive multifocal intraocular lens. *J Cataract Refract Surg* 1996; **22:** 1097–101.

Chapter 18 Wound complications in clear-cornea cataract surgery: causes, prevention and management

Matteo Piovella and Fabrizio I Camesasca

INTRODUCTION

Although clear-cornea cataract surgery dates back to the days of Albrecht von Graefe, its introduction in the present era of phacoemulsification (phaco) and foldable intraocular lenses (IOLs) is credited to Fine in 1992.[1] Clear corneal incision has become progressively successful on account of the safety and predictability of induced astigmatism and limited complications. Several authors have confirmed its role in controlling and stabilizing astigmatism.[2–4]

The elimination of conjunctival incision and of continuous sclerocorneal suture made possible by clear corneal incision reduces surgical time and enhances procedure standardization. At present, clear corneal incision represents the best available wound for the latest advances in cataract surgery: temporal incision allowing easy access even to the most difficult, deep-socketed eyes, and use of topical anesthesia.

WOUND CONSTRUCTION IN CLEAR CORNEAL INCISION

The first step in constructing a wound is choosing between diamond and metal blades. Cuts made using metal blades are less accurate but, as they meet more resistance from the cornea, the incision can be created gradually with the planned segments. However, the cicatrization of an incision made with a metal blade may be hampered by its irregularity. Diamond blades make for a faster, more regular cut; nevertheless, there is less opportunity to change the direction of the cut if it has been planned incorrectly. This may easily lead to a short tunnel. Diamond

blade incisions are less forgiving, particularly if the blade sides are sharp.

Even if the standardization of cataract surgical techniques tends to smooth out the differences among eyes, the surgeon must always remember that each eye is unique. Therefore, a simple technical approach like the constant use of the same level of magnification at the beginning of surgery will help the surgeon to understand the type of eye he is facing, i.e. small eye or long eye. A long or short eye means different—longer or shorter—ocular curvature, and thus the same incision width will exert a different influence on the final astigmatism. A shorter eye also means a shallower anterior chamber which requires careful incision to prevent damage to the anterior capsule, iris, etc.

Currently accepted techniques for clear corneal wound construction share the common goal of creating a valve seal mechanism as well as the reduction of induced astigmatism. The hydrostatic valve seal is reached when the surface architecture of the incision is square. Ernest demonstrated that a square tunnel is the most effective solution in maintaining the valve seal mechanism.[5] The ideal tunnel size is between 2.8 and 3.2 mm, a neutral size that induces no measurable astigmatism.[6,7]

Three basic incision techniques with self-sealing properties can be considered with diamond blades. A classic incision involves a 'preincision', i.e. vertical cut that creates a vertical step of 250–350 μm in the cornea. This step helps to expose the corneal stroma, detect the appropriate corneal plane for the horizontal part of the incision and prevent the roof of the incision from sliding. The incision must then be continued between the superficial half and one-third of the corneal stroma, following the corneal curvature for at least 1 mm. The blade then pushes down the cornea and continues forwards to create an inner lip (responsible for the valve seal mechanism) before entering the anterior chamber. Thus the total tunnel length is greater than 2 mm.

The second technique is similar to a classic incision but without preincision. With this method, the corneal stroma is not exposed and the incision depends greatly on the surgeon's experience and sensitivity.

The third technique, the hinged incision, was developed in the light of the theoretical goal of a longer, square tunnel, maintaining the incision well away from the optical axis. This technique requires a preincision (500–600 μm) far from the optical axis, in the gray zone of the limbus.[5,8–10] After this deeper preincision, the rest of the incision is made in a similar fashion to the classic incision, although there is a parallel component of some 3 mm. Hinged incisions are most capable of withstanding an applied external force.[11]

CLEAR CORNEAL WOUNDS AND IOLS

The wound constitutes the way out for the lens and the way in for the IOL. Wound construction is therefore closely related to the type and features of the IOL to be used. According to the theoretical model, to prevent the incision from stretching, the minimum size of the incision is determined by the perimeter of the IOL or the complex IOL-insertion instrument.[12] Another factor to take into consideration is corneal elasticity: the wound can increase in size by approximately 15–20% before tearing.[13–15] Consequently, the minimum size of the incision may be calculated by dividing the perimeter of the insertion complex by two and multiplying the resulting figure by 0.85%.

Let us consider a freshly made, unstretched incision. A polymethylmethacrylate (PMMA) IOL resembles the profile of the wound, so if the incision is the same size as the diameter of the lens, inserting the IOL should not stretch the incision. In practice, a rigid IOL has a certain thickness and the perimeter is slightly larger than twice the diameter (Fig 18.1). If the surgeon plans to insert a foldable IOL, the limitation is constituted by the perimeter of the complex folded IOL-insertion instrument (Figs 18.2 and 18.3). The section of the complex is almost circular and the wound profile is inevitably distorted. In this case, the minimum incision size to prevent the incision from stretching is not determined solely by the complex perimeter, on account of the inevitable fishmouth effect and consequent gaping of the wound. Thus the diameter of the unstretched wound must be 6% larger than the diameter of a PMMA IOL (Fig 18.4), but 57%

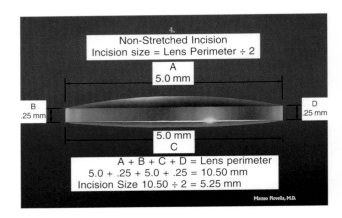

Figure 18.1. *Rigid IOL dimensions.*

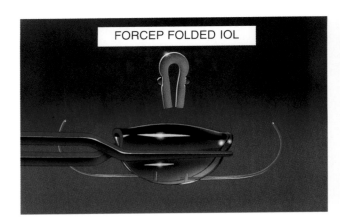

Figure 18.2. *Forceps-folded IOL.*

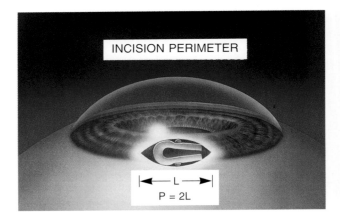

Figure 18.3. *Perimeter of the complex folded IOL-insertion instrument.*

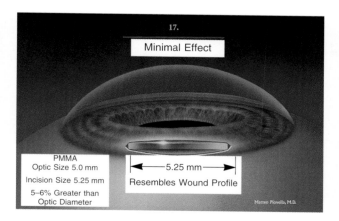

Figure 18.4. *Insertion of a rigid IOL: effect on incision size.*

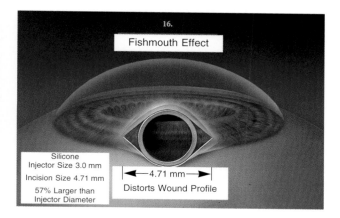

Figure 18.5. *Cartridge for silicon IOL insertion: fishmouth effect.*

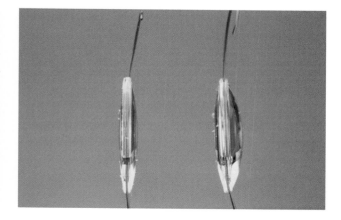

Figure 18.6. *+20.00 diopters IOLs made of silicone with different refractive index have different thicknesses.*

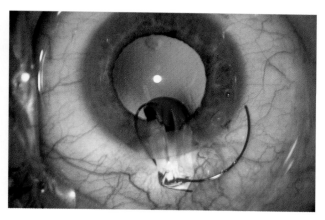

Figure 18.7. *The MemoryLens® does not require folding instruments.*

larger than the perimeter of the folded IOL-insertion instrument (Fig 18.5).

Therefore, a carefully planned wound requires a wider incision to allow the IOL to be inserted quickly and easily even if conditions are not ideal, such as in the event of an IOL that is not folded symmetrically.

Another critical piece of information that must be available to the surgeon is the power of the IOL to be inserted. A lens with a high power will require greater wound enlargement before insertion, unless it is a lens style that is designed for constant central thickness at all optical powers.

For limited widening (about 20%), a precalibrated blade may be used. Before widening, the preincision must be evaluated. Finally, the surgeon must bear in mind that the thickness of the IOL varies according to the power of the IOL, the refractive index, and the material from which it is made (Fig 18.6).

Therefore, insertion of an IOL through a 3.2-mm incision will seriously stretch the wound and can result in a loss of watertight properties. A stretched wound means stretched corneal stroma and Descemet's membrane. Phaco also enlarges the incision, and the size of the keratome may not correspond to the size of the final incision.[16]

Instrument maneuvering is also important in the interaction with the wound size. Tunnel distortion may occur in torsion of the complex folded IOL-insertion instrument. A thermoplastic lens, such as the MemoryLens, which does not need to be kept folded by an instrument during insertion, is the only foldable lens that does not require the optic and inserter to be placed in the tunnel at the same time. Furthermore, this particular lens is always correctly folded before insertion (Fig 18.7), given that it is pre-rolled by the manufacturer.

WOUND COMPLICATIONS: PREVENTION AND MANAGEMENT

Below are considered the most frequent complications related to wound construction: tunnel length and related problems, stretch, burn, and astigmatism.

TUNNEL CONSTRUCTION

Corneas vary in size, curvature and resistance to pressure and cut. A peripheral arcus is commonly present in older patients and may complicate corneal visualization. A tunnel of the proper width and length can be constructed using a precalibrated diamond or metal blade.

Preincision

A preincision must be made at the periphery of the clear cornea. A precalibrated diamond blade allows the best precut. The surgeon should precut during apnea to avoid an irregular wound profile caused by diaphragm motion. An irregular preincision may lead to an uneven incision. If the preincision is irregular, widening the incision may be dangerous.[17] Therefore, it is recommended to check the depth of the incision microscopically to detect which side offers the best opportunities for widening at the proper depth, i.e. in the event that one lip of the incision has been torn due to a superficial precut and trauma during phaco. In this case, the side with the preserved lip should be widened for lens insertion.

Tunnel size

Corneal folds and limitations in phaco probe motion are indications of an excessively long tunnel. A long tunnel enhances the hydrostatic valve seal mechanism. Pressure on the external side of the incision will not cause the wound to leak but it will increase intraocular pressure and push up the inner lip of the incision, further increasing the wound's valve seal properties. However, a long tunnel restricts phaco probe motion, and potentiates sleeve infusion compression and the risk of reduced infusion and corneal burn. Phaco requires angling the probe deep into the nucleus: if the tunnel is long, this will generate corneal folds, obscuring the surgeon's view of the anterior chamber. Particularly in a small eye, a long tunnel means that the phaco probe is closer to the visual axis, with the risk of greater damage to the corneal endothelium. Finally, a long tunnel

hampers in-the-bag IOL insertion, mostly of its distal loop.

A tunnel may be considered short in the event of leakage during surgery and this may occur even in the hands of an experienced surgeon. Pressure on the incision may easily cause the lip to open up on the outer side of the incision, with consequent leakage. Wound leak may be observed during phaco, requiring a higher infusion bottle to maintain the anterior chamber. A short tunnel would be safer with a properly placed suture, to prevent postoperative wound leak, iris prolapse, etc.[5]

Tunnel evaluation

In small eyes, the anterior chamber must be entered carefully to avoid the knife puncturing the anterior capsule. Immediate tunnel evaluation is mandatory. As soon as the incision has been made, the surgeon should assess whether the wound is likely to leak, as well as if it is necessary to place a suture at the end of surgery. In view of the fact that the wound may be stretched during surgery, the wound valve seal mechanism should also be evaluated at the end of surgery. Stromal hydration of the wound at the end of surgery may help to increase the valve seal mechanism.

WOUND BURN

The infusion flow rate has the important role of safeguarding the fluid balance in the anterior chamber and also influences phaco probe cooling. An excessively long tunnel, the surgeon's imperfect knowledge of phaco machine parameters, as well as any maneuver or situation leading to a constriction of the phaco sleeve and a consequent decrease of the infusion, may cause wound burn. Sleeve constriction may be the result of excessive elevation, lowering or lateralization of the phaco probe. This is especially true in deep-socketed eyes when working at the 12 o'clock position. A lateral clear corneal incision prevents the occurrence of this kind of complication.

Imperfect knowledge of phaco machine parameters may lead to wound burn because of excessive heating due to a prolonged use of high ultrasound (US) power. The choice of a low flow rate (12–16 ml/min) phaco technique, together with phaco in extremely dense nuclei requiring up to 100% US power, may all lead to inadequate cooling of the phaco probe. With new-generation phaco machines, US power should be set at 50–60% and increased only if necessary.

Sleeve aging may also cause wound burn: resterilization weakens sleeves, with consequent loss in elasticity and the ability to maintain a constant inflow. Disposable sleeves must be used once only.

Damage to the endothelial cells following phaco with clear corneal incision has been reported.[18] Our personal experience indicates that after topical anesthesia, lateral clear corneal incision and phaco, the density of the central corneal endothelial cells is reduced but the two most sensitive parameters of endothelial damage (coefficient of variation and percentage of hexagonal cells) are not significantly influenced.[19] Therefore, even if the necessary caution is always recommended, especially in eyes with a low preoperative endothelial cell count, phaco through clear corneal incision can be considered to be safe with respect to the endothelium.

WOUND STRETCH

A clear corneal incision may be stretched during phacoemulsification or the insertion of an IOL. Phaco will always cause the incision to stretch and widen.[16] The amount of stretching that a tissue can withstand before lacerating varies according to the consistency, strength and elasticity of the tissue. Differences between patients can be expected. A stretched incision means the potential loss of the valve seal mechanism. Safe surgery requires a safe strategy, i.e. a precise incision made with a precalibrated knife. Standardizing wounds means standardizing the stretching imparted by surgery. An incision of the correct size will result in minimal tissue damage after the IOL has been inserted.[20] An incision of up to 4.0 mm, varying with the IOL, is a safe option: it is large enough for the IOL to be inserted without causing stretching or jeopardizing the valve seal mechanism.

Using a shooter in a small (3.2–3.5-mm) wound may not only stretch the wound but also cause corneal stromal molding of the two lips of the incision, since it adapts to the shooter's circular section. The corneal tissue will maintain this curvature for some time and result in a partial loss of the valve seal mechanism.[1] Detecting a leakage during the reconstruction of the anterior chamber at the end of surgery is essential in deciding whether a suture is required. The risk of endophthalmitis, suggested as being more frequent in clear corneal incision, has proved to be comparable to that observed with scleral incision.[21]

INDUCED ASTIGMATISM

It has been demonstrated that clear-corneal cataract surgery does not bring about significant changes in central cornea astigmatism when compared to other types of incisions.[2–4] After cataract surgery, the cornea is nearly always flattened along the incision meridian.[6,11] Reducing the width of the incision, creating a watertight wound and eliminating sutures has led to a considerable reduction of induced astigmatism, leaving the surgeon with the problem of managing preoperative astigmatism by means other than the incision. Much energy and effort has been expended in this area, mostly through changing the meridian of incision. In practice, moving the incision also means surgery in uncomfortable positions and reduced surgical wound construction standardization.

The astigmatism management strategy we recommend is that of standardizing wounds. This means knowing the average astigmatism induced by the personal standard incision. To develop predictability in the creation of wounds, the surgeon must standardize wounds in the most straightforward way. Once the mean induced astigmatism is reasonably predictable, managing preoperative astigmatism can be left to specific keratotomy at the end of surgery, according to well-developed protocols.[1]

CONCLUSIONS

Effectively standardizing the procedure shortens the learning curve and offers better results to less experienced surgeons. The recommended size of a clear corneal temporal incision is 3.2 mm, enlarged to 4 mm for IOL insertion, as may be necessary with certain lens implants.

SMALL EYES

Short tunnels are more likely in small eyes, so the incision must begin closer to the limbus. In this case, a clear corneal incision will have a greater influence on the final astigmatism, on account of the smaller corneal curvature rays. Greater care is required when penetrating the chamber in order to prevent damage to the anterior capsule, because the anterior chamber is less deep.

LONG EYES

In comparison, long or larger eyes mainly offer surgical advantages. The anterior chamber is wider, the clear corneal incision arc has a lesser influence and the distance between the inner lip of the incision and the visual axis is greater.

REFERENCES

1 Fine HI, Fichman RA, Grabow HB. *Clear-corneal Cataract Surgery and Topical Anesthesia* (Thorofare, NJ: Slack Inc., 1993).

2 Müller-Jensen K, Barlinn B. Long-term astigmatic changes after clear corneal cataract surgery. *J Cataract Refract Surg* 1997; **23:** 354–7.

3 Poort-van Nouhijs HM, Hendrickx KHM, van Marle F, Boesten I, Beekhuis WH. Corneal astigmatism after clear corneal and corneoscleral incisions for cataract surgery. *J Cataract Refract Surg* 1997; **23:** 758–60.

4 Joo CK, Han HK, Kim JH. Computer-assisted videokeratography to measure changes in astigmatism induced by sutureless cataract surgery. *J Cataract Refract Surg* 1997; **23:** 555–61.

5 Ernest PH, Lavery KT, Kiessling LA. Relative strength of scleral corneal and clear-corneal incisions constructed in cadaver eyes. *J Cataract Refract Surg* 1994; **20:** 626–9.

6 Samuelson SW, Koch DD, Kuglen CC. Determination of maximal incision length for true small-incision surgery. *Ophthalmic Surg* 1991; **22:** 204–7.

7 Hayashi K, Hayashi H, Nakao F, Hayashi F. The correlation between incision size and corneal shape changes in sutureless cataract surgery. *Ophthalmology* 1995; **102:** 550–6.

8 Mackool RJ, Russell RS. Strength of clear-corneal incisions in cadaver eyes. *J Cataract Refract Surg* 1996; **22:** 721–5.

9 Ernest PH, Neuhann T. Posterior limbal incision. *J Cataract Refract Surg* 1996; **22:** 78–84.

10 Langermann (ASCRS 1994). Architectural design of a self-sealing corneal tunnel, single-hinge incision. *J Cataract Refract Surg* 1994; **20:** 84–8.

11 Ernest PH, Fenzl R, Lavery KT, Sensoli A. Relative stability of clear-corneal incisions in a cadaver eye model. *J Cataract Refract Surg* 1995; **21:** 39–42.

12 Kent DG, Paul TR, Patterson JE, Apple DJ. Intraocular lens perimeter determines its minimum incision size. *Arch Ophthalmol* 1998; in press.

13 Yamada H. Nervous and sense systems. In: Yamada H, Evans FG, eds. *Strength of Biological Materials* (Baltimore: MA: Williams and Wilkins Company, 1970) 238–43.

14 Bryant MR, Szerenyi K, Schmotzer H, McDonnell PJ. Corneal tensile strength in fully healed radial keratotomy wounds. *Invest Ophthalmol Vis Sci* 1994; **35:** 3022–31.

15 Wilson ED. Larger wound preferred over stretching tissue. *Ocul Surg News Int Edn* 1995; **6**(3): 49.

16 Steinert RF, Deacon J. Enlargement of incision width during phacoemulsification and folded intraocular lens implant surgery. *Ophthalmology* 1996; **103:** 220–5.

17 Radner W, Amon M, Malliger R. Diamond-tip versus blunt-tip caliper enlargement of clear corneal incisions. *J Cataract Refract Surg* 1997; **23:** 272–6.

18 Oshima Y, Tsujikawa K, Oh A, Harino S. Comparative study of intraocular lens implantation through 3.0 mm temporal clear corneal and superior scleral tunnel self-sealing incisions. *J Cataract Refract Surg* 1997; **23:** 347–53.

19 Piovella M, Camesasca FI, Gratton I. Morphometric analysis of endothelial cells after phacoemulsification with topical anesthesia and lateral clear-corneal incision. *Ophthalmology* 1996; **103**(suppl): 140.

20 Kohnen T, Lambert RJ, Koch DD. Incision sizes for foldable intraocular lenses. *Ophthalmology* 1997; **104:** 1277–86.

21 Weindler J, Spang S, Jung WK, Ruprecht KW. Bacterial anterior chamber contamination with foldable silicone lens implantation using a forceps and an injector. *J Cataract Refract Surg* 1996; **22**(suppl 2): 1263–6.

Chapter 19 **Intraocular lens power calculations in difficult cases**

Jack T Holladay

INTRODUCTION

The indications for intraocular lens implantation following cataract or clear lensectomy have significantly increased. These expanded indications result in more complicated cases such as patients with a scleral buckle, silicone in the vitreous, previous refractive surgery, piggy-back intraocular lenses in nanophthalmos, positive and negative secondary piggy-back intraocular lenses and speciality lenses, such as multifocal and toric intraocular lenses. Techniques for determining the proper intraocular lens and power are presented.

Several measurements of the eye are helpful in determining the appropriate intraocular lens power to achieve a desired refraction. These measurements include central corneal refractive power (K-readings), axial length (biometry), horizontal corneal diameter (horizontal white to white), anterior chamber depth, lens thickness, preoperative refraction and age of the patient. The accuracy of predicting the necessary power of an intraocular lens is directly related to the accuracy of these measurements.[1,2]

THEORETICAL FORMULAS

Fyodrov first estimated the optical power of an intraocular lens using vergence formulas in 1967.[3] Between 1972 and 1975, when accurate ultrasonic A-scan units became commercially available, several investigators derived and published the theoretical vergence formula.[4–9] All of these formulas were identical[10] except for the form in which they were written and the choice of various constants such as retinal thickness, optical plane of the cornea, and optical plane of the intraocular lens. These slightly different constants accounted for less than 0.50 D in

the predicted refraction. The variation in these constants was a result of differences in lens styles, A-scan units, keratometers, and surgical techniques among the investigators.

Although several investigators have presented the theoretical formula in different forms, there are no significant differences except for slight variations in the choice of retinal thickness and corneal index of refraction. There are six variables in the formula: (1) corneal power (K); (2) axial length (AL); (3) intraocular lens power (IOL); (4) effective lens position (ELP); (5) desired refraction (DPostRx); and (6) vertex distance (V). Normally, intraocular lens power is chosen as the dependent variable and solved for using the other five variables, where distances are given in millimeters and refractive powers given in diopters:

$$IOL = \frac{1336}{AL - ELP} - \frac{1336}{\dfrac{1336}{\dfrac{1000}{\dfrac{1000}{DPostRx} - V} + K} - ELP}$$

The only variable that cannot be chosen or measured preoperatively is the effective lens position. The improvements in intraocular lens power calculations over the past 30 years are a result of improving the predictability of ELP. Fig. 19.1 illustrates the physical locations of the variables. The optical values for corneal power (K_{opt}) and axial length (AL_{opt}) must be used in the calculations to be consistent with current ELP values and manufacturers' lens constants.

The term 'effective lens position' was recommended by the FDA in 1995 to describe the position of the lens in the eye, since the term anterior chamber depth (ACD) is not anatomically accurate for lenses in the posterior chamber and can lead to confusion for the clinician.[11] The ELP for intraocular lenses before 1980 was a constant of 4 mm for every lens in every patient (first-generation theoretical

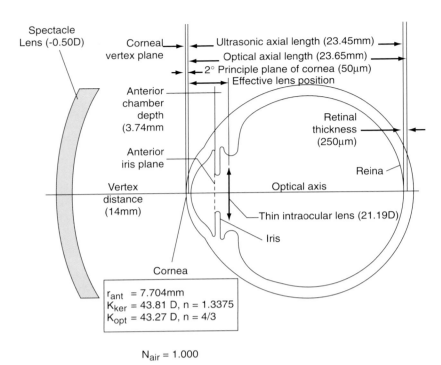

Figure 19.1. *Standardized pseudophakic schematic eye (thin intraocular lens). The values shown are the mean values for a pseudophakic eye: keratometric power of the cornea (K_{ker}), net optical power of the cornea (K_{opt}), and anterior radius of the cornea (r_{ant}). The optical axial length is 200 μm longer than the ultrasonically measured axial length, and the desired postoperative refraction is −0.50 D. With use of these values, the required thin intraocular lens power is 21.19 D at an effective lens position of 5.25 mm.*

formula). This value actually worked well in most patients because the majority of lenses were implanted by iris clip fixation, in which the principal plane averages approximately 4 mm posterior to the corneal vertex. In 1981, Binkhorst improved the prediction of ELP by using a single-variable predictor, the axial length, as a scaling factor for ELP (second-generation theoretical formula).[12] If the patient's axial length was 10% greater than normal (23.45 mm), he would increase the ELP by 10%. The average value of ELP was increased to 4.5 mm because the preferred location of an implant was in the ciliary sulcus, approximately 0.5 mm deeper than the iris plane. Also, most lenses were planoconvex, similar to the shape of the iris-supported lenses. The average ELP in 1996 has increased to 5.25 mm. This increased distance has occurred primarily for two reasons: the majority of implanted intraocular lenses are biconvex, moving the principal plane of the lens even deeper into the eye; and the desired location for the lens is in the capsular bag, which is 0.25 mm deeper than the ciliary sulcus.

In 1988, we proved[13] that using a two-variable predictor, axial length and keratometry, could significantly improve the prediction of ELP, particularly in unusual eyes (third-generation theoretical formula). The original Holladay 1 formula was based on the

geometric relationships of the anterior segment. Although several investigators have modified the original two-variable Holladay 1 prediction formula, no comprehensive studies have shown any significant improvement resulting from using only these two variables.

In 1995, Olsen published a four-variable predictor that used axial length, keratometry, preoperative anterior chamber depth and lens thickness.[14] His results did show improvement over the current two-variable prediction formulas. The explanation is very simple. The more information we have about the anterior segment, the better we can predict ELP. This explanation is a well-known theorem in prediction theory, where the more variables that can be measured describing an event, the more precisely one can predict the outcome.

In a recent study,[15] we discovered that the anterior segment and posterior segment of the human eye are often not proportional in size, causing significant error in the prediction of ELP in extremely short eyes (<20 mm). We found that even in eyes shorter than 20 mm, the anterior segment was completely normal in the majority of cases. Because the axial lengths were so short, the two-variable prediction formulas severely underestimated ELP, explaining part of the large hyperopic prediction errors with current two-variable

Table 19.1

Clinical conditions demonstrating the independence of the anterior segment and axial length.

Anterior segment size	Axial length		
	Short	Normal	Long
Small	Small eye Nanophthalmos	Microcornea	Microcornea + Axial myopia
Normal	Axial hyperopia	Normal	Axial myopia
Large	Megalocornea + Axial hyperopia	Megalocornea	Large eye Buphthalmos + Axial myopia

prediction formulas. After recognizing this problem, we began to take additional measurements on extremely short and extremely long eyes to determine if the prediction of ELP could be improved by knowing more about the anterior segment. Table 19.1 shows the clinical conditions that illustrate the independence of the anterior segment and the axial length.

For 3 years, we gathered data from 35 investigators around the world. Several additional measurements of the eye were taken, but only seven preoperative variables (axial length, corneal power, horizontal corneal diameter, anterior chamber depth, lens thickness, preoperative lens thickness, preoperative refraction and age) have been found to be useful for significantly improving the prediction of ELP in eyes ranging from 15 to 35 mm.

The improved prediction of ELP is not totally due to the formula, but is also a function of the technical skills of the surgeons who are consistently implanting the lenses in the capsular bag. A 20 D intraocular lens that is 0.5 mm axially displaced from the predicted ELP will result in approximately a 1.0 D error in the stabilized postoperative refraction. However, when piggy-back lenses totaling 60 D are used, the same axial displacement of 0.5 mm will cause a 3 D refractive surprise; the error is directly proportional to the implanted lens power. This direct relationship with the lens power is why the problem is much less evident in extremely long eyes, since the implanted intraocular lens is either low plus or minus to achieve emmetropia following cataract extraction.

The Holladay 2 formula and the interim results of the 35 investigators were presented at the June

ASCRS meeting in Seattle in 1996. Once these additional measurements become routine among clinicians, a new flurry of prediction formulas using seven or more variables will emerge, similar to the activity following our two-variable prediction formula in 1988.[13] The standard of care will reach a new level of prediction accuracy for extremely unusual eyes, just as it has for normal eyes. Calculations on patients with axial lengths between 22 and 25 mm and with corneal powers between 42 and 46 D will benefit from current third-generation formulas (Holladay 1,[13] SRK/T[16] and Hoffer Q[17]). In cases outside this range, the Holladay 2 should be used to ensure accuracy.

NORMAL CORNEA WITH NO PREVIOUS KERATOREFRACTIVE SURGERY

CLEAR LENSECTOMY FOR HIGH MYOPIA AND HYPEROPIA

The intraocular power calculations for clear lensectomy are no different than the calculations when a cataract is present. The patients are usually much younger, however, and the loss of accommodation should be discussed thoroughly. The actual desired postoperative refraction should also be discussed, since a small degree of myopia (−0.50 D) may be desirable to someone with no accommodation, to reduce their dependence on spectacles.

This procedure is usually reserved for patients who are outside the range for other forms of refractive surgery. Consequently, the measurements of axial length, keratometry, etc., are usually quite different from those in typical cataract patients, because of their degree of refractive error. In most of the cases with high myopia, the axial lengths are extremely long (>26 mm). In cases of high hyperopia, the axial lengths are very short (<21 mm).

In patients with myopia exceeding 20 D, removing the clear lens often results in postoperative refractions near emmetropia with no implant. The exact result depends on the power of the cornea and the axial length. The recommended lens powers usually range from −10 D to +10 D in the majority of these cases. The correct axial length measurement is very difficult to obtain in these cases because of the abnormal anatomy of the posterior pole. Staphylomas are often present in these eyes, and the macula is often not at the location in the posterior pole where the A-scan measures the axial length. In these cases it is recommended that a B-scan be performed to locate the macula (fovea) and recheck the measurement determined by A-scan. I have personally seen 3–4 D surprises resulting from the fact that the macula was on the edge of the staphyloma, and the A-scan measured to the deepest part of the staphyloma. Such an error results in a hyperopic surprise because the distance to the macula is much shorter than the distance to the center of the staphyloma. The third-generation theoretical formulas yield excellent results if the axial length measurement is accurate and stable.

In patients with hyperopia exceeding +8 D, the axial lengths are often less than 21 mm and require lens powers that exceed the normal range (>34 D). In these cases, piggy-back lenses are necessary to achieve emmetropia.[15] The only formula available at this time in these eyes is the Holladay 2. If the required lens power is less than or equal to 34 D, then the piggy-back lenses are not required and third-generation theoretical formulas may be used.

PIGGY-BACK INTRAOCULAR LENSES TO ACHIEVE POWERS ABOVE 34 D

Patients with axial lengths less than 21 mm should be calculated using the Holladay 2 formula. In these cases, the size of the anterior segment has been shown to be unrelated to the axial length.[15] In many of these cases the anterior segment size is normal and only the posterior segment is abnormally short. In a few cases, however, the anterior segment is small and proportional to the short axial length (nanophthalmos). The

differences in the size of the anterior segment in these cases can cause an average of 5 D hyperopic error with third-generation formulas because they predict the depth of the anterior chamber to be very shallow. Use of the newer formula can reduce the prediction error in these eyes to less than 1 D.

Accurate measurements of axial length and corneal power are especially important in these cases because any error is magnified by the extreme dioptric powers of the intraocular lenses. Placement of both lenses in the bag with the haptics aligned is essential. Inadvertent placement of one lens in the bag and the other in the sulcus can cause a 4 D refractive surprise.

PATIENTS WITH PREVIOUS KERATOREFRACTIVE SURGERY (RK, PRK, AND LASIK)

BACKGROUND

The number of patients who have had keratorefractive surgery (radial keratotomy (RK), photorefractive keratectomy (PRK), or laser-assisted in situ keratomileusis (LASIK)) has been steadily increasing over the past 20 years. With the advent of the excimer laser, these numbers are predicted to increase dramatically. Accurate determination of their corneal power is difficult and is usually the determining factor in the accuracy of the predicted refraction following cataract surgery. Providing this group of patients with the same accuracy with intraocular lens power calculations as we have provided our standard cataract patients presents an especially difficult challenge for the clinician.

PREOPERATIVE EVALUATION

Corneal evaluation

At present, far more patients have had RK than PRK and LASIK combined. Also, our long-term follow-up of RK patients is much greater. The long-term studies of RK patients reveal that some have hyperopic shifts in their refraction and develop progressive against-the-rule astigmatism.[18] The long-term refractive changes in PRK and LASIK are unknown, except for the regression effect following attempted PRK corrections exceeding 8 D. Whichever procedure the patient has had, the stability or instability of the refraction must be determined. This determination includes daily fluctuations from morning to night as well as long-term changes over the past few years. Each of these factors must be used in determining the desired postoperative target refraction and to prepare the patient for the visual changes and realistic expectations following the procedure.

In all of these cases, biomicroscopy, retinoscopy, corneal topography and endothelial cell counts are recommended. These first three tests are primarily directed at evaluating the amount of irregular astigmatism. This determination is extremely important preoperatively because the irregular astigmatism may be contributing to the reduced vision as well as the cataract. The irregular astigmatism may also be the limiting factor in the patient's vision following cataract surgery. The endothelial cell count is necessary to recognize any patients with low cell counts from the previous surgery who may be at higher risk for corneal decompensation or prolonged visual recovery.

The potential acuity meter (PAM), super pinhole and hard contact lens trial are often helpful as secondary tests in determining the respective contribution to reduced vision by the cataract and the corneal irregular astigmatism. The patient should also be informed that only the glare from the cataract will be eliminated; any glare from the keratorefractive procedure will essentially remain unchanged.

Methods of determining corneal power

Accurate determination of the central corneal refractive power is the most important and difficult part of the entire intraocular lens power calculation process. The explanation is quite simple. Our current instruments for measuring corneal power make too many incorrect assumptions with corneas that have irregular astigmatism. The cornea can no longer be compared to a sphere centrally, the posterior radius of the cornea is no longer 1.2 mm steeper than the anterior corneal radius, etc. Because of these limitations, the calculated method and the trial hard contact lens method are most accurate, followed by corneal topography, automated keratometry and finally manual keratometry.

Calculation method

For the calculation method, three parameters must be known: the K-readings and refraction before the keratorefractive procedure and the stabilized refraction after the keratorefractive procedure. It is important that the stabilized postoperative refraction be measured before any myopic shifts from nuclear sclerotic cataracts occur. It is also possible for posterior subcapsular cataracts to cause an apparent myopic shift, similar to capsular opacification, where the patient wants more minus in the refraction to make the letters appear smaller and darker. The concept which we described in 1989 subtracts the change in refraction due to the keratorefractive procedure at the corneal plane from the original K-readings before the procedure to arrive at a calculated postoperative K-reading.[19] This method is usually the most accurate because the preoperative K-values and refraction are usually accurate to ±0.25 D. An example calculation to illustrate the calculation method is given.

Example:
Mean preoperative K =
   42.50 @ 90° and 41.50 @ 180° = 42.00 D
Preoperative refraction =
   −10.00 + 1.00 × 90°, vertex = 14 mm
Postoperative refraction =
   −0.25 + 1.00 × 90°, vertex = 14 mm

Step 1. Calculate the spheroequivalent refraction for refractions at the corneal plane (SEQ_c) from the spheroequivalent refractions at the spectacle plane (SEQ_s) at a given vertex, where:

a) SEQ = sphere + 0.5 (cylinder)

b) $SEQ_c = \dfrac{1000}{\dfrac{1000}{SEQ_s} - \text{vertex (mm)}}$

Calculation for preoperative spheroequivalent refraction at corneal plane:

a) $SEQ_R = -10.00 + 0.5 \times (1.00) = -9.50\,D$

b) $SEQ_c = \dfrac{1000}{\dfrac{1000}{-9.50} - 14} = -8.38\,D$

Calculation for postoperative spheroequivalent refraction at corneal plane:

a) $SEQ_R = -0.25 + 0.5 \times (1.00) = +0.25\,D$

b) $SEQ_c = \dfrac{1000}{\dfrac{1000}{+0.25} - 14} = +0.25\,D$

Step 2. Calculate the change in refraction at the corneal plane:

Change in refraction =
preoperative SEQ_c – postoperative SEQ_c
Change in refraction =
–8.38 – (+0.0.25) + –8.68 D

Step 3. Determine calculated postoperative corneal refractive power:

Mean postoperative K = mean preoperative
K – change in refraction at corneal plane
Mean postoperative K = 42.00 – 8.68 = 33.32 D

This value is the calculated central power of the cornea following the keratorefractive procedure. For intraocular lens programs requiring two K-readings, this value would be entered twice.

Trial hard contact lens method

The trial hard contact lens method requires a plano hard contact lens with a known base curve and a patient whose cataract does not prevent them from being refracted to approximately ±0.50 D. This tolerance usually requires a visual acuity of better than 20/80. The patient's spheroequivalent refraction is determined by normal refraction. The refraction is then repeated with the hard contact lens in place. If the spheroequivalent refraction does not change with the contact lens, then the patient's cornea must have the same power as the base curve of the plano contact lens. If the patient has a myopic shift in the refraction with the contact lens, then the base curve of the contact lens is stronger than the cornea by the amount of the shift. If there is a hyperopic shift in the refraction with the contact lens, then the base curve of the contact lens is weaker than the cornea by the amount of the shift.

Example:
The patient has a current spheroequivalent refraction of +0.25 D. When a plano hard contact lens with a base curve of 35.00 D is placed on the cornea, the spherical refraction changes to –2.00 D. Since the patient had a myopic shift with the contact lens, the cornea must be weaker than the base curve of the contact by 2.25 D. Therefore, the cornea must be 32.75 D (35.00 – 2.25), which is slightly different from the value obtained by the calculation method. In equation form, we have:

Spheroequivalent refraction *without* hard contact
lens = +0.25 D

Base curve of plano hard contact lens = 35.00 D
Spheroequivalent refraction *with* hard contact
lens = –2.00 D
Change in refraction = –2.00 – (+0.25) =
–2.25 D (myopic shift)
Mean corneal power = base curve of plano
hard contact lens + change in refraction
Mean corneal power = 35.00 + –2.25 D
Mean corneal power = 32.75 D

Note: this method is limited by the accuracy of the refractions, which may be limited by the cataract.

Corneal topography

Current corneal topography instruments measure more than 5000 points over the entire cornea and more than 1000 points within the central 3 mm. This additional information provides greater accuracy, compared to keratometers, in determining the power of corneas with irregular astigmatism. The computer in topography instruments allows the measurement to account for the Stiles–Crawford effect, actual pupil size, etc. These algorithms allow a very accurate determination of the anterior surface of the cornea.[20] They provide no information, however, on the posterior surface of the cornea. In order to accurately determine the total power of the cornea, the power of both surfaces must be known.

In normal corneas that have not undergone keratorefractive surgery, the posterior radius of curvature of the cornea averages 1.2 mm less than the anterior surface. In a person with an anterior corneal radius of 7.5 mm using the Standardized Keratometric Index of Refraction of 1.3375, the corneal power would be 45.00 D. Several studies have shown that this power overestimates the total power of the cornea by approximately 0.56 D. Hence, most intraocular lens power calculations today used a net index of refraction of 1.3333 (4/3) and the anterior radius of the cornea to calculate the net power of the cornea. With use of this lower value, the total power of a cornea with an anterior radius of 7.5 mm would be 44.44 D. This index of refraction has provided excellent results in normal corneas for intraocular lens power calculations.

Following keratorefractive surgery, the assumptions that the central cornea can be approximated by a sphere (no significant irregular astigmatism or asphericity) and that the posterior corneal radius of curvature is 1.2 mm less than the anterior radius are no longer true. Corneal topography instruments can account for the changes in the anterior surface, but are unable to account for any differences in the relationship with the posterior radius of curvature. In RK, the mechanism of having a peripheral bulge and central flattening apparently causes similar changes in both the anterior and posterior radii of curvature, so that use of the net index of refraction for the cornea (4/3) usually gives fairly accurate results, particularly for optical zones larger than 4–5 mm. In RKs with optical zones of 3 mm or less, the accuracy of the predicted corneal power diminishes. Whether this inaccuracy is due to the additional central irregularity with small optical zones or the difference in the relationship between the front and back radii of the cornea is unknown at this time. Studies measuring the posterior radius of the cornea in these patients will be necessary to answer this question.

In PRK and LASIK, the inaccuracies of these instruments in measuring the net corneal power are almost entirely due to the change in the relationship between the radii of the front and back of the cornea, since the irregular astigmatism in the central 3-mm zone is usually minimal. In these two procedures, the anterior surface of the cornea is flattened, with little or no effect on the posterior radius. Use of a net index of refraction (4/3) will lead to overestimation of the power of the cornea by 14% of the change induced by the PRK or LASIK; that is, if a patient had a 7 D change in the refraction at the corneal plane from a PRK or LASIK with spherical preoperative *K*-values of 44 D, the actual power of the cornea is 37 D and the topography instruments will give 38 D. If a 14 D change in the refraction has occurred at the corneal plane, the topography instruments will overestimate the power of the cornea by 2 D.

In summary, the corneal topography instruments do not provide accurate central corneal power following PRK, LASIK and RKs with optical zones of 3 mm or less. In RKs with larger optical zones, the topography instruments become more reliable. The calculation method and hard contact lens trial are always more reliable.

Automated keratometry

Automated keratometers are usually more accurate than manual keratometers in corneas with small optical zone (≤3 mm) RKs, because they sample a smaller central area of the cornea (nominally 2.6 mm). In addition, the automated instruments often have additional eccentric fixation targets that provide more information about the paracentral cornea. When a measurement error on an RK cornea is made, the instrument almost always gives a central corneal power that is greater than the true refractive power of the cornea. This error occurs because the

samples at 2.6 mm are very close to the paracentral knee of the RK. The smaller the optical zone and the greater the number of the RK incisions, the greater the probability and magnitude of the error. Most of the automated instruments have reliability factors that are given for each measurement, helping the clinician to decide on the reliability in the measurement.

Automated keratometry measurements following LASIK or PRK yield accurate measurements of the front radius of the cornea because the transition areas are far outside the 2.6-mm zone that is measured. The measurements are still not accurate, however, because the assumed net index of refraction (4/3) is no longer appropriate for the new relationship between the front and back radii of the cornea after PRK or LASIK, just as with the topographic instruments. The change in central corneal power, as measured by the keratometer, resulting from PRK or LASIK must be increased by 14% to determine the actual refractive change at the plane of the cornea. Hence, the automated keratometer will overestimate the power of the cornea proportionally to the amount of PRK or LASIK performed.

Manual keratometry

Manual keratometers are the least accurate in measuring central corneal power following keratorefractive procedures, because the area that they measure is usually larger than that measured by automated keratometers, at 3.2 mm in diameter. Therefore, measurements in this area are extremely unreliable for RK corneas with optical zones ≤4 mm. The one advantage with the manual keratometer is that the examiner is actually able to see the reflected mires and the amount of irregularity present. Seeing the mires does not help get a better measurement, but does allow the observer to discount the measurement as unreliable.

The manual keratometer has the same problem with PRK and LASIK as topographers and automated keratometers, and is therefore no more accurate. The manual keratometer will overestimate the change in the central refractive power of the cornea by 14% following PRK and LASIK.

Choosing the desired postoperative refraction target

Determination of the desired postoperative refractive target is no different than in other patients with cataracts, in whom the refractive status and the presence of a cataract in the other eye are the major determining factors. A complete discussion of the avoidance of refractive problems with cataract surgery is beyond the scope of this chapter, and is given in Holladay and Rubin.[21] A short discussion of the major factors follows.

If the patient has binocular cataracts, the decision is much easier because the refractive status of both eyes can be changed. The most important decision is whether the patient prefers to be myopic and read without glasses, or near emmetropic and drive without glasses. In some cases the surgeon and patient may choose the intermediate distance (–1.00 D) as the best compromise. Targeting for monovision is certainly acceptable, provided the patient has successfully utilized monovision in the past. Trying to produce monovision in a patient who has never experienced this condition may cause intolerable anisometropia and require further surgery.

Monocular cataracts allow fewer choices for the desired postoperative refraction, because the refractive status of the other eye is fixed. The general rule is that the operative eye must be within 2 D of the non-operative eye in order to avoid intolerable anisometropia. In most cases this means matching the other eye or targeting for up to 2 D nearer emmetropia; that is, if the non-operative eye is –5.00 D, then the target would be –3.00 D for the operative eye. If the patient is successfully wearing a contact lens in the non-operative eye or has already demonstrated his ability to accept monovision, then an exception can be made to the general rule. It should always be stressed, however, that, should the patient be unable to continue wearing a contact lens, the necessary glasses for binocular correction may be intolerable, and additional refractive surgery may be required.

Special limitations of intraocular lens power calculation formulas

As discussed previously, the third-generation formulas (Holladay 1, Hoffer Q and the SRK/T) and the new Holladay 2 are much more accurate than previous formulas in unusual eyes. Older formulas such as the SRK1, SRK2 and Binkhorst 1 should not be used in these cases. None of these formulas will give the desired result if the central corneal power is measured incorrectly. The resulting errors are almost always in the hyperopic direction following keratorefractive surgery, because the measured corneal powers are usually greater than the true refractive power of the cornea.

To further complicate matters, the newer formulas often use keratometry as one of the predictors to estimate the effective lens position of the intraocular lens. In patients who have had keratorefractive surgery, the corneal power is usually much flatter than normal and certainly flatter than before the keratorefractive procedure. In short, a patient with a 38 D cornea without keratorefractive surgery would not be expected to be similar to a patient with a 38 D cornea with keratorefractive surgery. Newer intraocular lens power calculation programs are now being developed to handle these situations and will improve predictability in these cases.

INTRAOPERATIVE EVALUATION

Intraoperative visualization and corneal protection

Intraoperative visualization is usually more difficult in patients with previous RK than in the normal cataract patient and is somewhat similar to that in severe arcus senilis or other conditions that cause peripheral corneal haze. The surgeon should be prepared for this additional difficulty by making sure that the patient is lined up so that the cataract can be visualized through the optical zone. This usually means lining up the microscope perpendicular to the center of the cornea, so that the surgeon is looking directly through the optical zone at the center of the cataract. When the peripheral cortex is removed, the eye can be rotated so that visualization of the periphery is through the central optical zone. It is also prudent to coat the endothelium with viscoelastic to minimize any endothelial cell loss, since the keratorefractive procedure may have caused some prior loss.

Intraoperative autorefractor/retinoscopy

Large refractive surprises can be avoided by intraoperative retinoscopy or hand-held autorefractors. These refractions should not be relied upon, however, for fine-tuning the intraocular lens power, since there are many factors at surgery that may change in the postoperative period. Factors such as the pressure from the lid speculum, axial position of the intraocular lens, and intraocular pressure may cause the intraoperative refraction to be different than the final stabilized postoperative refraction. If the intraoperative refraction is within 2 D of the target refraction, no lens exchanges should be considered unless intraoperative keratometry can also be performed.

POSTOPERATIVE EVALUATION

Refraction on the first postoperative day

On the first postoperative day following cataract surgery, patients who previously have had RK usually have a hyperopic shift, similar to that on the first postoperative day following their RK. This phenomenon is primarily due to the transient corneal edema that usually exaggerates the RK effect. These patients also exhibit the same daily fluctuations during the early postoperative period after their cataract surgery as they did after the RK. Usually, this daily shift is in a myopic direction during the day, due to the regression of corneal edema after awakening in the morning.[22] Because the refractive changes are expected and vary significantly among patients, no lens exchange should be contemplated until after the first postoperative week or until after the refraction has stabilized, whichever is longer.

Very few results of cataract surgery following PRK and LASIK are available. In the few cases that have been reported, the hyperopic shift on the first day and daily fluctuations appear to be much less, similar to those in the early postoperative period following these procedures. In most cases the stability of the cornea makes these cases no different than patients who have not had keratorefractive surgery.

Long-term results

The long-term results of cataract surgery following RK are very good. The long-term hyperopic shifts and development of against-the-rule astigmatism over time following cataract surgery should be the same as in the long-term studies following RK. The problems with glare and starburst patterns are usually minimal because the patients have had to adjust to these unwanted optical images following the initial RK. If the patient's primary complaint before cataract surgery is glare and starbursts, it should be made clear to the patient that only the glare due to the cataract will be removed by surgery, and the symptoms that are due to the RK will remain unchanged.

Long-term results following PRK and LASIK are non-existent. Since there are no signs of hyperopic drifts or development of against-the-rule astigmatism

in the 5-year studies following PRK, one would not expect to see these changes. However, the early studies following RK did not suggest any of these long-term changes either. Only time will tell whether central haze, irregular astigmatism, etc. will be problems that develop in the future.

PATIENTS WITH PREVIOUS SCLERAL BUCKLING AND/OR SILICONE IN THE VITREOUS CAVITY

Patients who have undergone scleral buckling usually have an increase in their axial length by an average of 0.8 mm, which usually results in an approximate 2.4 D myopic shift. This value may range from 0 mm to 2.0 mm, depending on the location and tension on the encircling band. If no silicone oil has been placed in the vitreous cavity, then measurement of the axial length is no different than in patients with high myopia. Choice of the target postoperative refraction is also no different than in the normal patient, although many of these patients prefer myopia, since in many cases this has been the refraction for most of their life.

If the patient does have a longer axial length in the eye with the scleral buckle, matching the refraction to the other eye will require a weaker-power intraocular lens. Although the patient may experience aniseikonia (image size disparity, larger in the eye with the buckle), they will usually adjust to this difference within 2–3 weeks. If the lens power is chosen to eliminate image size disparity, by using a stronger lens to make the patient more myopic so that the spectacle has more minus, the image sizes are nearly the same (iseikonia). The problem is that the anisometropia (unequal refractive errors) induces a prism difference that causes diplopia when reading. The patient cannot adjust to the diplopia and either the spectacles must be slabbed-off, a contact lens must be worn, a secondary piggy-back intraocular lens must be implanted or a lens exchange must be performed.

If silicone has been placed in the vitreous cavity, the case becomes much more complex. An accurate axial length cannot be measured with silicone in the vitreous cavity. The oil is so dense that the ultrasound echoes rarely come from the retina because they are so attenuated. The measured axial length is far too short, even when the measurement is adjusted for the ultrasound speed in silicone oil. It is recommended that the axial length from the other eye be used in these cases, and 0.8 mm added to this length of the cataractous eye if a scleral buckle has been performed. If both eyes have silicone in the vitreous cavity and preoperative axial lengths were not measured, then one simply uses a standard lens power, adjusting up or down depending on the patient's most recent refraction before any surgery. Many retina surgeons are now measuring the axial length before using silicone oil, to avoid this dilemma.

If the axial length is known in the eye with silicone, then the intraocular lens power can be determined in the normal manner except for adjusting for the index of refraction difference between silicone and vitreous. It is recommended that planoconvex intraocular lenses be used in these cases to minimize the effect of the silicone reducing the effective power of the back surface of the intraocular lens. When planoconvex lenses are used, the average additional power required with silicone in the vitreous cavity is approximately 3–5 D. If a lens with power on the posterior surface is used, then the required power is much greater and ranges from 5 to 10 D, depending on the power of the back surface.

An additional benefit of the planoconvex lens is that it minimizes the change in refraction if the silicone oil is removed. It is best to leave the patient near plano if it is possible that the silicone intraocular lens will be removed, since the shift when the oil is removed will always be in a myopic direction. The formulas for calculating the exact lens power, with an accurate axial length and silicone in the vitreous cavity, are too complex for this discussion, but several computer programs now have the appropriate formulas to perform this calculation exactly. Unfortunately, in many of these cases the best-corrected vision is poor, so that exact calculations result in very little additional benefit to the patient.

INTRAOCULAR LENS POWER CALCULATIONS USING K-VALUES AND PREOPERATIVE REFRACTION

FORMULA AND RATIONALE FOR USING PREOPERATIVE REFRACTION VERSUS AXIAL LENGTH

In a standard cataract removal with intraocular lens implantation, the preoperative refraction is not very helpful in calculating the power of the implant, because the crystalline lens will be removed, so that dioptric power is being removed and then replaced. In cases where no power is being removed from the eye, such as secondary implants in aphakia, a piggy-back intraocular lens in pseudophakia or a minus intraocular lens in the anterior chamber of a phakic patient, the necessary intraocular lens power for a desired postoperative refraction can be calculated from the corneal power and preoperative refraction—the axial length is not necessary. The formula for calculating the necessary intraocular lens power is given below.[23]

$$IOL = \frac{1336}{\dfrac{1336}{\dfrac{1000}{\dfrac{1000}{PreRx} - V} + K} - ELP} - \frac{1336}{\dfrac{1336}{\dfrac{1000}{\dfrac{1000}{DPostRx} - V} + K} - ELP}$$

where ELP is expected lens position in mm (distance from corneal vertex to principal plane of intraocular lens, IOL is intraocular lens power in diopters, K is net corneal power in diopters, PreRx is preoperative refraction in diopters, DPostRX is the desired postoperative refraction in diopters, and V is the vertex distance in mm of refractions.

EXAMPLE CASES SHOWING CALCULATION OF THE INTRAOCULAR LENS POWER FROM PREOPERATIVE REFRACTION

As mentioned above, the appropriate cases for using the preoperative refraction and corneal power include: (1) secondary implant in aphakia, (2) secondary piggy-back intraocular lens in pseudophakia, and (3) a minus anterior chamber intraocular lens in a high myopic phakic patient. In each of these cases, no dioptric power is being removed from the eye, so the problem is simply to find the intraocular lens at a given distance behind the cornea effective lens position that is equivalent to the spectacle lens at a given vertex distance in front of the cornea. If emmetropia is not desired, then an additional term, the desired postoperative refraction, must be included. The formulas for calculating the predicted refraction and the back-calculation of the effective lens position are given in the reference and will not be repeated here.[23]

Example: secondary implant for aphakia

The patient is 72 years old and is aphakic in the right eye and pseudophakic in the left eye. The right eye can no longer tolerate an aphakic contact lens. The capsule in the right eye is intact and a posterior chamber intraocular lens is desired. The patient is −0.50 D in the left eye and would like to be the same in the right eye.

Mean keratometric K = 45.00 D
Aphakic refraction = +12.00 sphere @ vertex of 14 mm
Manufacturer's ACD lens constant = 5.25 mm
Desired postoperative refraction = −0.50 D

Each of the values above can be substituted in the refraction formula above, except for the manufacturer's ACD and the measured K-reading. The labeled values on intraocular lens boxes are primarily for lenses implanted in the bag. Since this lens is intended for the sulcus, 0.25 mm should be subtracted from 5.25 mm to arrive at the equivalent constant for the sulcus. The ELP is therefore 5.00 mm. The K-reading must be converted from the measured keratometric K-reading (n = 1.3375) to the net K-reading (n = 4/3), for the reasons described previously under corneal topography. The conversion is performed by multiplying the measured K-reading by the following fraction:

$$\text{Fraction} = \frac{(4/3) - 1}{1.3375 - 1} = \frac{1/3}{0.3375} = 0.98765$$

Mean refractive K = mean keratometric K × Fraction
Mean refractive K = (45.00 × 0.98765) = 44.44 D

With use of the mean refractive K, aphakic refraction, vertex distance, ELP for the sulcus and the desired postoperative refraction, the patient needs a 22.90 D intraocular lens. A 23 D intraocular lens would yield a predicted refraction of −0.57 D.[23]

Example: secondary piggy-back intraocular lens for pseudophakia

In patients with a significant residual refractive error following the primary intraocular lens implant, it is often easier surgically and more predictable optically to leave the primary implant in place and calculate the secondary piggy-back intraocular lens power necessary to achieve the desired refraction. This method does not require knowledge of the power of the primary implant or the axial length. This method is particularly important in cases where the primary implant is thought to be mislabeled. The formula works for plus or minus lenses, but negative lenses are just becoming available at this time.

The patient is 55 years old; he had a refractive surprise after the primary cataract surgery and was left with a +5.00 D spherical refraction in the right eye. There is no cataract in the left eye and he is plano. The surgeon and the patient both desire him to be −0.50 D, which was the target for the primary implant. The refractive surprise is felt to result from a mislabeled intraocular lens that is centered in the bag and would be very difficult to remove. The secondary piggy-back intraocular lens will be placed in the sulcus. This is very important, since placement of the second lens in the bag several weeks after the primary surgery is very difficult. More importantly, it may displace the primary lens posteriorly, reducing its effective power and leaving the patient with a hyperopic error. Placement of the lens in the sulcus minimizes this posterior displacement:

Mean keratometric K = 45.00 D
Pseudophakic refraction = +5.00 sphere @ vertex of 14 mm
Manufacturer's ACD lens constant = 5.25 mm
Desired postoperative refraction = −0.50 D

With use of the same-style lens and constant as in the previous example, and modification of the K-reading to net power, the formula yields a +8.64 D intraocular lens for a −0.50 D target. The nearest available lens is +9.0 D, and would result in −0.76 D. In these cases, extreme care should be taken to ensure that the two lenses are well centered with respect to one another. Decentration of either lens can result in poor image quality and can be the limiting factor in the patient's vision.

Example: primary minus anterior chamber intraocular lens in a high myopic phakic patient

The calculation of a minus intraocular lens in the anterior chamber is no different than the aphakic calculation of an anterior chamber lens, except that the power of the lens is negative. In the past these lenses have been reserved for high myopia that could not be corrected by RK or PRK. Since most of these lenses fixate in the anterior chamber angle, concerns of iritis and glaucoma have been raised. Nevertheless, several successful cases have been reported with good refractive results. Because successful LASIK procedures have been performed in myopia up to −20.00 D, these lenses may be reserved for myopia exceeding this power in the future. Interestingly, the power of the negative anterior chamber implant is very close to the spectacle refraction for normal vertex distances:

Mean keratometric K = 45.00 D
Phakic refraction = −20.00 sphere @ vertex of
   14 mm
Manufacturer's ACD lens constant = 3.50 mm
Desired postoperative refraction = −0.50 D

Use of an ELP of 3.50 and modification of the K-reading to net corneal power yields −18.49 D for a desired refraction of −0.50 D. If a −19.00 D lens is used, the patient would have a predicted postoperative refraction of −0.10 D.

REFERENCES

1 Holladay JT, Prager TC, Ruiz RS, Lewis JW. Improving the predictability of intraocular lens calculations. *Arch Ophthalmol* 1986; **104:** 539–41.
2 Holladay JT, Prager TC, Chandler TY, Musgrove KH, Lewis JW, Ruiz RS. A three-part system for refining intraocular lens power calculations. *J Cataract Refract Surg* 1988; **13:** 17–24.
3 Fedorov SN, Kolinko AI, Kolinko AI. Estimation of optical power of the intraocular lens. *Vestnk Oftalmol* 1967; **80:** 27–31.
4 Fyodorov SN, Galin MA, Linksz A. A calculation of the optical power of intraocular lenses. *Invest Ophthalmol* 1975; **14:** 625–8.
5 Binkhorst CD. Power of the prepupillary pseudophakos. *Br J Ophthalmol* 1972; **56:** 332–7.
6 Colenbrander MC. Calculation of the power of an iris clip lens for distant vision. *Br J Ophthalmol* 1973; **57:** 735–40.
7 Binkhorst RD. The optical design of intraocular lens implants. *Ophthalmic Surg* 1975; **6:** 17–31.
8 van der Heijde GL. The optical correction of unilateral aphakia. *Trans Am Acad Ophthalmol Otolaryngol* 1976; **81:** 80–8.
9 Thijssen JM. The emmetropic and the iseikonic implant lens: computer calculation of the refractive power and its accuracy. *Ophthalmologica* 1975; **171:** 467–86.
10 Fritz KJ. Intraocular lens power formulas. *Am J Ophthalmol* 1981; **19:** 414–15.
11 Holladay JT. Standardizing constants for ultrasonic biometry, keratometry and intraocular lens power calculations. *J Cataract Refract Surg* 1997; **23:** 1356–70.
12 Binkhorst RD. *Intraocular Lens Power Calculation Manual. A Guide to the Author's TI 58/59 IOL Power Module,* 2nd edn (New York: Richard D. Binkhorst, 1981).
13 Holladay JT, Prager TC, Chandler TY, Musgrove KH, Lewis JW, Ruiz RS. A three-part system for refining intraocular lens power calculations. *J Cataract Refract Surg* 1988; **14:** 17–24.
14 Olsen T, Corydon L, Gimbel H. Intraocular lens power calculation with an improved anterior chamber depth prediction algorithm. *J Cataract Refract Surg* 1995; **21:** 313–19.
15 Holladay JT, Gills JP, Leidlein J, Cherchio M. Achieving emmetropia in extremely short eyes with two piggy-back posterior chamber intraocular lenses. *Ophthalmology* 1996; **103:** 1118–23.
16 Retzlaff JA, Sanders DR, Kraff MC. Development of the SRK/T intraocular lens implant power calculation formula. *J Cataract Refract Surg* 1990; **16:** 333–40.
17 Hoffer KJ. The Hoffer Q formula: a comparison of theoretic and regression formulas. *J Cataract Refract Surg* 1993; **19:** 700–12.
18 Holladay JT, Lynn M, Waring GO, Gemmill M, Keehn GC, Fielding B. The relationship of visual acuity, refractive error and pupil size after radial keratotomy. *Arch Ophthalmol* 1991; **109:** 70–6.
19 Holladay JT, IOL calculations following RK. *Refract Corneal Surg J* 1989; **5**(3): 203.
20 Lowe RF, Clark BA. Posterior corneal curvature. *Br J Ophthalmol* 1973; **57:** 464–470.
21 Holladay JT, Rubin ML. Avoiding refractive problems in cataract surgery. *Surv Ophthalmol* 1988; **32**(5): 357–60.
22 Holladay JT. Management of hyperopic shift after RK. *Refract Corneal Surg J* 1992; **8:** 325.
23 Holladay JT. Refractive power calculations for intraocular lenses in the phakic eye. *Am J Ophthalmol* 1993; **116:** 63–6.

Chapter 20 Emmetropization at cataract surgery

Thomas Kohnen and Markus J Koch

A predictable postoperative refraction following cataract extraction is one major goal of modern cataract surgery. Therefore precise calculation of intraocular lens (IOL) power and predictable surgically induced changes to the eye is mandatory. Prior to cataract surgery, most of our patients have a refractive error, either resulting from myopization caused by cataract development or as a primary myopic, hyperopic or astigmatic refractive error. Surgical intervention provides a possibility to influence the postoperative refraction at the time of cataract extraction.

Myopia and hyperopia can be corrected with an IOL of the appropriate power, and astigmatism can be controlled with cataract incision or additional surgical interventions, astigmatic keratotomy,[1] or with the use of toric IOLs.[2]

In the early days of IOL implantation, a lens with a standardized power was chosen, and this resulted in a high rate of postoperative ametropia. Today, an almost perfect refractive outcome can be achieved by implantation of an IOL with appropriate power. The improvement in surgical techniques has stabilized the accuracy of the procedure, especially small-incision surgery with foldable IOL implantation, as it induces minimal shape changes in the human eye. New IOL materials provide us with the opportunity to obtain planned refractive results after cataract removal.

FUNDAMENTAL THOUGHTS

An important question before cataract surgery in each patient should be 'What is the optimal postoperative refraction for the eye of this patient?'

In 1981, Christophe Huber, a Swiss ophthalmologist, proposed that slight myopic astigmatism would be an advantage for the postoperative refractive outcome. The shape, rather than the size, of the blurred retinal image changes as Sturm's conoid moves over the retina. Consequently, myopic astigmatism would be the optimal refraction after IOL implantation. The induced corneal ametropia is a spherocylinder with a very low equivalent power, and increases the depth of focus.[3]

Various authors follow different concepts of postoperative refractive outcome planning. The most common approach to postoperative refraction for patients with monofocal IOLs is a slightly simple myopic astigmatism. This would provide a good depth of focus postoperatively, and a slightly myopic refractive outcome of approximately −0.25 to −0.5 per 180° with a spherical equivalent of −0.5 D has a potential 'safety gap' towards emmetropia. Avoidance of undercorrection or postoperative hyperopia is desired because the latter is much less tolerated by most patients than a low myopic postoperative refraction. Some patients require a specific postoperative refraction (e.g. myopic patients who desire postoperative unaided prefer reading ability and would like to wear spectacles for far and medium distance as they have done for their whole life).

IOL CALCULATION

At the outset of IOL implantation, a standardized IOL power of 19.5 D was chosen; in some cases the power changed by an estimate to enhance postoperative refractive outcome. However, in approximately 20% of cases, a postoperative refractive error of ±2 D occurred. In 1967, almost 20 years after the first IOL implantation by Ridley,[4] the first formula to calculate IOLs was proposed by Fyodorov. The delay in obtaining accurate IOL calculation formulas during the early years of IOL history was caused by the inability to measure the axial length of the eye. This became possible in the 1970s with the introduction of ultrasound echography. Mathematical formulas to

Table 20.1

Formulas to calculate IOL power to determine the postoperative IOL power.

First generation
Fyodorov
Colenbrander
Hoffer
van der Heijde
Thijssen
Binkhorst
SRK

Second generation
Hoffer
Binkhorst II
Holladay I
SRK-II

Third generation
Hoffer Q
Haigis
Holladay (II, R)
SRK/T
Naeser
Norrby

calculate IOL power are derived either from theoretical models of the eye's optic or from regression statistics applied to the postoperative refractive outcome of cataract surgery. First-generation (Table 20.1) theoretical formulas, such as the Fyodorov,[5] Collenbrander,[6] Hoffer,[7] van der Heijde[8] or Binkhorst,[9] besides axial lengths and keratometer readings, required a constant value for the anterior chamber depth (ACD) IOL position. In the first-generation regression formulas (SRK), the ACD was replaced by an A-constant specific for each IOL style. At that time it was recommended that each surgeon should develop his own personalized A-constant for each IOL style.

Second-generation formulas (Table 30.1) appeared in the early 1980s, when Hoffer and Binkhorst independently replaced the constant ACD in their respective formulas with one that varied based on the axial length (AL). Hoffer[10] used an ACD prediction formula for posterior chamber lenses based on a study which showed that the measured postoperative ACD was directly proportional to the AL of the eye (ACD = 0.292AL −2.93). The Binkhorst II formula altered the constant ACD as a function of the AL (ACD = AL/23.45 × ACD).[11] The SRK regression formula was changed to SRK-II with a modification to the A-constant; it was increased in 1.0 D steps when the AL was less than 22 mm (+1), 21 mm (+2), or 20 mm (+3), and decreased by 0.5 D if longer than 24.5 mm.[12]

Third-generation formulas (Table 20.1), which are now used, vary the ACD based on the patient's AL and corneal curvature and have included additional measurements to increase the accuracy of IOL calculation.

The accuracy of IOL calculation depends on four factors:

1) accuracy of the biometric data (AL and corneal power)
2) accuracy of IOL power quality control
3) accuracy of the IOL position in the eye
4) accuracy of the IOL power formulas used to obtain desired lens power.

Third-generation formula calculations (Table 20.1) have increased precision and safety in reaching postoperative emmetropia.[13–15] Not only refinements of formulas used to calculate the appropriate power of an IOL for each specific patient,[16] but also improvements in the design and standardization of measurements (corneal power and ultrasound biometer) and surgical refinements in cataract surgery and IOL implantation, have increased the accuracy of IOL calculation.

STANDARDIZATION OF MEASUREMENTS (ULTRASOUND BIOMETER, CORNEAL CURVATURE)

The two most important values for IOL calculation are AL and average corneal power; accordingly, measurement errors for these two values will cause the greatest deviations from the desired refraction. A double check of these two values for each patient before IOL implantation is recommended.

The AL of the eye is generally measured using A-scan ultrasound (Fig. 20.1). The average velocity of ultrasound varies between a normal eye, an eye of unusual AL (deviation from 23.45 mm) and a cataractous eye. Therefore, either a corrected AL factor should be used to determine the average velocity, or ultrasonic biometers which use gates should be used to increase the accuracy of AL measurements. Recently, new ultrasound machines have been developed to decrease the standard deviation of the measurements to 0.1 mm. Also,

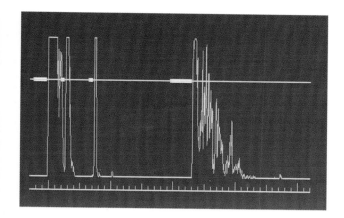

Figure 20.1. *Ultrasound echography (A-scan) of an eye to determine axial length (AL), phakic anterior chamber depth and phakic lens thickness.*

techniques to determine the AL have been refined by B-scan measurements.[17] New methods, e.g. laser interferometry, might replace ultrasonography in the future, because accuracy can be greater.

The average corneal power is usually determined by keratometry. Unfortunately, the diameter of the optical zone measured varies from 2.4 to 3.2 mm among different manufacturers, and not all manufacturers use the standardized keratometric index of refraction (1.3375). More information on the corneal power, topography and curvature is obtained by computerized videokeratography (CVK). As an additional improvement for IOL calculation, recently computerized videokeratography-derived curvature values were shown to be either slightly less accurate[18] or more accurate[19,20] as compared to standard keratometry values in predicting IOL power. Nevertheless, CVK provides important data in eyes with abnormal or surgically altered corneal surfaces.[18] The exact evaluation of corneal shape and height will most likely provide more accuracy and better results of corneal curvature and power for IOL calculations and will become an additional measurement to increase the predictability of IOL calculation.

SURGICAL REFINEMENTS IN IOL IMPLANTATION

With the development of continuous curvilinear capsulorhexis, safe and secure IOL implantation into the capsular bag has become the standard for cataract surgery. The capsular bag is the most anatomic position for an IOL and is a very predictable place for good and constant refractive results.

VARIOUS IOL MATERIALS

IOLs can be grouped into rigid and foldable lenses. If the main chemical components are analyzed, IOL materials can be divided into two groups: acrylate/methacrylate polymers and silicone elastomers (Fig. 20.2).

The first group contains rigid polymethylmethacrylate (PMMA) IOLs and the so-called 'soft acrylic and hydrogel' IOLs. Foldable acrylate/methacrylate polymers have been developed by altering the side-groups of the standard methacrylate polymer backbone.[21] Because of the various components, they differ in refractive indices, water content, folding and unfolding behavior and surface properties (Fig. 20.2). The second group of IOLs are made of foldable polysiloxanes. The silicone–oxygen backbone confers mechanical flexibility, and the appendant organic groups, e.g. methyl and phenyl, determine properties such as refractive index, mechanical strength and clarity. Obviously, the advantages of small incisions for cataract surgery—low induced astigmatism, fewer postoperative complications, possibly less inflammation and quicker rehabilitation of the patient—have encouraged surgeons to increasingly use foldable IOLs.[22]

VARIOUS IOL DESIGNS

The refractive power of an IOL varies with its form and point of implantation. The optics of IOLs within the normal range of implantation (10–30 D) are designed as biconvex or planoconvex models. Today's standard for PMMA IOLs is a single-piece lens design, whereas foldable IOLs are either three-piece (J-loop, C-loop) or plate haptic designs. The angulation of the haptics towards the lens induces a different localization of the lens cardinal point in the bag or the sulcus. These two main technical points of design, in addition to the IOL material (Table 20.2), which also changes the thickness of the lens, induce varying anterior chamber depths postoperatively and should be considered for each type of lens to allow the calculation of the correct IOL for implantation.

Special situations, such as scleral fixated IOLs, anterior chamber lenses or phakic implants (such as

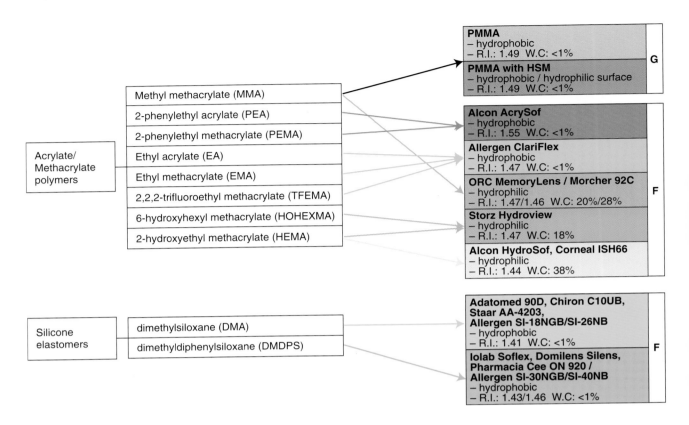

Figure 20.2. *The major components of rigid and foldable IOL optics. Some currently available IOLs are shown. The hydrophilicity of the IOL depends on the water contact angle in air; the lower this value, the more hydrophilic the IOL surface. PMMA, polymethylmethacrylate; HSM, heparin surface modification; R, rigid; F, foldable; RI, refractive index; WC, Water content. (Reproduced from Kohnen[22] with permission.)*

the Baikoff angle fixated or the Worst–Fechner iris claw anterior chamber IOLs, and posterior chamber IOLs (deformable intraocular refractive corrective lens or intraocular contact lens (ICL)) require separate calculation modalities, which can be obtained in advanced IOL calculation programs.[16]

REFINEMENTS OF IOL CALCULATING FORMULAS

IOL power calculations have tremendously improved in accuracy over the past two decades, and at present the standard of care is that at least 50.0% of patients are within ±0.5 D of predicted refraction, 90.0% within ±1.00 D, and 99.9% within ±2.00 D.[23,24] In a recent publication, the average standard deviation of the predicted refraction in a larger series of patients was

Table 20.2

Refractive index of IOL optic materials.

Lens	Refractive index
Human lens	1.39
AMO silicone (SI18/26)	1.41
Starr/Chiron silicone	1.41
Pharmacia/Iovision silicone	1.43
Alcon IOGEL	1.43
AMO silicone (SI30/40)	1.46
Allergan/Ioptex AcryLens (AR40)	1.47
Storz Hydroview	1.47
PMMA	1.49
Alcon AcrySof	1.55

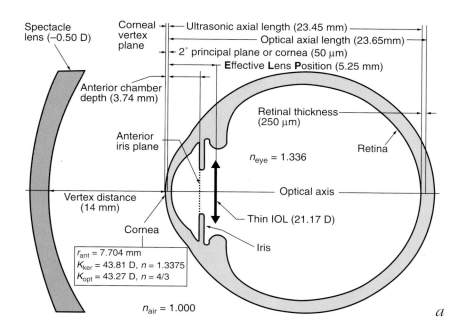

Figure 20.3. *(a) Standardized pseudophakic schematic eye (thin IOL). (b) Standardized pseudophakic schematic eye (thick IOL). Reproduced from Holladay,[16] with permission.*

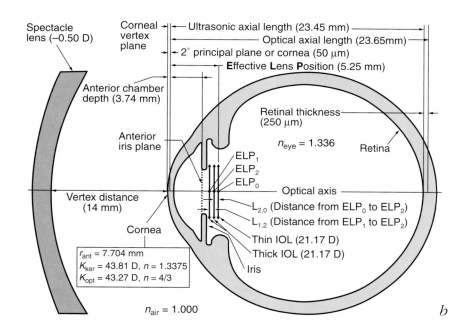

0.8–0.9 D, which meant that at least 80% of patients obtained a postoperative refraction which varied by less than 1 D from the calculated refraction.[25]

Third-generation formulas use additional measurements and different mathematical models to calculate refraction; these include variable anterior pseudophakic chamber depth, preoperative estimation of the lens haptic plane, ray tracing and vergence calculation.[16,26,27] Several additional factors are used for back-calculating the lens power and estimating the postoperative refraction (Fig. 20.3). In general, the measurements which have been identified as determining the postoperative IOL power the most are AL, corneal power, horizontal corneal diameter, phakic

Table 20.3
The most important measurements in determining the postoperative IOL power in the concept of Holladay.[16]

Axial length
Corneal power
Horizontal corneal diameter
Phakic anterior chamber depth
Phakic lens thickness
Preoperative refraction
Age

anterior chamber depth, phakic lens thickness, preoperative refraction and age[16] (Table 20.3).

IOL CALCULATION IN SPECIAL SITUATIONS

PEDIATRIC CATARACT

IOL calculation in cases of pediatric cataract is performed with new, third-generation formulas as in high hyperopia, because infant eyes are usually short. However, the refractive outcome in patients younger than 6 years will change over time because the eye is growing. Two main methods of choosing an IOL for pediatric patients exist:

• Make the eye emmetropic at the time of surgery and thereby treat amblyopia immediately, followed later by an IOL exchange because of increasing myopia.
• Undercorrection of the eye at the time of surgery (treated with glasses or contact lenses) which might result in emmetropization when the eye is further grown.

HIGH HYPEROPIA AND MYOPIA

For very short ALs, third-generation formulas seem to be better than older ones, but still not sufficient, especially because of the disproportional anterior segment in these eyes.[14]

Results of cataract surgery in highly myopic eyes with axial lengths of 31.0 mm or greater with implantation of low- or negative-power IOLs have been reported for a group of 32 eyes without any operative or postoperative complication except opacification of the posterior capsule. The use of the SRK II formula

with an individual surgeon's factor showed good predictability of the refractive target.[28] However, better formulas without the use of a personalized correction factor have yet to be developed.

PIGGY-BACK LENSES

Calculating and achieving emmetropia after cataract surgery is difficult in extremely short eyes (AL less than 20 mm). Measurement errors show greater effects in these cases and can sometimes be induced by the predetermined calibration for 23.5-mm eyes and velocities in most ultrasound axiometers which lead to wrong time coding for the different velocities of anterior chamber, lens, and vitreous body. IOLs of more than 34 diopters are not commonly available and have to be customized. In the USA these IOLs have only recently been approved by the US Food and Drug Administration. Implantation of multiple IOLs with parallel haptics has become an alternative in these situations, but the lens calculation, even with third-generation formulas, is not yet exact. Formulas which also distinguish between different types of short eyes show better but not sufficient performance.[14] Hyperopic surprises, therefore, are a common problem, especially because of the unpredictable position of the lenses and their induced different ACDs.[15] Additional measurements of the anterior segments—such as corneal white to white measurements—can help to distinguish the different types of eyes and lead to a better prediction of postoperatrive lens position. This will probably result in smaller prediction errors.

Refractive surprises still occur in these patients and lens exchanges may be necessary. Whether an additional third lens would be a better alternative has not yet been explored. A new experimental type of piggy back lens with an exchangeable self-centering second optic could make this task of lens exchange easier.[29] It consists of a primary IOL with 10° angulated haptics which is implanted in the capsule bag and a secondary IOL with 15° posterior haptic angulation which is implanted directly beneath the iris in the ciliary sulcus. This second IOL is then rotated 90° towards the first IOL's haptics and fixated between the haptics and optic of the primary IOL. A system of two IOLs has the advantage of higher refractive powers and exchangeability in cases of refractive surprise or change in refraction, as in children.

OTHERS

Other aspects, such as silicone oil after vitreoretinal surgery, have added a new facet not only in biometry but also for the calculation of the postoperative refractive outcome. The oil leads to a postoperative hyperopic shift of about 4 diopters. This should be considered when calculating IOLs if a long-term tamponade with silicone oil is planned; in cases of later removal of the oil, the lens should be chosen according to the formulas only.[30] IOL calculations for eyes in other special situations, such as refractive surgery, are covered in Chapter 19.

MULTIFOCAL INTRAOCULAR LENS

Loss of accommodation is a major disadvantage of any kind of lens extraction. The use of multifocal IOLs (MIOLs) allows an enlarged depth of focus and a reduction in the need for glasses postoperatively, especially if the fellow eye is emmetropic or will be operated on with the same MIOL soon after. The need to wear glasses will decrease after implantation in both eyes, especially by reaching emmetropia and avoiding postoperative refractive errors.[31] Foldable silicone refractive MIOLs, in comparison to monofocal IOLs, demonstrate no difference distance visual acuity, but the uncorrected and distance-corrected near acuities are significantly better. Compared to monofocal IOLs, contrast acuity and contrast sensitivity are found to be lower at low contrast levels and high spatial frequency (20 cpd) because of similar projection of several pictures at various focal points on the retina. However, bilateral multifocal implantation improves functional results.[32] The optic design of the Array-MIOL (Allergan Medical Optics), with an increased weighting for the distance focus and an aspheric surface, produces less scattering light than bifocal IOLs or diffractive MIOLs, in which 18% of the light energy cannot be used by the retina.[33]

The full advantage of increased depth of focus in MIOLs can best be obtained after binocular implantation and perfect lens calculation for emmetropia.

CONTROL AND MANIPULATION OF THE POSTOPERATIVE ASTIGMATISM

The variety of surgical techniques and their effects on postoperative astigmatism have been studied in detail. The preservation of corneal sphericity and the reduction of induced or pre-existing postoperative astigmatism is the aim of surgical planning and techniques. Several options for modulating astigmatism are available,

including incision parameters (size, configuration and construction, location and closure), astigmatic keratotomy, scleral flap recession and resection, toric IOL implantation and postoperative medical treatment.[34]

The influence of different surgical procedures on the astigmatic result increases depending on the location of the procedure and the size of the tissue gape, which induces more astigmatism in corneal than in scleral incisions[35] by flattening the meridian of incision and steepening the meridian 90° away.[36-39] Small CCIs have fewer surgical complications and less induced astigmatism, which leads to better early visual acuity and rehabilitation.[40,41] Temporal incision was found to be more stable in comparison to the 12 o'clock position for limbal and scleral incisions, resulted in higher wound strength and induced less astigmatism.[39] These effects increased postoperatively and were highly significant after 8 months.

To control astigmatism at the time of cataract extraction we have developed a nomogram for our surgery (Table 20.4).[34]

IOL EXCHANGE

With modern IOL implantation into the capsular bag a maximal shift of about ±1 diopter can be expected over the course of the postoperative period. This can be caused by remaining viscoelastic substances that lead to a shift of the cardinal point of the IOL in the postoperative period. Therefore, a change of the IOL should be performed rapidly if there is a substantial refractive error after the operation and if the patient is considerably unhappy. After the error has been found, the IOL can be recalculated. In our experience, most of the calculation errors are due to incorrect AL or corneal power measurements. An additional calculation for a sulcus-implanted lens should be performed before reimplantation in cases of posterior capsular rupture and inability to implant the exchanged IOL into the capsular bag.

SUMMARY

Todays' standard of care of aphakia in the industrialized countries is extracapsular cataract extraction and posterior chamber IOL implantation. Unfortunately, it is not yet possible to calculate the exact refractive power of the crystalline lens to be removed and replaced with an IOL of appropriate power. Therefore, other parameters are measured and formulas are used to predict the desired IOL power as accurately as possible. With different incision location and configuration, postoperative astigmatism can be controlled.

REFERENCES

1 Kershner RM. Clear corneal cataract surgery and the correction of myopia, hyperopia, and astigmatism. *Ophthalmology* 1997; **104**: 381–9.

2 Shimizu K, Misawa A, Suzuki Y. Toric intraocular lenses: correcting astigmatism while controlling axis shift. *J Cataract Refract Surg* 1994; **20**: 523–6.

3 Huber C. Einfacher myopischer Atigmatismus, ein Akkommodationsersatz nach Linsenimplantation. *Klin Monatsbl Augenheilkd* 1981; **178**: 284–8.

4 Ridley H. Intraocular acrylic lenses. *Trans Ophthalmol Soc UK* 1952; **LXXI**: 617–21.

5 Fyodorov SN, Kolinko AI. Estimation of optical power of the intraocular lens. *Vestn Oftalmol* 1967; **80**: 27–31.

6 Collenbrander MC. Calculation of the power of an iris clip lens for distant vision. *Br J Ophthalmol* 1973; **57**: 735–40.

7 Hoffer KJ. Mathematics and computers in intraocular lens calculation. *Am Intraocul Implant Soc J* 1975; **1**: 4–5.

8 van der Heijde GL. A nomogram for calculating the power of the prepupillary lens in aphakic eye. *Bibliotheca Ophthalmol* 1975; **83**: 273–5.

9 Binkhorst CD. The optical design of intraocular lens implants. *Ophthalmic Surg* 1975; **6**: 17–31.

10 Hoffer KJ. The effect of axial length on posterior chamber lens and posterior capsule position. *Curr Concepts Ophthalmic Surg* 1984; **1**: 20–2.

11 Binkhorst RD. Biometric A scan ultrasonography intraocular lens power calculation. In: Emery JE, ed. *Current Concepts in Cataract Surgery* (St Louis: CV Mosby, 1978) 175–82.

12 Sanders DR, Retzlaff J, Kraff MC. Comparison of the SRK II formula and other second generation formulas. *J Cataract Refract Surg* 1988; **14**: 136–41.

13 Hoffer KJ. The Hoffer Q formula: a comparison of theoretic and regression formulas. *J Cataract Refract Surg* 1993; **19**: 700–12.

14 Holladay JT, Gills JP, Leidlein J, Chericho M. Achieving emmetropia in extremely short eyes with two piggyback posterior chamber intraocular lenses. *Ophthalmology* 1996; **103**: 1118–23.

15 Norrby NE, Koranyi G. Prediction of intraocular lens power using the haptic plane concept. *J Cataract Refract Surg* 1997; **23**: 254–9.

16 Holladay JT. Standardizing constants for ultrasonic biometry, keratometry, and intraocular lens power calculations. *J Cataract Refract Surg* 1997; **23**: 1356–70.

17 Berges O, Puech M, Assouline M, Letenneur L, Gastellu-Etchegory M. B-mode guided vector-A-mode biometry versus A-mode biometry to determine axial length and intraocular lens power. *J Cataract Refract Surg* 1998; **24**: 529–535.

18 Husain SE, Kohnen T, Maturi R, Er H, Koch DD. Computerized videokeratography and keratometry in determining intraocular lens calculations. *J Cataract Refract Surg* 1996; **22**: 362–6.

19 Cuaycong M, Gay C, Emery J, Haft E, Koch D. Comparison of the accuracy of computerized videokeratography and keratometry for use in intraocular lens calculations. *J Cataract Refract Surg* 1993; **19**(S): 178–81.

20 Assouline M, Briat B, Kaplan-Messas A, Renrad G, Pouliquen Y. Analyse videokératoscopique informatisée et chirurgie de la cataracte par phacoemulsification. Calcul prédicatif de la puissane de l'implant intraoculaire. *J Fr Ophthalmol* 1997; **20**: 411–17.

21 Christ FR, Buchen SY, Deacon J, et al. Biomaterials used for intraocular lenses. In: Wise DL, Tranto DL, Altobelli DE, Yaszemski MJ, Gresser JD, Schwartz ER, eds. *Encyclopedic Handbook of Biomaterials and Bioengineering*, Vol. 2, Part B. *Applications* (New York: Marcel Dekker, Inc 1995) 1261–313.

22 Kohnen T. The variety of foldable intraocular lens materials. *J Cataract Refract Surg* 1996; **22**: 1255–8.

23 Holladay JT, Prager TC, Ruiz RS et al. improving the predictability of intraocular lens power calculations. *Arch Ophthalmol* 1986; **104**: 539–41.

24 Holladay JT, Musgrove KH, Prager TC, et al. A three-part system for refining intraocular lens power calculations. *J Cataract Refract Surg* 1988; **14**: 17–24.

25 Hoffman PC, Hütz WW, Eckardt HB. Bedeutung der Formelauswahl für die postoperative Refraktion nach Katarakt-Operation. *Klin Monatsbl Augenheilkd* 1997; **211**: 168–77.

26 Naeser K. Intraocular lens power formula based on vergence calculation and lens design. *J Cataract Refract Surg* 1997; **23**: 1200–7.

27 Haigis W. Biometrie. In: Straub W, Kroll P, Küchle HJ, eds. *Augenärztliche Untersuchungsmethoden* (Stuttgart: Enke, 1995) 255–304.

28 Kohnen S, Brauweiler P. First results of cataract surgery and implantation of negative power intraocular lenses in highly myopic eye. *J Cataract Refract Surg* 1996; **22**: 416–20.

29 Mittelviefhaus H. Piggyback intraocular lens with exchangeable optic. *J Cataract Refract Surg* 1996; **22**: 676–81.

30 Grinbaum A, Treister G, Moisseiev J. Predicted and actual refraction after intraocular lens implantation in eyes with silicone oil. *J Cataract Refract Surg* 1996; **22**: 726–9.

31 Pieh S, Weghaupt H, Rainer G, Skorpik C. Sehschärfe und Brillentrageverhalten nach Implantation einer diffraktiven Multifokallinse. *Klin Monatsbl Augenheilkd* 1997; **210**: 38–42.

32 Eisenmann D, Jacobi FK, Dick B, Jacobi K. Die 'Array'-Silikon-Multifokallinse: Erfahrungen nach 150 Implantationen. *Klin Monatsbl Augenheilkd* 1996; **208**: 270–2.

33 Simpson MJ. The diffractive multifocal intraocular lens. *Eur J Implant Refract Surg* 1989; **1**: 115–21.

34 Kohnen T, Koch DD. Methods to control astigmatism in cataract surgery. *Curr Opin Ophthalmol* 1996; **7**: 75–80.

35 Olsen T, Dam-Johansen M, Bek T, Hjortdal JO. Corneal versus scleral tunnel incision in cataract surgery. *J Cataract Refract Surg* 1997; **23**: 337–41.

36 Koch DD, Lindstrom RL. Controlling astigmatism in cataract surgery. *Semin Ophthalmol* 1992; **7**: 224–33.

37 Kohnen T. Corneal shape changes and astigmatic aspects of scleral and corneal tunnel incisions. *J Cataract Refract Surg* 1997; **23**: 301–2.

38 Kohnen T, Mann PM, Husain SE, Abarca A, Koch DD. Corneal topographic changes in induced astigmatism resulting from superior and temporal scleral pocket incisions. *Ophthalmic Surg Lasers* 1996; **27**: 263–9.

39 Anders N, Pham DT, Antoni HJ, Wollensak J. Postoperative astigmatism and relative strength of scleral tunnel incisions: a prospective clinical trial. *J Cataract Refract Surg* 1997; **23**: 332–6.

40 Lyle WA, Jin GJC. Prospective evaluation of early visual and refractive effects with small clear corneal incisions for cataract surgery. *J Cataract Refract Surg* 1996; **22**: 1456–60.

41 Masket S, Tennen DG. Astigmatic stabilization of 3.0 mm temporal clear corneal cataract incisions. *J Cataract Refract Surg* 1996; **22**: 1451–5.

Chapter 21 **New foldable intraocular lenses**

Tobias H Neuhann

The idea of using folding intraocular lenses (IOLs) for aphakia correction was first discussed almost 40 years ago, following implantation of the first polymethylmethacrylate (PMMA) lens.[1] Elastomeric materials that return to their original configurations after folding were needed to overcome some of the problems of rigid lenses.

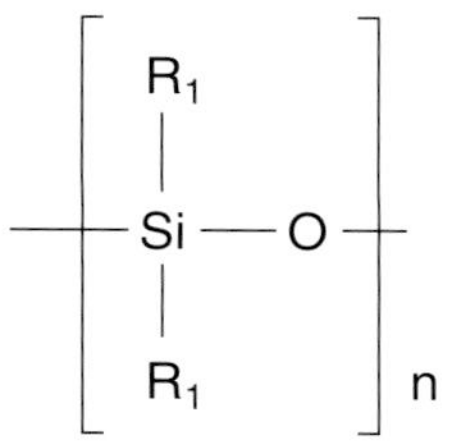

SILICONE IOLS

Even though silicone was not the first foldable material to be used in IOL surgery, positive experiences with solid cross-linked silicone in contact lenses, scleral buckles and glaucoma shunts, as well as implants in other medical fields, formed the basis for its successful application in cataract surgery. Heart valves, breast implants, hydrocephalic shunts and other implants demonstrated excellent human biocompatibility for silicone. Silicones are polymers composed of silicone–oxygen chains containing organic groups such as vinyl, methyl or phenyl groups. These groups are essential for the characteristics of these polysiloxanes, such as mechanical stability, glass transforming temperature, tensile strength, elongation, modulation transfer function, optical transparency and refractive index. The first silicone lens was implanted in 1984 by Mazzocco[2] (Figs. 21.1–21.3).

Today, we look back on 15 years of clinical experience with silicone lenses in ophthalmology. Theoretically, there is a multitude of 'silicone polymers' (Fig. 21.1);[3] however, polydimethylsiloxane (PDMS) (Fig. 21.2) and polydimethyldiphenylsiloxane (Fig. 21.3) as used in IOL technology demonstrate inertia, i.e. they are not only non-toxic but also non-inflammatory, non-mutagenic, non-sensitizing and non-irrigating in the intraocular environment. The components are proven, pure, stable to the degradative agents, and do not leach into the intraocular environment as has been supposed.[4]

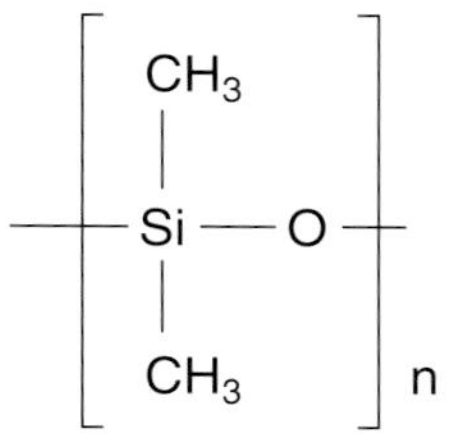

Figure 21.1. *Structural formula of polysiloxane.*

Figure 21.2. *If R_1 groups are methyl groups, the elastomer is called polydimethylsiloxane (PDMS).*

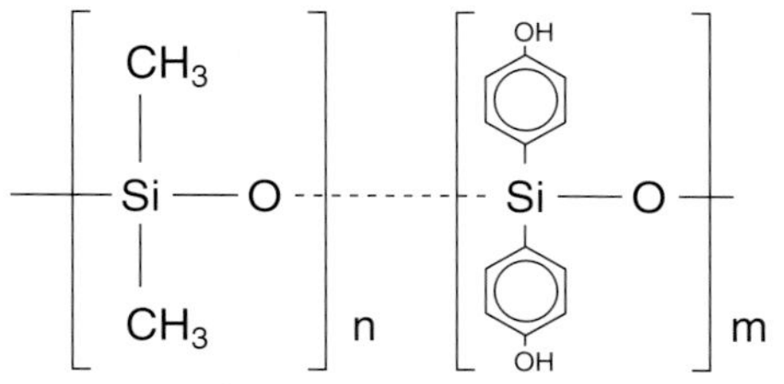

Figure 21.3. *If R_1 groups are n methyl and m phenyl groups, the elastomer is a second-generation silicone with a higher refractive index, polydimethyldiphenylsiloxane (PDMDPS).*

Polymer structure has been further developed, and foldable silicone IOLs can be produced with a large variety of chemical, physical and mechanical properties. These include silicone-plate lenses,[2] and one-piece

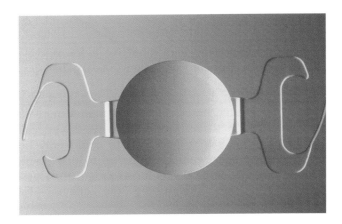

Figure 21.9. *Accommodating lens (courtesy of J.S. Cumming).*

ciliary muscle and the zonular apparatus, with the haptics fixated in the capsular bag. This new silicone IOL is presently undergoing clinical trials in Germany, is manufactured by Medevec and is distributed by Acrimed (Fig. 21.9).

EXPLANTATION OF SILICONE LENSES

With the increased number of foldable lens implants, the number of necessary explantations through a small incision also gains in importance. The advantage of all polysiloxanes used in ophthalmology is that they can be cut inside the eye.

Typical reasons for explantation are incorrect lens power, intolerance of the multifocal design, anisometropia with aniseikonia, IOL damage during the implantation process and intra- and postoperative IOL displacement.

Therefore, knowledge of certain lens characteristics is helpful and important, especially refractive index and central corneal thickness. Lenses of high refractive index or with a constant central thickness can be cut and exchanged more easily than thicker ones. Furthermore, owing to its surface characteristics, silicone does not form bonds with the lens capsule, so that even years after implantation these lenses can be well explanted without traumatizing the zonule or the capsule. However, the hydrophobic surface characteristics of silicone lenses may constitute a disadvantage when silicone oil needs to be instilled into the posterior segment or in cases with capsular shrinkage syndrome requiring IOL exchange.

To retain the advantages of a small incision during explantations of silicone lenses, the IOL must be divided into two 3-mm pieces, since an intraocular refolding of silicone lenses in water is not possible, as they are slippery and resist folding attempts.[22]

NEW BUT NOT FOLDABLE

The bitoric IOL was developed by H.-R. Koch and manufactured by Dr Schmidt Intraokularlinsen in Germany. The disk-shaped PMMA implant consists of two toric lenses of the same power, both with one planar and one toric side, which counter-rotate to produce a variable degree of astigmatic power. The direction of the haptic defines the position of the cylindrical axis, and two additional lines in the optical periphery allow an exact intraocular positioning. The range of this 6-mm toric IOL is outstanding: 12.5 or 13.4 mm in diameter; spherical power between −3.0 D and +30 D combined with cylindrical power from +1.0 D to +12.0 D.

ACRYLIC IOLs

A new group of foldable IOLs are the flexible acrylic lenses. These cross-linked copolymers of methacrylate and acrylate esters were developed especially for IOLs; they are thermoplastic and contain a UV filter. The synthetic strategy with this material is to combine a monomer that will provide a higher refractive index than is possible with silicone, and a monomer with a relatively long hydrocarbon side-chain to provide flexibility. These lenses belong to the same family of acrylic–methacrylic polymers as PMMA.[23]

These lenses have the following characteristics.

THERMOPLASTICITY

While silicone IOLs reach their glass transforming temperature at approximately −100 °C, that of presently available acrylic lenses covers a range from +12 °C to +20 °C. This affects IOL folding as well as unfolding of the implants. The folding process of this type of implant may be somewhat more difficult at low room temperature compared to that of a corresponding silicone IOL, however, the unfolding of an acrylic IOL in the capsular bag is considerably slower and more controlled than is the case with the comparable silicone IOL.[24] As a consequence, surgery may be terminated while the implant has not unfolded completely.

TACKINESS

The surface quality is closely related to the manufacturing process and is also temperature-dependent.[25] The warmer the material, the more sensitive and tacky the surface.

A positive consequence of this tackiness is a mechanical adhesiveness between lens capsule and IOL, which, in turn, leads to reduction of secondary cataract. Clinical experience shows that capsule opacification with acrylic lenses rarely has an impact on vision; Nd:YAG laser capsulotomy is significantly reduced with these lenses.[26]

A disadvantage of this tackiness, however, is that a multitude of small particles may stick to the lens surface and be pressed into the material with the implantation instruments, where they remain forever, since they are not absorbed.[27,28] For these reasons, injector implantation or disposable implantation forceps are gaining increasing importance in the context of these lenses (Fig. 21.10).[29]

REFRACTIVE INDEX

The refractive index (RI) of acrylic lenses ranges from 1.47 to 1.55, compared to 1.41–1.46 for silicone and 1.49 for PMMA. The role of RI is graphically represented in Fig. 21.4.

WATER CONTENT

The characteristic for pure foldable acrylic lenses is a water content below 2%.

SILICONE OIL TOLERANCE

The surface characteristics of acrylic lenses make them appear more suitable for surgical procedures in the posterior segment, since with application of silicone oil the border layer between the IOL and silicone oil does not impair the intraoperative view of the posterior segment surgeon, as compared with silicone lenses; for the latter, this can only be achieved with installation of adhesive viscoelastics.[30]

CHEMICAL STRUCTURE

Fig. 21.11 shows the basic formula of acrylic lens materials. The chemical relationship to the known

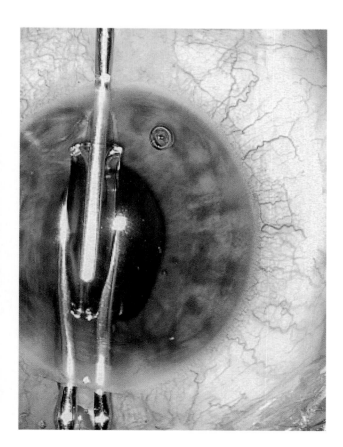

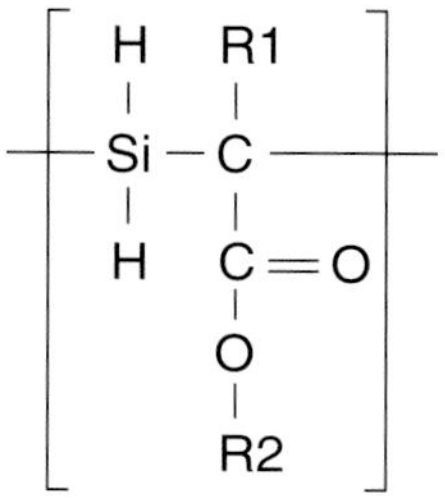

Figure 21.10. *Explantation of an acrylic lens.*

Figure 21.11. *Basic formula of acrylic IOL material.*

and proved polymethylacrylate (PMA) and PMMA is obvious.

With PMA:

$R_1 = (H)n$
$R_2 = (CH_3)n$

With PMMA:

$R_1 = (CH_3)n$
$R_2 = (CH_3)n$

THE LENSES

The AR40 from Allergan—a three-piece IOL—contains:

$R_1 = (CH_3)m,o$ *and* $(H)n$
$R_2 = (CH_2–CH_3)m,n$ *and* $(CH_2–CF_3)o$

This implant was first introduced in 1994, first with a polypropylene haptic and modified C-loop by Loptex as ACR360. After the merger of this company with Allergan, the clinical data were evaluated.[25] The results led to the use of a different haptic material and design as well as to the development of an injector (Figs 21.12 and 21.13).

The lens characteristics are as follows:

Specific gravity (g/ml):	1.17
Refractive index:	1.47
Tensile strength (lb/in²):	843
Elongation (%):	205
Glass transforming temp. (°C):	+12
Optic:	true 6 mm
Haptics:	extruded PMMA

The MA30BM (Fig. 21.14), manufactured by Alcon, is a three-piece IOL. This lens is the 'little brother' of the MA60BM:

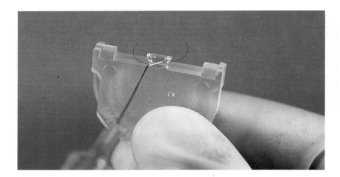

Figure 21.12. *AR40, Allergan, folded.*

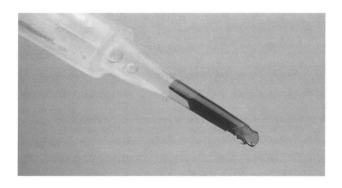

Figure 21.13. *Injector with IOL. The rolled implant is stained blue for reasons of representation. The cartridge is transparent.*

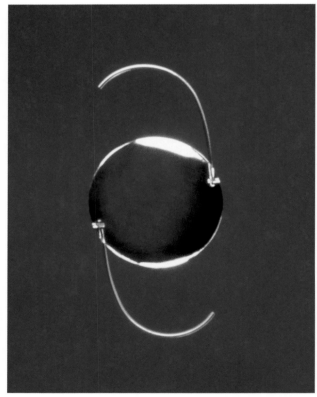

Figure 21.14. *MA30BM, Alcon.*

R_1 = (CH$_3$)m,o or (H)n
R_2 = (CH$_2$–CH$_2$–phenol ring)m,n,o

This phenol ring increases the refractive index and can be compared with the phenol ring in the structural formula of PDMDPS in terms of meaning and purpose.

The material has been implanted since 1991 with excellent results. The recently observed 'glistenings'[31] do not affect patients' visual acuity, or glare and contrast sensitivity, or biocompatibility, and are non-progressive.

The advantages of this material with the highest refractive index available are its high biocompatibility,[32] significant reduction of posterior capsular opacification[33] and lens epithelial cell proliferation, and its excellent modulation transfer function (MTF), combined with the ease of implantation.

A new one-piece lens design started clinical evaluation in 1998.

The lens characteristics are as follows:

Specific gravity (g/ml):	1.12
Refractive index:	1.554
Tensile strength (lb/in²):	344
Elongation (%):	285
Glass transforming temp. (°C):	+18
Optic:	true 5.5 mm
Haptics:	extruded PMMA

Other specifics of acrylic lenses

MTF is an objective measure to describe optical resolution of an IOL. It depends on refractive index, homogeneity and transparence of the lens material as well as on the smoothness of the optic surface.[28] The

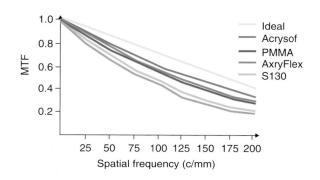

Figure 21.15. *MTF curves of different IOL materials.*

MTF measures the efficiency of light transfer. The data are plotted as modulation versus spatial frequency, which is measured in cycles/mm. For comparison, the MTF or PMMA serve as a reference curve, as it has remained closest to the theoretical ideal lens until today (Fig. 21.15).

EXPLANTATION OF ACRYLIC LENSES

Explantation of acrylic lenses, performed for the same reasons as given for silicone lenses, provides special opportunities: if the difference between the intraocular temperature of approximately 36–37 °C and the glass transforming temperature is sufficiently great, the IOL can be refolded intraocularly. If, in addition, the tensile strength is rather low, which may also be the reason for an explantation in some cases due to tearing of the optic during folding or implantation or because of haptic damage,[11] the 6-mm optic can be cut into two halves, similar to a silicone IOL, and exchanged through the small incision.[34]

LOW-WATER ACRYLIC-HYDROGEL AND POLYHEMA IOLs

The third group of new IOLs, hydrogels, is summarized under the above title.

As hydrogel has demonstrated excellent performance in contact lenses on the one hand and its chemical structure indicates a close relationship to PMMA on the other, it was among the first material to be tried as an alternative to PMMA.[35] Hydrogel is a copolymer of methacrylate esters containing one hydroxyl group in the side-chain.[36]

The implants are based on the same formula as PMMA and acrylic (Fig. 21.11).

With PMMA:

R_1 = (CH$_3$)n
R_2 = (CH$_3$)n

With p-HEMA (polyhydroxyethylmethacrylate):

R_1 = (CH$_3$)n
R_2 = (CH$_2$–CH$_2$–OH)n

The OH group leads to hydrophilicity, which seems to be extremely important for biocompatibility.

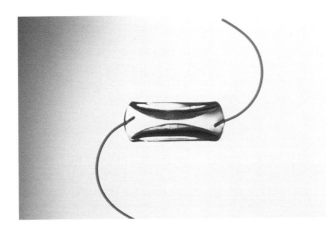

Figure 21.16. *MemoryLens, ORC.*

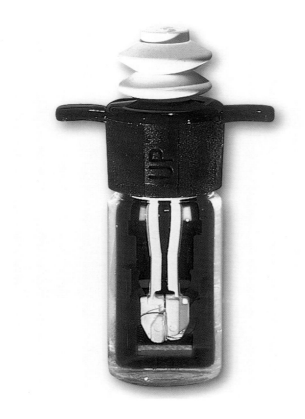

Figure 21.17. *MemoryLens inside the container.*

As early as 1976, Epstein implanted the first hydrogel IOLs in South Africa. Mehta, Blumenthal and Amon followed with further developments and reports.[37-42]

MONOFOCAL LENSES

The introduction of the MemoryLens™ (Figs 21.16 and 21.17), a three-piece IOL from the Optical Radiation Corporation (ORC), in 1989 brought about the beginning of the age of these new low-water acrylic hydrogels. Like mere acrylic lenses, this implant unites the numerous advantages of the rigid PMMA lens and the folding option, thus contributing to a reduced intraoperative traumatization and quicker rehabilitation.[43] The lens material consists of a cross-linked copolymer of methylmethacrylate (MMA), which is the hydrophobic portion, 2-hydroxyethylmethacrylate (HEMA), which is the hydrophilic portion, ethylene glycol dimethacrylate (EGDMA), which is the cross-linker, and a benzophenone group for UV blocking.

The thermoplastic properties of this material are the prerequisites for the specific delivery system of this lens: the prefolded IOL maintains its rolled form owing to a cooling chain. The mean required incision size is 3.8 mm and no special instrumentation is needed for insertion into the eye. The glass transforming temperature is +25 °C; nevertheless, the IOL surface is not resistant against injuries caused by the instruments.[44] The intraocular temperature of approximately 36 °C causes this implant to unfold very slowly and gently. The clinical results are comparable with those of PMMA.[45] An implant with a 5.5-mm optic and PMMA loops will soon be available.

The lens characteristics are as follows:

Water content (%):	20
Specific gravity (g/ml):	1.19
Refractive index:	1.47
Tensile strength (lb/in²):	4897
Elongation (%):	30
Glass transforming temp. (°C):	+25
Optic:	true 6 mm HEMA–MMA–MOBP–EDGMA
Haptics:	polypropylene

The Hydroview™ H60M—a second-generation lens—from Storz is a unique one-piece IOL with UV blocker (Fig. 21.18). The hydrogel contains HEMA, 6-hydroxyethylmethacrylate (HOHEXMA) and 1,6-hexanedioldimethacrylate (HDDA). The lens is therefore hydrophilic. To this optic, blue PMMA haptics are chemically bonded by means of an interpenetrating polymer network formed during the manufacturing process.[46]

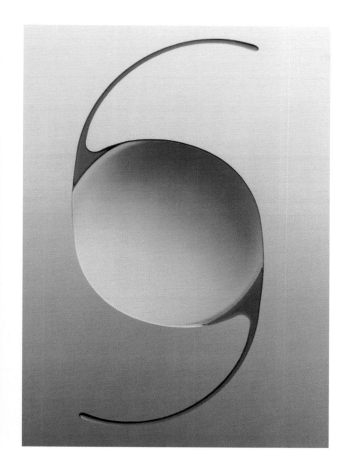

Figure 21.18. *Hydroview (H60M), Storz.*

It is delivered in a newly designed container which combines a folder mechanism and a preimplantation hydration system.

The lens has been under clinical evaluation since 1994. Preliminary 3-year follow-up results from a joint US, Australian and European study show that this lens is safe, centers well and provides only few complications. The complications reported so far include limited posterior capsular opacification and lens epithelial cell growth on the IOL surface, probably induced by the lens' biocompatibility and water content.

The lens characteristics are as follows:

Water content (%):	18.7
Specific gravity (g/ml):	1.12
Refractive index:	1.47
Tensile strength (lb/in²):	300
Elongation (%):	100
Glass transforming temp. (°C):	75 ±5
Optic:	true 6 mm
Haptics:	bonded blue PMMA

The Acrystal from Laboratoires IOL Technologie, France, is a new one-piece IOL brought onto the market in 1996 which is composed of two monomers: HEMA and MMA.

This hydrophilic acrylic forms a three-dimensional network presenting characteristic properties, especially with regard to mechanical aspects. The cohesion of the material is achieved via strong chemical links, and a chromophor group acts as UV light absorber.

Lens and material are under clinical trial; the company offers a series of designs and variations (Acrystal, Acrystal angulé, Tripode, Acrybag, Stabibag, Vision Multifocal).

The lens characteristics are as follows:

Water content (%):	38
Specific gravity (g/ml):	1.118
Refractive index:	1.47
Tensile strength (lb/in²):	
Elongation (%):	
Glass transforming temp. (°C):	
Optic:	true 6 mm
Haptics:	various shapes in one piece

Acrigel from Corneal in France was introduced in 1995. This new lens is also made of a new hydrophilic acrylic hydrogel and a mixture of hydrophobic and hydrophilic monomers, including a UV absorber. The hydrophobic monomers add strength to the materials; there is improved tensile strength when compared with pure hydrogel. The material characteristics are quite similar to those of silicone. Two monomers form part of the lens material: HEMA and MMA.

Six-month postoperative follow-up data on 50 patients demonstrating the excellent biocompatibility of this lens were presented at the 1997 ESCRS congress in Prague (S. Raab-Cumpelik and T.H. Neuhann).

Visional SMP in Switzerland supplies a corresponding material in Galand Acrygel. This IOL is also a single-piece construction with excellent centration, dimensions based on biometric measurements and a uniplanar configuration which allows a small optic without side-images. Two hundred cases with 1-year of follow-up are on file.

The lens characteristics are as follows:

Water content (%):	25.6
Specific gravity (g/ml):	1.15
Refractive index:	1.465
Tensile strength (lb/in²):	300
Elongation (%):	420
Glass transforming temp. (°C):	
Optic:	true 6 mm biconvex
Haptics:	one-piece closed loop

The BioComFold IOL (Fig. 21.19) is a new implant from Morcher in Germany and was first implanted in 1994. This IOL is composed of the following two monomers: HEMA (12%) and MMA (88%).

The device is undergoing clinical evaluation and shows good clinical results.

The lens characteristics are as follows:

Water content (%):	28
Specific gravity (g/ml):	1.18
Refractive index:	1.46
Tensile strength (lb/in²):	
Elongation (%):	
Glass transforming temp. (°C):	−15
Optic:	true 6 mm
Haptics:	blue PMMA

The Collamer IOL and the Intraocular Contact Lens (ICL) were developed by STAAR AG Switzerland (Fig. 21.20). This new hydrophilic hydrogel, which is a p-HEMA containing approximately 33% water, 3,4-benzophenone (cross-linked UV blocker) also contains 0.2% porcine collagen.

Porcine connective tissue was chosen because the amino acid compositions of collagens of humans and pigs are similar and highly biocompatible. Because of the highly cross-linked structure of the material, this collagen cannot become subject to biodegradation. The refractive index is 1.47, and the ICL and the Collamer IOL for aphakia, the designs using this material, have been under clinical investigation since 1994 and deliver very good results.[47]

Another new interesting one-piece design, the HE26C (FIg. 21.21), was recently launched by Domilens, Germany. The lens is also produced by Visional SMP Switzerland and has similar properties to Galand Acrygel.

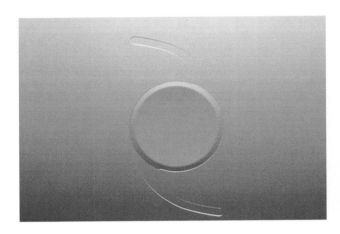

Figure 21.19. *BioComFold (95B), Morcher.*

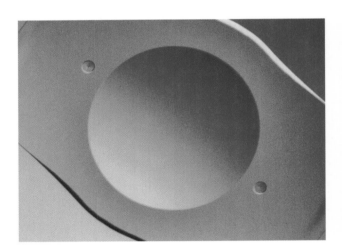

Figure 21.20. *ICL, STAAR AG.*

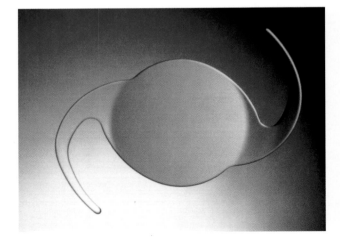

Figure 21.21. *HE26C, Domilens.*

EXPLANTATION OF LOW-WATER ACRYLIC AND POLY-HEMA LENSES

Extensive knowledge of the lens characteristics is mandatory for a successful and atraumatic explantation or exchange.

The high glass transforming temperature of the Memory IOL generally only allows explantation after enlargment of the incision to 6 mm. However, the author has successfully performed intraocular refolding and explantation of a Memory lens through a 4.5-mm incision, using prewarmed balanced salt solution (BSS) and prewarmed viscoelastics in a case with unwanted postoperative refraction.

The Hydroview and Acrigel lenses have a similar tensile strength to the AcrySof. They are suitable both for bisection or refolding and exchange through a small incision.

The Collamer IOL and the ICL show their unique properties also during explantation: both lenses refold automatically into the initial incision and thus can be explanted as a whole. The prerequisite with both implants is that they are held approximately in the middle of their longitudinal axis with straight forceps in such a way that the passage through the step incision is opened without the lens tearing at the same time.

CONCLUSIONS

Today's IOL market can be described as follows: although foldable IOLs made of a variety of materials have been available since 1984 in Europe, Japan and the USA, rigid PMMA IOLs are still preferred, but to an ever-decreasing extent.[48,49]

The distinct trend towards foldables, and especially the large new family of acrylics, can no longer be neglected. Acrylic lenses, as well as low-water acrylics and polyHEMA IOLs, have shown a biocompatibility at least as good as that of PMMA or silicone and at the same time are chemically closely related to the still generally favored PMMA.

Taking also into account that small-incision cataract surgery clearly renders better results[50] accompanied by quicker postoperative rehabilitation,[8] there is no doubt that the future belongs to foldable IOLs.

The clinical application of foldable IOLs will not overtake that of rigid PMMA until the turn of the millenium. Two important reasons will be the close chemical relationship of the new acrylics to PMMA and their excellent biocompatibility.[51]

REFERENCES

1 Dreifus M, Wichterle O, Lim D. Intrakameraln: cocky z hydrokoloidnich akrylatu. *CS Optalmologic* 1960; **16:** 154–9.

2 Mazzocco TR, Davidson BM. Insertion technique and clinical experience with silicone lenses. In: Mazzocco TR, Rajacich GM, Epstein E, eds. *Soft Implant Lenses in Cataract Surgery* (Thorofare, NJ: Slack, 1986) 97–106.

3 Christ FR, Fencil DA, Van Gent S, Knight PM. Evaluation of the chemical, optical, and mechanical properties of elastomeric intraocular lens materials and their clinical significance. *J Cataract Refract Surg* 1989, **15:** 176–84.

4 Buchen SY, Richards SC, Solomon KD, et al. Evalution of the biocompatibility and fixation of a new silicone intraocular lens in the feline model. *J Cataract Refract Surg* 1989; **15:** 545–53.

5 Menapace R, Radax U, Vass C, Amon M, Papapanos P. In-the-bag implantation of the PhacoFlex SI-30 high-refractive silicone lens through self-sealing sclerocorneal and clear corneal incisions. *Eur J Implant Refract Surg* 1994; **6**(suppl).

6 Egan CA, Kottos PJ, Francis IC. Prospective study of the SI-40NB foldable silicone intraocular lens. *J Cataract Refract Surg* 1996; **22**(suppl 2): 1272–6

7 Utrata PJ, Brown DC. STAAR Elastimide three-piece silicone IOL. In: Martin RG, Gills JP, Sanders DR eds. *Foldable Intraocular Lenses* (Thorofare, NJ: Slack, 1993) 117.

8 Neduhann T, Neuhann Th. Die 'Clear Cornea Incision' für die Phakoemulsifikation. In: Robert et al., eds, 7. *DGII Kongreß* (Heidelberg: PRO EDIT, 1993) 100–3.

9 Menapace R, Radax U, Vass C, Amon M, Papapanos P. No-stitch, small incision cataract surgery with flexible intraocular lens implantation. *J Cataract Refract Surg* 1994; **20:** 534–42.

10 Yang S, Makker H, Christ FR. Accelerated ultraviolet aging of intraocular lens optic materials: a 50 year simulation. *J Cataract Refract Surg* **23:** 940–7.

11 Milazzo S, Turnt P, Artin B, Charlin JF. Long-term follow-up of three-piece, looped, silicone intraocular lenses. *J Cataract Refract Surg* 1996; **22**(suppl 2).

12 Grabow HB. The clear corneal incision. In: Fine IH, Fichman RA, Grabow HB. eds. *Clear-Corneal Cataract Surgery and Topical Anesthesia* (Thorofare, NJ; Slack, 1993) 50–1.

13 Kohnen T, Magdowski G, Koch DD. Oberflächenqualität faltbarer Intraocularlinsen aus Silikon—Eine rasterelektronenmikroskopische Studie. *Klin Monatsbl Augenheilkd* 1995; **207:** 215–82.

14 Mamalis N, Phillips B, Kopp CH, Crandall AS, Olson RJ. Neodymium:YAG capsulotomy rates after phacoemulsification with silicone posterior chamber intraocular lenses. *J Cataract Refract Surg* 1996; **22**(suppl 2): 1296–302.

material is a hydrogel with 38% water content, and can best be described as soft and elastic. HEMA can be combined with a variety of copolymers which affect the water content, and optical, mechanical and biological properties of the materials. Lenses composed of copolymers of HEMA include the Memory lenses composed of HEMA and MMA co-monomers and the Hydroview lens composed of HEMA and hydroxyhexylmethacrylate co-monomers. Although the Memory and Hydroview lenses are hydrophilic, the water content is relatively low and the mechanical properties are closer to those of so-called acrylic lenses such as AcrySof, in that they are pliable rather than elastic. These lenses are marketed by their respective companies as hydrogel lenses, whilst, as mentioned, other European companies have chosen to market similar low water content lenses as acrylic lenses.

Hydrogels can be described as polymeric materials which exhibit the ability to swell in water and retain a significant fraction of water within their structure but which will not dissolve in water. The term therefore encompasses a large number of different chemical compounds, both natural and synthetic. Synthetic hydrogels include poly(hydroxyalkyl methacrylates and acrylates), poly(acrylamides and methacrylamides), poly(N-vinyl-2-pyrolidone), polyelectrolyte complexes, and poly(vinyl alcohol). These compounds have different properties which are influenced by the water content, and chemical, anionic, cationic or neutral nature of the polymer. PolyHEMA is a soft hydrophilic acrylic hydrogel material developed for biomedical use, and has a long history of use as a biomaterial and as an intraocular lens implant. Ophthalmic surgeons often use the terms polyHEMA and hydrogel interchangeably, but the properties of different hydrogels may vary considerably, as indeed may the different copolymers of hydrogels containing polyHEMA. Hydrogels and, in particular, polyHEMA have several potential advantages compared to PMMA as an intraocular lens material, including a hydrophilic surface, improved biocompatibility, thermal stability and optical properties, and mechanical properties that allow a lens to be folded and inserted through small incisions.[4]

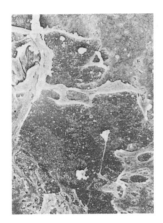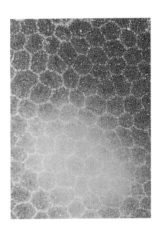

Figure 22.2. *Scanning electron micrograph of the endothelium of a rabbit cornea after 15 s of contact with a PMMA IOL on the left and with a polyHEMA IOL on the right.*

interfacial tension is the difference in surface energy of a material and its surrounding environment. In the case of a hydrophilic material in an aqueous environment, the interfacial tension will be extremely low, and this is thought to be one of the major reasons why these materials are well tolerated by biological tissues. The hydrophilic surface of hydrogels is also the primary reason why these materials produce minimal damage on contact with the endothelium and other cellular surfaces. Endothelial contact with hydrophobic PMMA and other materials is known to cause severe cellular damage by a process of adherence of the cells to the surface of the lens optic.[5] The actual contact adhesion force between biomaterials and the endothelium has been measured and found to be far less in hydrogel materials than with polymethylmethacrylate.[6] An intraocular hydrogel lens, when compared in a quantitative fashion to a PMMA intraocular lens, was found to cause minimal endothelial cell damage on contact with the endothelium (Fig. 22.2).[7]

HYDROPHILIC SURFACE

Perhaps the major difference between hydrogels and alternative materials is their hydrophilic nature. The

BIOCOMPATIBILITY

A polymer can be termed biocompatible if it does not produce any adverse effects in the surrounding biological tissues when implanted and maintains its

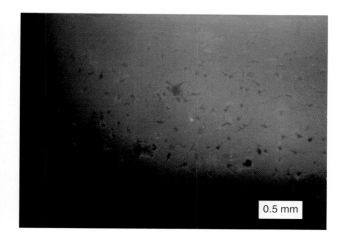

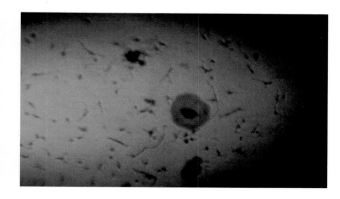

0.5 mm

Figure 22.3. *High-power slit lamp photograph of a patient with a PMMA implant (below) and a polyHEMA implant (above) 3 weeks following surgery. The comparison demonstrates the lack of foreign body giant cells on the polyHEMA lens. (Courtesy of Professor Y. Majima.)*

desired function and form without degradation by the particular biological environment at the site of implantation. The potential of polyHEMA as a more biocompatible material has been confirmed by in vitro laboratory studies,[8] animal studies,[9] and clinical trials.[10] The incidence of foreign body giant cells on polyHEMA is considerably reduced compared to PMMA (Fig. 22.3).[11] The cellular reaction to an intraocular lens may be used as an index of biocompatibility of an implant. Typically, early adhesion of small cells, probably lens epithelial cells, may be observed on the lens optic following implantation of

an intraocular lens. These cells diminish with time but in some cases are replaced by cellular proliferation visible on the optic as pseudophakic precipitates. The pseudophakic precipitates, which consist of fibrinous precipitates, mononuclear inflammatory cells and giant cells, have been associated with clinical signs of poor tolerance and may represent an immune reaction to the presence of an implant.[12,13] Lens epithelial cell adhesion and proliferation on polyHEMA is reduced compared to more hydrophobic materials such as PMMA. This phenomenon appears to be related at least in part to the water content of 38% and surface energy, as other hydrogels with lower water content may not exhibit the same lack of cellular adhesion. This would explain the recent observations concerning low water content hydrogels such as the Hydroview lens from Storz, which is a copolymer of HEMA and hydroxyhexylmethacrylate. These materials appear to encourage growth of a monolayer of lens epithelial cells, with proliferation of cells from the anterior capsule onto the optic. Giant cells representing an immunoproliferative response, however, are uncommon, indicating biocompatibility, but the cellular interaction is considered to be less desirable than that of higher water content hydrogels such as polyHEMA.

One of the advantages of polyHEMA over other hydrogels is its stability to varying conditions of pH, temperature and tonicity. PolyHEMA has the thermal stability and resistance to UV degradation that is characteristic of methacrylate polymers. PolyHEMA will undergo all the chemical reactions of the hydroxyl and ester groups but is only capable of hydrolysis in conditions of high alkalinity and temperature far beyond those encountered in a normal biological environment. PolyHEMA has a smaller pore size than higher water content hydrogels. Therefore, the possibility of protein or drug interactions and tissue ingrowth is less with HEMA than with other higher water content hydrogel materials. The pores of 38% polyHEMA are as small as 5–20 Å, but pores 10 times larger occur in higher water content hydrogels. The pores are, therefore, so minute that to imagine a sponge-like architecture is misleading. In fact, large molecules such as proteins probably do not penetrate the matrix significantly. Similarly, viruses and bacteria cannot enter the matrix. There is, however, a free exchange of small, water-soluble electrolytes such as sodium and potassium between the water component of the lens and the aqueous. Hydrogels do have the potential to undergo calcification. This propensity is more pronounced in the macroporous forms and is also related to the species and site of implantation.[14,15] All materials implanted as IOLs have had unusual changes reported, e.g. the discoloration of silicone lenses,[16] vacuoles or glistenings in acrylic lenses[17] and the reports of internal crazing or crystallization in PMMA intraocular lenses. Similarly, there have been isolated reports of calcification of hydrogel implants in Europe.[18] These appear to be unique occurrences of inorganic precipitation due to a particular combination of local factors, including pH, Ca^{2+} and phosphate, possibly related to intracameral medications. Lens factors include the possibility of an incompletely polymerized lens blank or impurities such as methacrylic acid which could theoretically encourage such a phenomenon. Loss of fluid from a vial during sterilization could also result in a supersaturated solution which could encourage precipitation. Patient factors which could be relevant include metabolic abnormalities or a localized *Propionibacterium acnes* reaction as a primary process, with the involvement of the lens being a secondary phenomenon. A hydrogel intraocular lens (IOGEL model no. PC12 and 1103) manufactured from polyHEMA has been implanted since 1983 in over 24 000 patients worldwide. Multinational studies have demonstrated that the lens is well tolerated, and patients have achieved postoperative visual acuity equivalent to that obtained with PMMA intraocular implants.[19–21] The lens has been implanted over a period of 15 years and there has been no discoloration or degradation of the material.

THERMAL STABILITY

PMMA and hydrophobic acrylic lenses cannot be autoclaved and require chemical or gas methods of sterilization. Concerns exist regarding ethylene oxide sterilization of products, due to the potential toxicity of ethylene oxide residues and the existence of resistant organisms.[22] In comparison, polyHEMA is a thermostable compound and can be autoclaved repeatedly without significantly altering its properties. Autoclaving is, therefore, a rapid, safe and effective method of sterilization of a hydrogel intraocular lens. The adherence of bacteria to an implant at the time of implantation is an important characteristic of intraocular lenses with regard to maintaining sterility and reducing the chance of intraocular infection. The adhesion of *Staphylococcus epidermidis* to different

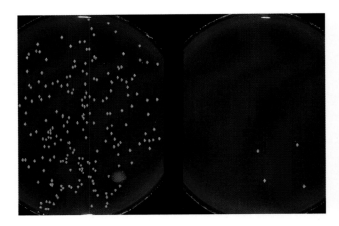

Figure 22.4. *Comparison of residual adherent* Staphylococcus epidermidis *colonies cultured from a polyHEMA lens on the left and a PMMA lens on the right after exposure of the lenses to the same concentration of organisms.*

intraocular lenses has been measured and found to be significantly less with polyHEMA than with PMMA (Fig. 22.4).[23] Almost all commercial polymers contain additives of various types, including residual monomer, catalyst and solvent. In particular, monomer in significant concentrations is known to be toxic and has the potential for leaching, following implantation.[24]

The monomer content of several PMMA IOLs analysed by gas–liquid chromatography (GLC) was found to be 0.8%. By the same method of analysis, the residual monomer in hydrogel IOLs was below the detectable limit of 0.004%. This is because the permeability and water content of a hydrogel makes it possible to extract all impurities, such as unreacted monomer and initiator fragments, during processing of the hydrogel lens.

OPTICAL PROPERTIES

An intraocular lens has to be optically clear and capable of manufacture with a precision surface with a resolution of at least 100 line pairs/mm in air. When analysed, the resolution of a hydrated hydrogel lens in an aqueous medium is 84 line pairs/mm. A PMMA lens with a resolution of 276 line pairs/mm in air has a

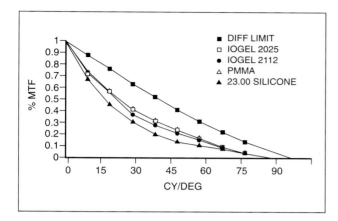

Figure 22.5. *Graph displaying the modulation transfer function expressed as a percentage at different spatial frequencies, expressed as cycles per degree, for the optics of a theoretical ideal diffraction limited intraocular lens (IOL), two polyHEMA IOLs, and a silicone IOL. All lenses have the same dioptric power of 23.00 D in aqueous.*

similar resolution in aqueous of 94 line pairs/mm. A comparison of the resolution of an ideal diffracted limited lens with a PMMA, silicone and hydrogel optic showed no significant difference in the modulation transfer function between PMMA and hydrogel materials (Fig. 22.5). The limiting factor in resolution of the materials depends on the quality of manufacture and is not related to the different refractive indices. PolyHEMA has a water content of 38%, a refractive index of 1.44, and no inherent UV absorption. A lower refractive index may be desirable for an implant once it is implanted, as the surface is less reflective (Fig. 22.6). The highly reflective surface of PMMA and other implants may be disturbing to some patients. The incorporation of a bonded UV absorber, either a benzophenone or a benzotriazole, has been shown to be possible, and the refractive index and tensile strength can be increased by the addition of a suitable co-monomer. PolyHEMA is transparent to YAG laser radiation at a wavelength of 1064 mm and, furthermore, has been found to be relatively resistant to damage by the YAG laser.[25,26] Intraocular lenses composed of different biomaterials were subjected to YAG laser, at varying energy levels, focused on the optical surface of the lenses. The damage to the hydrogel lenses was confined to localized pitting, with less marking being noted than on PMMA or silicone lenses (Fig. 22.7). This is due to the resilience and stress-free nature of the gel-like structure, which is unlike the

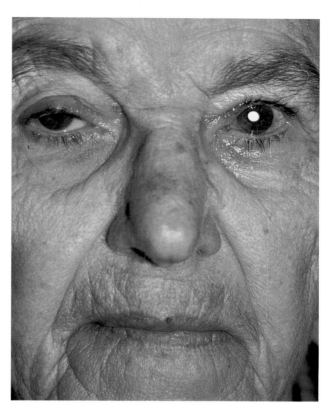

Figure 22.6. *Photograph of a patient demonstrating the typical bright reflection from the surface of a PMMA lens. This phenomenon is much less common in patients with lower refractive index hydrogel lenses.*

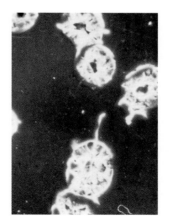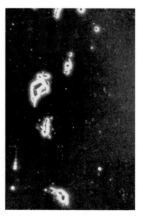

Figure 22.7. *Scanning electron micrograph of the surface of a PMMA lens on the left and a polyHEMA lens on the right after applying a YAG laser at the same energy level of 2.0 MJ directly to the surface.*

more stressed and rigid structure of materials such as PMMA and glass. When incubated with cultured endothelial cells, hydrogel IOLs subjected to high YAG laser energy levels showed no sign of toxicity.

MECHANICAL PROPERTIES

A prosthesis to replace a hip joint would have to be composed of a hard, rigid and extremely durable material. The normal crystalline lens, however, is a fragile, gel-like structure containing significant quantities of water. When hydrated, polyHEMA is soft, flexible and hydrophilic, similar to the normal crystalline lens. The mechanical strength of polyHEMA is such that it can be handled and implanted without tearing and can maintain itself in the desired position in the eye. Hydrogels in their dehydrated state can be lathed or moulded to a precision optic with a variety of supporting structures, similar to existing PMMA IOLs. Lenses can be manufactured by computer-controlled lathes and milling machines and then tumble polished. This method of manufacture achieves a precision and finish superior to other methods of manufacture. Scanning electron microscopy of a polyHEMA hydrogel lens compared to a moulded three-piece silicone lens showed the hydrogel lens to be smooth without the edge flash and irregularities at the optic–haptic junction which can occur in moulded three-piece designs (Fig. 22.8). Hydrated hydrogel lenses can be folded for insertion through a small incision without altering their physical or optical properties.

Folding experiments to examine the effect of folding on different foldable intraocular lenses demonstrated no detectable damage or creases in the surface of polyHEMA lenses and no change in the optical resolution following folding.[27] A hydrogel lens designed to be inserted in the dehydrated state for later re-expansion would have to be composed of a high water content hydrogel. The higher the water content of a hydrogel material, the higher the expansion ratio but the lower the refractive index. An intraocular lens with a low refractive index requires a thicker optic. When one examines the water content expansion ratios and refractive indexes of available hydrogels, it becomes apparent that a smaller incision is more feasible by folding a lower water content hydrogel such as polyHEMA than by inserting a dehydrated high water content material. A dehydrated hydrogel is as damaging to the endothelium as PMMA, and the sterilization and purification of a dehydrated hydrogel are also

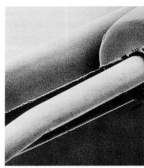

Figure 22.8. *Scanning electron micrograph comparing the edge appearance of a lathe, cut tumble polished, IOGEL 2000S hydrogel implant to that of a moulded, three-piece silicone implant.*

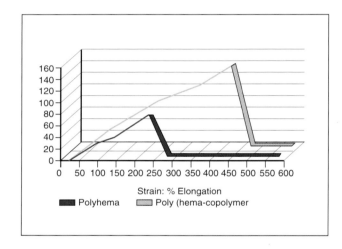

Figure 22.9. *Graph of the tensile strength of a copolymer of HEMA and a hydrophobic co-monomer demonstrating a twofold increase in the tensile strength and elongation at break of the material. The resultant polymer had a refractive index of 1.46 and a water content of 27%.*

problematic. Nevertheless, the expansile properties of hydrogels offer another mechanism for insertion through small incisions. HEMA can be polymerized with a large number of relatively hydrophobic co-monomers to modify the water content and mechanical properties. The refractive index can be increased to 1.46 and the tensile strength increased two-fold by copolymerizing HEMA with a long-chain copolymer such as ethoxyethylmethacrylate. Reducing the water content to 27% increases the refractive index and mechanical strength and results in a thinner optic with greater resistance to damage during folding (Fig. 22.9).

This facilitates insertion through a small incision and is a strategy employed by companies such as Storz and IOLTECH. The resultant copolymers of HEMA are lower water content hydrogels and may not have the same biocompatibility as pure polyHEMA.

CHEMISTRY OF HYDROGELS

Hydrogel polymers are typically prepared by bulk polymerization or with a small amount of aqueous diluent, using ethylene glycol dimethacrylate as a cross-linking agent. Temperature-sensitive initiators are commonly utilized and the polymerization environment must be carefully controlled to avoid incomplete polymerization with excessive residual monomer. Water baths are commonly used to avoid thermal overload, which can result in a lens blank with intrinsic stress. Of particular concern is the use of highly purified monomer and the avoidance of contamination with methacrylic acid to maintain a neutral polymer. The polymer obtained in this fashion is a glassy material similar in many ways to PMMA. Unlike PMMA, however, when exposed to water, polyHEMA absorbs approximately two-thirds of its own weight of water to form a three-dimensional stable network with the consistency of an elastic gel. The amount of water absorbed expressed as a percentage of the weight of the hydrated gel is known as the equilibrium water content and has a profound effect on the permeability, mechanical properties, surface properties and biocompatibility of the resulting material. Alternative methods of polymerization include solution polymerization, cast-moulding, and gamma irradiation.

HYDROGEL LENS DESIGNS

HISTORY

Hydrogel implants have been considered as an alternative to PMMA by several investigators for different reasons. Edward Epstein was the first person to use a hydrogel implant, as long ago as 1976. These posterior chamber implants composed of polyHEMA were inserted in the dehydrated state and sterilized with ethylene oxide. The major reason why Epstein considered hydrogel was the prospect that the soft

material would be better tolerated with respect to mechanical imperfections, which were not uncommon in intraocular lenses manufactured with the available technology at the time. Mehta implanted an iris-supported lens in 1978. Once again, he thought that the soft material would reduce the iris chafing encountered with this type of implant and method of fixation.

My personal interest in hydrogel implants was motivated by the prospect of improved biocompatibility and the ability to fold these implants for small-incision cataract surgery. This interest led me to the development of the IOGEL series of hydrogel lenses manufactured from polyHEMA, which I first implanted in August 1983. These posterior chamber fully hydrated implants were autoclaved and the soft, flexible lens was folded and inserted through 3.5-mm incisions following phacoemulsification.[28]

Michael Blumenthal also used hydrogel lenses, generally with a higher water content than that of polyHEMA; he inserted a dehydrated lens, to take advantage of the expansile properties of this material once hydrated. His designs included a relatively thick, disk-shaped implant. Albert Galand and Camille Budo also implanted similar disk-shaped hydrogel lenses manufactured from polyHEMA and implanted with an intercapsular technique. Because of the higher refractive index, these were considerably thinner and required an exacting technique, as retraction of the capsular flap could result in decentration.

Steven Siepser designed several single-piece high water content hydrogel lenses, but to my knowledge these were not implanted. The basic concept was to insert the implants in a dehydrated state through a small incision following phacoemulsification. 3M developed a three-piece hydrogel implant, based on this concept, but clinical studies were discontinued.

DESIGNS

Foldable lenses can be classified according to the material composition or the design structure. The latter can be helpful in considering currently available hydrogel lenses.

Plate haptic hydrogel lenses

The IOGEL PC12 and 1103 lenses from Alcon were plate haptic hydrogel lenses. These lenses are easy to insert but the fixation is not as reliable as with

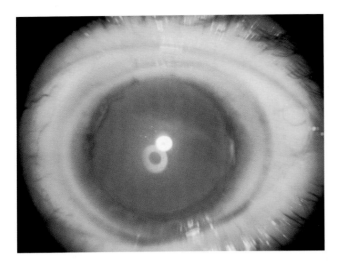

Figure 22.10. *Photograph of a patient with an IOGEL PC12 plate haptic hydrogel lens implanted over 10 years previously. The posterior capsule remained clear and the patient corrected to 20/20.*

conventional PMMA lenses. The lens proved to be well tolerated and was implanted in thousands of patients (Fig. 22.10). With all plate haptic lenses there is a need to avoid early YAG laser capsulotomy. Reports from the USA of dislocation following early (less than 3 months) YAG laser capsulotomy limited the widespread use of the IOGEL[29] lens, but post-YAG dislocation can be avoided if early and large YAG laser capsulotomies are avoided.[30] A polyHEMA plate haptic design (ISH66) is available from Corneal (Fig. 22.11), and a HEMA/MMA copolymer plate haptic design (92C) with a water content of 28% is available from Morcher. Modified plate haptic hydrogel lenses include the Acrybag lens from IOLTECH (Fig. 22.12) in France, which incorporates holes in the plate to encourage fixation, as well as the Tripode and Stabibag designs (Figs 22.13 and 22.14) from the same company. These lenses are marketed as acrylic lenses but are examples of a low water content copolymer of HEMA described in more detail above.

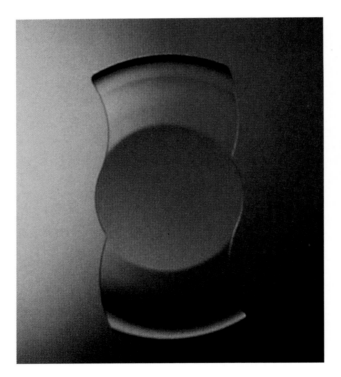

Figure 22.11. *Photograph from a graphic of a polyHEMA plate haptic lens (model ISH66) available from Corneal.*

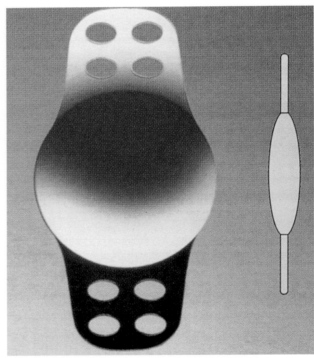

Figure 22.12. *Photograph from a graphic of a modified plate haptic hydrogel lens (Stabibag), incorporating holes in the flange, available from IOLTECH. The hydrogel is a low water content copolymer of HEMA and is marketed as an acrylic lens.*

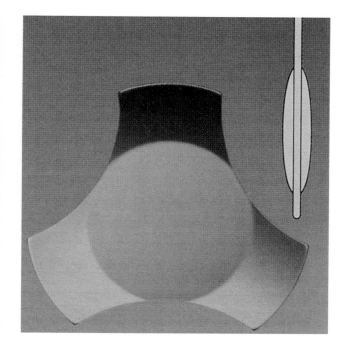

Figure 22.13. *Photograph from a graphic of the Tripode hydrogel–acrylic lens available from IOLTECH.*

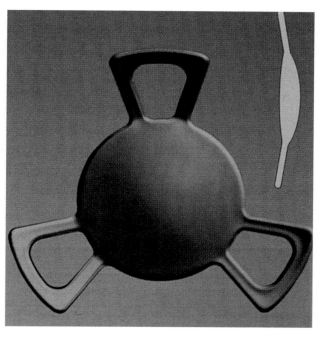

Figure 22.14. *Photograph from a graphic of the Acrybag hydrogel–acrylic lens available from IOLTECH.*

Loop haptic hydrogel lenses

Hydrogel lenses with conventional PMMA or polypropylene loops are available from several manufacturers. The Memory lens from Mentor (U940A) has a haptic composed of a copolymer of HEMA and MMA with a water content of 20% and polypropylene loop haptics (Fig. 22.15). At certain temperatures, acrylic polymers change from a rigid state and become more pliable. This property is termed the glass transition temperature and can affect the folding properties of an intraocular lens. PolyHEMA has a very low glass transition temperature and, unlike with other acrylic lenses, the foldability is not altered in the range of temperatures experienced in a clinical environment. Copolymerizing HEMA with other monomers such as MMA can affect the glass

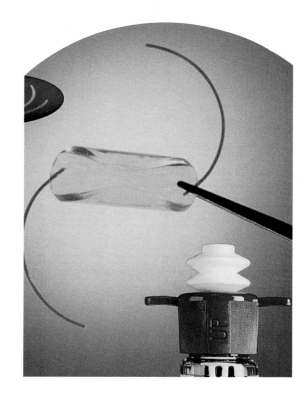

Figure 22.15. *Photograph from a graphic of the Memory lens (UA940A) available from Mentor. The lens is a copolymer of HEMA and MMA and initially required cooling and warming chambers for folding and retention of the folded state. The lens is now supplied cooled and prefolded and can be inserted without folding instruments.*

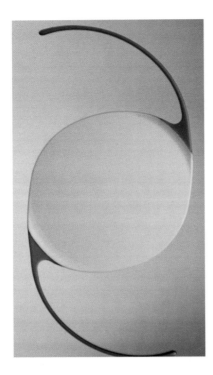

Figure 22.16.
Photograph of the Storz Hydroview (H60M). The lens is a conventional one-piece design with a low water content (18%) hydrogel optic bonded to PMMA haptics.

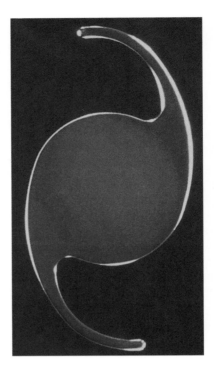

Figure 22.17.
Photograph of the Hydrosof polyHEMA lens available from Alcon. This lens is an example of a single-piece hydrogel lens with a hybrid haptic which combines features of a plate haptic and a conventional loop-style lens.

transition temperature so that the material can be flexible at body temperature but relatively rigid when cooled. The Memory lens utilizes this phenomenon to maintain the lens in a prefolded state when cooled. Following insertion, the increase in temperature allows the lens to spontaneously unfold.

Morcher produces a similar three-piece hydrogel lens (92S) composed of a copolymer of HEMA and MMA with a water content of 28%. The Hydroview lens from Storz (H60M) (Fig. 22.16) is a one-piece design with PMMA haptics and an optic composed of a copolymer of HEMA and hydroxyhexylmethacrylate with a water content of 18%. The PMMA haptics are bonded intimately to the optic during polymerization by an interpenetrating polymer network. The conventional PMMA loops provide reliable fixation but could compromise the ability to insert the lens with an injector.

Hybrid haptic hydrogel lenses

These lenses have hybrid haptics combining features of plate haptic and conventional loop-style lenses. The entire lens is made from the same foldable material, retaining the ease of insertion of

a single-piece soft lens whilst achieving early fixation and stability similar to that of conventional loop haptics.

I developed a modification of the original IOGEL lens, the IOGEL 2000 series, now manufactured by Alcon as the Hydrosof lens (SH30GC).[31] The lens is manufactured from medical grade polyHEMA with an intrinsic water content in the order of 38% by weight and incorporates a benzotriazole UV absorber. The optic of the lens is 5.5 mm and merges via a crescentic flange into a terminal loop with an overall diameter of 12.00 mm (Fig. 22.17).

The design of the lens is based on a concept of minimum loop rigidity. A haptic which has sufficient rigidity to support the weight of a lens in aqueous within the capsular bag is considered adequate for modern cataract surgery. The surgical technique of phacoemulsification and capsulorhexis provides a different support environment for an implant than that achieved by extracapsular surgery in the early 1980s, when most of the criteria for loop rigidity were derived. Once fusion of the anterior and posterior capsule occurs around the optic and between the haptic and optic, the position of an implant is maintained and it is not necessary for a flexible haptic to further resist the compressive force

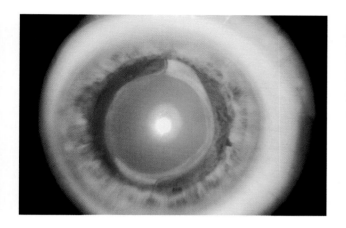

Figure 22.18. *Photograph of a patient with an IOGEL 2000 series implant 12 months following surgery. The fusion between the leaflets of the anterior and posterior capsule in the interval between the optic and haptic is visible and responsible for the fixation and stability of an IOL implant.*

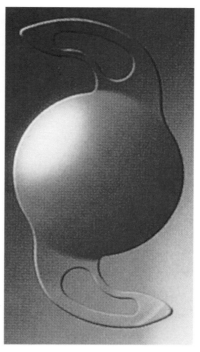

Figure 22.19. *Photograph of a hybrid haptic lens designed by P. Sourdille and available from Corneal. The lens is a copolymer of polyHEMA with a water content of 26%.*

of the capsular bag (Fig. 22.18). The haptic of the new hydrogel intraocular lens design has sufficient rigidity to maintain centration in the early postoperative period, is compressible without distorting the capsular bag and avoids the posterior vaulting of previous flange-style designs. One-piece design is considered preferable to three-piece construction, and the fact that the entire lens is foldable allows the lens to be inserted with an injector system similar to that used for single-piece flexible footplate intraocular lenses.

Other hybrid haptic hydrogel lenses include a hydrogel lens manufactured by Corneal (Fig. 22.19) and the Acrystal lens produced by IOLTECH (Fig. 22.20).

CLINICAL EXPERIENCE

It is difficult to generalize about the clinical results achieved with hydrogel lenses, as the term describes a range of different designs and materials with varying chemical compositions and water contents. Nevertheless, there do appear to be common features in the clinical results experienced with this type of implant.

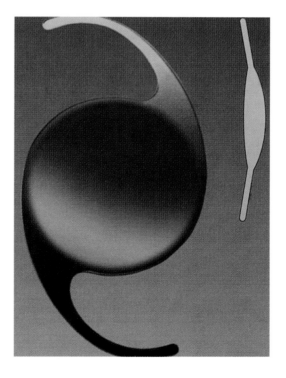

Figure 22.20. *Photograph from a graphic of the Acrystal hydrogel lens model manufactured by IOLTECH.*

INSERTION TECHNIQUES

A variety of techniques can be used to insert hydrogel lenses, including folding forceps and injectors. The folding characteristics are favourable in that the materials fold easily without marking and the surface is not sticky. The lenses unfold promptly but without the explosive elastic recoil which may be encountered with silicone lenses. Generally, the materials are not as strong as silicone or acrylic materials, and care must be taken to avoid sharp instrumentation. Attempts to insert polyHEMA lenses through an incision of inadequate length may result in a fracture of the optic. As described previously, lower water content hydrogels are more durable.

INFLAMMATORY COMPLICATIONS

Typically there is little if any inflammation in the postoperative period, and inflammatory complications such as postoperative uveitis, fibrin reaction or cystoid macular oedema are extremely rare with hydrogel lenses. The incidence of foreign body giant cells on polyHEMA and other hydrogels is considerably reduced compared to PMMA, which indicates that these materials are well tolerated. As mentioned previously, the adhesion of lens epithelial cells to a hydrogel varies with the water content, which would explain observations of a monolayer of lens epithelial cells, derived from the anterior capsule, on the optic in low water content hydrogels which is not seen in polyHEMA.

NON-INFLAMMATORY COMPLICATIONS

Non-inflammatory complications include decentration and significant opacification of the posterior capsule. The fixation characteristics of a hydrogel lens will, of course, vary with the design. The surfaces of hydrogels are non-adhesive, but intraocular lenses do not rely on adhesion to the capsule for fixation and stability. Past reports of decentration and even dislocation following YAG laser capsulotomy are related to the plate haptic design rather than being a feature of hydrogel materials. A three-piece or single-piece hydrogel lens with conventional loop haptics would be expected to have the same fixation and centration characteristics as a PMMA lens of similar construction.

Hybrid haptics such as the Hydrosof lens allow fixation similar to that encountered with conventional flexible loop haptics. The leaflets of the anterior and posterior capsule undergo early fusion in the interval between the haptic and the edge of the optic, ensuring stable fixation. The results of clinical trials demonstrated that the hybrid haptic is able to accommodate compression of the capsular bag and allows early, reliable fixation. The mean decentration of the implant measured by a photographic method was 0.22 mm in relation to the centre of the pupil. This was similar to that obtained by post-mortem studies of PPMA implants, where the mean decentration was 0.28 mm.

There are several factors which influence the rate of opacification of the posterior capsule and whether a capsulotomy may be necessary for an individual patient. Surgical factors of relevance include the size of the opening in the anterior capsule, the amount of residual anterior capsule, and the completeness of removal of cortical and residual lens epithelial cells. The properties of an intraocular lens which are thought to influence the rate of capsular opacification include the type of polymer from which the intraocular lens is fabricated and the haptic and optic design of an implant. Design features which are thought to be of relevance include the size of the optic of the implant, thickness of the optic, and curvature of the posterior surface of the implant. These factors have to be considered when considering the rate of opacification of the posterior capsule experienced with a particular implant including hydrogel designs. Hydrogel lenses, however, do appear to behave in a similar manner with respect to posterior capsule opacification, as early fibrosis of the posterior capsule is extremely rare. Later epithelial cell proliferation, however, is not uncommon and YAG laser capsulotomy may be required, usually 2 or 3 years following surgery for this phenomenon. The incidence of YAG laser capsulotomy is similar to that with PMMA but may be greater than that anticipated with hydrophobic acrylic lenses, where a more intimate adhesion of the posterior capsule or a well defined edge to the optic may delay epithelial cell proliferation.

VISUAL ACUITY

Patients who have had hydrogel lenses implanted have achieved excellent visual acuity. In studies published on polyHEMA lenses, the corrected acuity of all patients (excluding pre-existing macular disease) at latest follow-up was 20/40 or better in 100%, 20/30 or better in 95%, 20/25 to 20/20 or better in 85% and 20/15 or better in 15% of patients.[31] A more detailed analysis indicated that patients with polyHEMA lenses achieved better visual acuity, improved contrast sensitivity, and less glare disability when compared to a group of patients who received PMMA implants.[32] The visual performance of hydrogel lenses is therefore at least equivalent to that achieved with other materials.

FUTURE DIRECTIONS

In my view, the philosophy that a foldable lens should have merit beyond that of incision size is fundamental in considering new intraocular lens designs and materials. As such, the potential of hydrogels and polyHEMA in particular as more biocompatible materials has been confirmed, as discussed previously. It is encouraging to see the increasing acceptance of hydrogel lenses and, in particular, the different materials and designs that have become available in recent years. Our experience with this generation of hydrogel lenses should clarify what is the preferred water content and the influence of these factors on the biocompatibility of hydrogel materials. Therapeutic medications such as antibiotics

and antiproliferative agents can be added to a hydrogel lens for a slow release following implantation. This may be helpful in reducing endophthalmitis as well as in reducing the incidence of capsular opacification. Hydrogel lenses may be inserted dry and then allowed to expand, or folded for small-incision surgery. Perhaps in the future it will be possible to combine both these properties to achieve smaller incisions. Future designs will include modifications of single-piece designs with hybrid haptics as well as conventional-style lenses with loops composed of a low water content hydrogel. Multifocal optics have been incorporated into hydrogel lenses (Fig. 22.21) and there are accommodative or pseudo-accommodative designs incorporating hydrogels (Fig. 22.22).

The existing characteristics of hydrogels and the fact that the materials and design can be optimized, is the reason why hydrogel lenses are increasingly being considered as more physiological intraocular lenses and will be implanted in increasing numbers in the future.

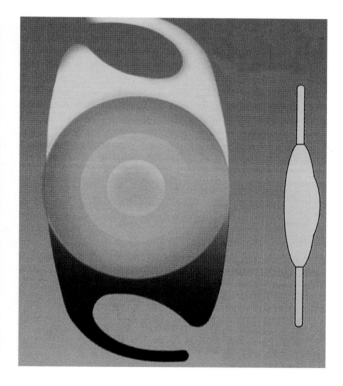

Figure 22.21. *Photograph from a graphic of a modified plate haptic hydrogel lens from IOLTECH which incorporates a multifocal optic.*

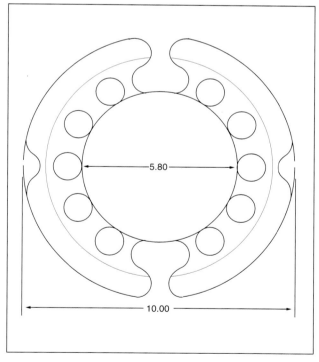

Figure 22.22. *Schematic diagram of a hydrogel disk lens manufactured by Morcher which is claimed to improve pseudo-accommodation following surgery. The lens is a copolymer of HEMA and MMA.*

REFERENCES

1 Barrett GD. Small incision lenses. In: *Proceedings of the XXVI International Congress of Ophthalmology*, Singapore, March 1990 (Elsevier Science Publishers, 1991) 25–7.

2 Shepherd JR. Induced astigmatism in small incision cataract surgery. *J Cataract Refract Surg* 1989; **15:** 85–8.

3 Ratner BD, Hoffman AS. *Synthetic Hydrogels for Biomedical Applications* ACS Symposium Series, No. 31 (Washington, DC: American Chemical Society, 1979).

4 Barrett GD. Hydrogels as an intraocular lens material. Acta XXV *Concil Ophthalmol* 1986; 1397–401.

5 Kaufman HE, Kartz J. Endothelial damage from intraocular lens insertion. *Invest Ophthalmol* 1976; **15:** 996–1000.

6 Blumenthal M, Yalon M. Interaction of soft and hard intraocular lenses with cat endothelium: in vivo studies. *Cornea* 1982; **1:** 129–32.

7 Barrett G, Constable IJ. Corneal endothelial loss with new intraocular lenses. *Am J Ophthalmol* 1984; **98:** 157–65.

8 Joo CK, Kim JH. Compatibility of intraocular lenses with blood and connective tissue cells measured by cellular deposition and inflammatory response in vitro. *J Cataract Refract Surg* 1992; **18:** 240–6.

9 Carlson KH, Cameron JD, Lindstrom RL. Assessment of the blood–aqueous barrier by fluorophotometry following poly(methyl methacrylate), silicone, and hydrogel lens implantation in rabbit eyes. *J Cataract Refract Surg* 1993; **19:** 9–15.

10 Pham DT, Wollensak J, Welzl-Hinterkorner E. Special indications for hydrogel IOLs. Small-incision technique with iridoplasty. *Eur J Implant Refract Surg* 1992; **4:** 25–27.

11 Amon M, Menapace R. Cellular invasion on hydrogel and poly(methyl methacrylate) implants. An in vivo study. *J Cataract Refract Surg* 1991; **17:** 774–9.

12 Bryan JA, Peiffer RL, Brown DT, Eifrig DE, Vollotton WW. Morphology of pseudophakic precipitates on intraocular lenses removed from human patients. *Am Intraocul Implant Soc J* 1985; **11:** 260–7.

13 Galin MA, Tuberville AW, Doston RS. Immunological aspects of intraocular lenses. *Int Ophthalmol Clin* 1982; **22:** 227–34.

14 Imai Y, Mashuhara E. Long term in vivo studies of poly(2-hydroxyethylmethacrylate). *J Biomaterials Res* 1982; **16:** 609–17.

15 Cerveny J, Sprinel L. The calcifications of poly(glycol methacrylate) gels in experimental and clinical practice. *Polymers Med* 1981; **XI:** 71–7.

16 Milauskas ART. Silicone lens implant discoloration in humans. *Arch Ophthalmol* 1991; **109:** 913–15.

17 Dhaliwal DK, Mamalis N, Olson RJ, et al. Visual significance of glistenings seen in the AcrySof intraocular lens. *J Cataract Refract Surg* 1996; **22:** 452–7.

18 Bucher PJM, Buchi ER, Daicker BC. Dystrophic calcification of an implanted hydroxyethylmethacrylate intraocular lens. *Arch Ophthalmol* 1995; **113:** 1431–5.

19 Barrett GD, Beasley H, Lorenzetti OJ, Rosenthal A. Multicentre trial of an intraocular hydrogel lens implant. *J Cataract Refract Surg* 1987; **13:** 621–6.

20 Menapace R, Amon M, Radax U. Evaluation of 200 consecutive IOGEL 1103 capsular-bag lenses implanted through a small incision. *J Cataract Refract Surg* 1992; **18:** 252–64.

21 Percival P. Prospective study comparing hydrogel with PMMA implants. *Ophthalmic Surg* 1989; **20:** 255–61.

22 Singh G, Bohnke M, von Domarus D, Draeger J. Toxicity of methods of implant material sterilisation on corneal endothelium. *Ann Ophthalmol* 1985; **17:** 727–30.

23 Ng EWM, Barrett GD, Bowman E. In vitro bacterial adherence to hydrogel and PMMA intraocular lenses. *J Cataract Refract Surg* 1996; **22:** 1331–5.

24 Holyk PR, Eifrig DE. Effect of monomeric methymethacrylate on ocular tissues. *Am J Ophthalmol* 1979; **88:** 385–95.

25 Keates RH, Sall KN, Kreter JK. Effect of the Nd:YAG laser on polymethylmethacrylate, HEMA copolymer, and silicone intraocular materials. *J Cataract Refract Surg* 1987; **13:** 401–9.

26 Joo CK, Kim JH. Effect of neodymium:YAG laser photodisruption on intraocular lenses in vitro. *J Cataract Refract Surg* 1992; **18:** 562–6.

27 Kohnen T, Magdowski G, Koch DD. Scanning electron microscopic analysis of foldable and hydrogel lenses. *J Cataract Refract Surg* 1996; **22:** 1342–50.

28 Barrett GD. My technique of IOGEL implantation. *Implants Ophthalmol* 1989; **3:** 45–7.

29 Levy JH, Pisacano AM, Anello RD. Displacement of bag-placed hydrogel lenses into the vitreous following neodymium:YAG laser capsulotomy. *J Cataract Refract Surg* 1990; **16:** 563–6.

30 Menapace R, Yalon M. Exchange of IOGEL hydrogel one-piece foldable intraocular lens for bag-fixated J-loop poly(methylmethacrylate) intraocular lens. *J Cataract Refract Surg* 1993; **19:** 425–30.

31 Barrett GD. A new hydrogel intraocular lens design. *J Cataract Refract Surg* 1994; **20:** 18–25.

32 Lowe KJ, Barrett GD. A comparison of visual function with PMMA and poly HEMA intraocular lenses. *Eur J Implant Refract Surg* 1995; **7:** 271–4.

Chapter 23 **Optical performance of foldable lenses**

Christian J Spaleck

FOLDABLE LENSES: RATIONALE

Although polymethylmethacrylate (PMMA) IOLs have been used with increasing success since Ridley's first implantation in 1949, in time surgeons have become aware of the limitations of this material:

- Despite excellent tissue tolerance, given its rigidity it can produce, in some cases, uveal irritation leading to chronic uveitis.[1–4]
- The large incision necessary to implant a rigid PMMA IOL does not comply with the incision size necessary to remove the cataract by phacoemulsification, which evolved as the state-of-the-art procedure.
- Physical and optical rehabilitation are delayed and then reproducibility of the refractive outcome is decreased by large incisions with induced astigmatism.[5–8]

In addition to faster rehabilitation, the advantages of small-incision surgery include less endothelial cell damage,[9–13] greater wound stability[9,14,15] and increased safety during surgery.[16,17] Foldable IOLs, therefore, are being used with increasing frequency.

The effect of folding on optical performance, however, has been questioned. The optical performance of foldable IOLs is measured by appropriate laboratory testing and by evaluation of clinical data.

LABORATORY TESTING

BACKGROUND

On the basis of chemical composition and physical behavior, contemporary foldable IOLs are subdivided into the groups shown in Table 23.1.

Information on foldable lenses in general must be interpreted with care, since there are great differences between individual generations of the same material.

TRANSMISSION, UV ABSORPTION

Spectral transmissions of visible light do not differ between PMMA and foldable IOL materials. No comparative study of the effectiveness of UV absorbers used in foldable IOL materials has been published. Since the cornea absorbs UV light up to 300 nm and the natural crystalline lens absorbs most of the light between 300 and 400 nm, the cutoff of UV absorbers in IOLs at 400 nm is critical to protect the retina against hazardous UV light after cataract removal.[21–23]

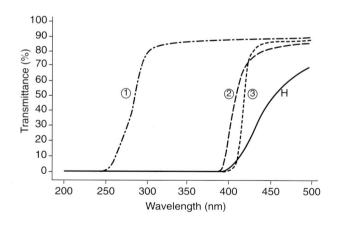

Figure 23.1. *UV and blue light transmission curves of: (1) a non-UV-absorbing PMMA IOL; (2) a silicone UV-absorbing IOL; (3) a PMMA UV-absorbing IOL; (H) the natural crystalline lens.[18]*

Table 23.1

Foldable intraocular lens materials.[18-20]

Material	Chemical composition	Refractive index	Tg (glass transition temperature (°C))	Incision size (mm)
Silicone elastomer	Polysiloxane, side-chains methyl, vinyl, phenyl Hydrophobic			
1st generation		1.41	<100	3.2–3.8
2nd generation		1.43–1.46	<100	3.0–3.2
Hydrogels	PolyHEMA, copolymers of MMA, HOHEXMA, HEMA Plasticizer: water Water content 20–38%			
1st generation		1.43	<0	3.5
2nd generation		1.47	<0–25	3.2–4.0
Foldable acrylics	Copolymers of PEA, PEMA, EA, EMA, TEFMA Water content <1%	1.47–1.55	11–25	3.0–3.8

MMA, methylmethacrylate; HOHEXMA, 6-hydroxyethylmethacrylate; HEMA, 2-hydroxyethylmethacrylate.

BIOCOMPATIBILITY, UV STABILITY

Extensive biocompatibility as well as UV stability evaluation of foldable IOL haptic and optic materials has been carried out. The new materials, i.e. second-generation silicone and hydrogels, as well as foldable acrylic materials, have shown the necessary properties for use in IOLs.[2,11,19,24-28]

OPTICAL PERFORMANCE: RESOLUTION EFFICIENCY, MODULATION TRANSFER FUNCTION (MTF)

Currently, two standards for assessing and describing the imaging quality of monofocal IOLs are in use:

- the standard ANSI Z80.7 1994, which superseded the standard ANSI Z80.7 1984 from the American National Standards Institute;
- the proposed ISO 11979–2 from the International Organization for Standardization.

These standards apply slightly different test configurations and approval limits: 60% resolution efficiency in air and 70% resolution efficiency in aqueous humor with wet cell, respectively, and 0.43 modulation at 100 line pairs/mm in the ISO eye model.

Although resolution is still used to describe the optical performance of IOLs in the more recent literature, the ISO MTF is preferred because it evaluates the IOL in the context of optics of the eye. MTF integrals

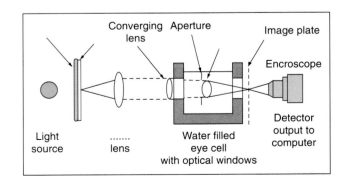

Figure 23.2. *ISO MTF measurement eye cell.*

or contrast at spatial frequencies of particular interest are found to be useful benchmarks of optical quality.[29–34]

For the ISO standard, a 3-mm aperture and 550-nm monochromatic light source are used.

MECHANICAL STABILITY, OPTICAL ABERRATIONS

Unlike rigid IOLs, foldable lenses are made of either elastomers or thermoplastic copolymers with glass

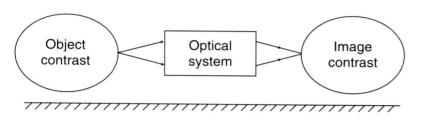

Figure 23.3. *The concept of optical transfer.*[18]

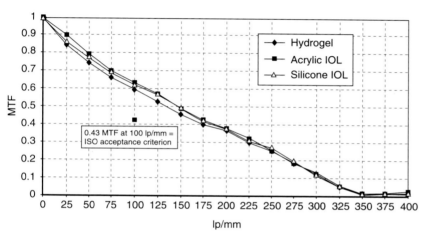

Figure 23.4. *ISO MTF curves of various foldable IOL lens materials, 20 D, 35 °C (unpublished observations).*

Table 23.2

Optical resolution of foldable IOLs.

Author	Year	Material tested	Method	Result
Holladay et al.[35,36]	1987	PMMA silicone, 1st generation	Resolution efficiency (USAF target test)	Silicone >70% in water (similar to PMMA)
Christ et al.[24]	1989	silicone, 1st generation silicone, 2nd generation	Resolution power	241.0 ± 49.1 lp/mm 236.4 ± 19.3 lp/mm
Kulnig et al.[37]	1987	PMMA silicone, 1st generation	Resolution efficiency (eye model)	1.6 (20/20 = 1.0) 1.3
Kulnig et al.[38]	1990	hydrogel, 1st generation silicone, 1st generation	Resolution efficiency (eye model)	1.0 (20/20 = 1.0) 1.3
Knorz et al.[39]	1993	PMMA silicone, 1st generation	MTF through an eye model	PMMA slightly better than silicone

lp, line pairs.

transition temperatures below or just below the room temperature. This means that foldable IOL's optic integrity depends on their hardness, impact resistance, elasticity, viscoelastic rheometry and stress–strain cycling behavior.

Thus foldable IOL optics may become deformed as a result of:

• folding
• instrument contact
• haptic compression due to capsular shrinkage.

All permanent optic deformations will result in decreased optical performance.

During the late 1980s, there were several reports concerning mechanical damage to foldable IOLs, which in most cases resulted from inadequate instrumentation or lack of surgeon experience.

Manipulation and implantation of foldable IOLs require a learning period and the use of appropriate instruments, which must be chosen with regard to the design and the mechanical properties of each individual foldable IOL style.

Silicone has been found to be very stable mechanically.[40] Early hydrogel material was described as being vulnerable to folding instruments.[38] Several articles have dealt with the brittle nature of foldable acrylic leading to cracking or marking[41] or even stress fractures necessitating explantation.[42,43] Warming acrylic lenses to 37 °C is recommended for ease of implantation.

Scanning electron or light microscopic analysis of acrylic and hydrogel IOLs prior to and after folding has revealed excellent surface quality, albeit with mild defects caused by folding or the forceps.[44,45]

Regarding acrylics, permanent optic damage appeared only after prolonged (>20 min) folding, and 60 min of folding did not affect the final MTF.[46] The optical quality of soft acrylic IOLs is not easily affected by deformation and implantation, unless extremely unphysiological manipulations are applied to the lens.

After implantation, foldable IOLs can demonstrate acute optical deformation when the haptics are compressed to 10 mm diameter, in similar fashion to the contraction of the postoperative lens capsule. The degree of this deformation depends mostly upon the elastic modulus of the optic material. Since silicone has a higher elastic modulus than the hydrogel and foldable acrylic materials at room temperature, silicone lenses have less acute optical deformation. The deformation also depends on the haptic design and material.

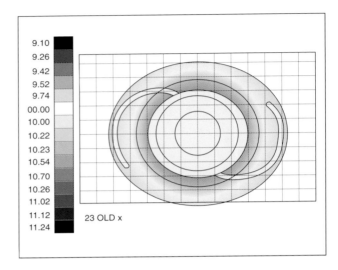

Figure 23.5. *Optical deformation of a silicone lens as a result of haptic compression to 10 mm (unpublished observations).*

Lenticular pseudophakic astigmatism caused by postsurgical haptic compression will probably only be transient for three-piece lenses. Plate haptic lenses made of silicone, however, might retain some degree of permanent pseudophakic lenticular astigmatism (unpublished observations).

CLINICAL OBSERVATIONS

VISUAL ACUITY, INDUCED ASTIGMATISM

Table 23.3 provides a comprehensive overview of clinical visual acuities achieved with different styles of foldable IOLs. Note that the studies are dissimilar and that the data cannot be genuinely compared.

The benefit of foldable lenses with regard to visual performance when compared with PMMA lenses is the result of the small-incision technique. Reduction or even elimination of surgically induced cylinder by sutureless scleral tunnel or clear corneal incisions has been well documented by a large number of investigators who have compared foldable IOLs with PMMA lenses.[5–9,14,51,56,63,81–84]

COLOR VISION, CONTRAST SENSITIVITY, GLARE

Early reports of color vision in eyes with PMMA IOLs revealed similar results to those of normal phakic eyes.[85,86] Color discrimination ability in eyes with silicone IOLs was found to be significantly better in the blue sensitivity test than for normal phakic eyes.[87] No reports regarding color perception with hydrogel or acrylic IOLs have been published.

Contrast sensitivity testing comparing PMMA to silicone material did not reveal statistically significant differences;[39,88] however, in eyes implanted with first-generation silicone IOLs contrast sensitivity may be lower than in eyes with conventional PMMA lenses.[89] In comparison of pseudophakic patients with PMMA, acrylic and silicone IOLs at 6 weeks after surgery, PMMA- and acrylic-implanted eyes had significantly better Regan-contrast sensitivity scores and less glare sensitivity.[90]

IN VIVO CHANGES OF FOLDABLE LENSES: DISCOLORATION, GLISTENING, SURFACE ADHESIONS

For first-generation silicone material, in vivo discoloration has been noted frequently, although significant functional changes have not been reported.[68,91,92]

Unlike silicone lenses, where impurities left by the filtration process can be found, glistenings in one particular foldable acrylic lens are more frequent and may develop over time. These are due to water vapor in the lens. Usually they reach a level of saturation after several months; visual acuity and contrast sensitivity are not affected for grade I glistenings[90] (Mehdorn E, personal communication). Lucke and Bopp, however, found that 17% of 171 eyes had glistenings grades I–III in healthy patients, and severe glistenings (grades II–III) in 37% of diabetics and in 38% of cases with accompanying vitreoretinal disorders (Lucke K, personal communication). It may be possible that an impaired blood–aqueous barrier might trigger water influx into the acrylic implanted material. The incidence of glistenings is also related to other factors such as sterilization and packaging: of 17 patients who received an acrylic lens, which was packaged in the now abandoned AcryPak, all has substantial functional impairment due to glistenings grades II to III.[28] The overall significance of this phenomenon has not been established.

The optical performance of foldable IOLs can also be influenced by interactions of the lens material with

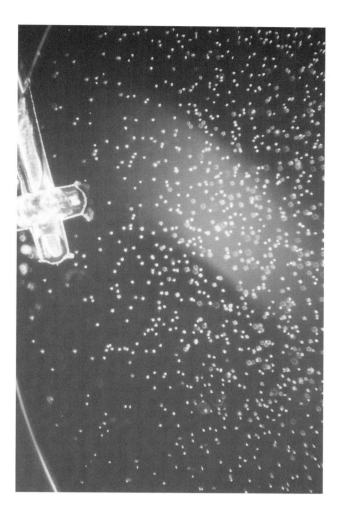

Figure 23.6. *Glistenings in a soft acrylic lens, grade II (courtesy of B. Dick).*

the intraocular environment. For example, dystrophic calcifications within and on the surface of polyHEMA IOLs have been observed.[93] Additionally, Amon and coworkers have reported a correlation between the surface energy of IOL materials and biocompatibility, and suggested this as an explanation for the higher incidence of cell reactions on hydrophobic IOL surfaces, such as silicone.[94,95] Moreover, regarding posterior segment surgery, either during fluid–air exchange or in the presence of silicone oil, silicone IOLs in eyes with open posterior capsules may interfere with fundus visualization.[96,97] Silicone lenses should be avoided in patients who are at high risk of subsequent retinal surgery.

Table 23.3
Visual outcome after implantation of various foldable IOL materials.

Author	Year	Lens style	Number of eyes	Maximum follow up (months)	UCVA (uncorrected visual acuity)	BCVA (best-corrected visual acuity)	Remarks
Stark et al.[47]	1983	PMMA PCIOLs	2524	14	NA	A = 88% bcA = 94%	
FDA grid							
Silicone							
Skorpik et al.[48]	1987	AA4004	50	7	NA	A = 80%	dec/dis = 6%
Neumann et al.[49]	1987	AA4004 AA4203	76	12	NA	A = 96% B = 58%	dec/dis = 11% CME = 3%
Levy and Pisacano[50]	1988	AA4004 AA4203	117	2	NA	A = 81% bcA = 96%	dec/dis = 2.5% CME = 5.8% YAG = 37.5%
Shepherd[51]	1989	AA4004 AA4203	99	3	A = 61%	A = 99%	
Neumann and Cobb[52]	1989	AA4203	76	NA	A = 79%	A = 94% C = 85%	dec/dis = 11%
		PhacoFlex	12	NA	A = 34%	A = 100% C = 17%	dec/dis = 25% YAG = 17%
Levy et al.[53]	1991	Different styles	83	2	NA	bcA = 92.2% bcB = 22.5%	YAG = 39.9%
Koch et al.[54]	1991	Different styles	50	3	D = 80%	D = 89%	
Brint et al.[6]	1991	SI-20	53	1.5	A = 92.5% B = 18.9%	A = 100% B = 66%	
Steinert et al.[5]	1991	SI-20	65	3	A = 70%	NA	
Grabow[55]	1991	AA4004	500	3	A = 83%	NA	
Martin et al.[56]	1992	SI-18	65	3	A = 69.4%	A = 77%	
Uusitalo et al.[14]	1993	SI-18	10	6	A = 90%	NA	
Ernest[57]	1993	SI-30	69	0.5	A = 78%	NA	
Lindstrom and Post[58]	1993	SI-18 SI-26	401	36	NA	bcA = 91%	
Steuhl et al.[59]	1994	SI-19	50	24	NA	mean = 0.6	
Menapace et al.[60]	1994	SI-19 SI-26	100	7.5	NA	A = 89% B = 52%	YAG = 4%
Menapace et al.[61]	1994	SI-30	70	3	NA	B = 58.6% bcB = 67.2%	dec/dis = 8.6%
Artaria et al.[62]	1994	AA4203	100	12	A = 75%	mean = 0.7	CME = 3%
Utrata et al.[63]	1994	AA4203	112	12	A = 68%	NA	
Oshika et al.[7]	1994	SI-30	93	6	A = 85.5% C = 42.9%	A = 100% C = 96.2%	CME = 2.1%

Study	Year	IOL	No.		Mo.	Visual acuity	Complications
Zehetmayer et al.[64]	1994	AA4203	54	NA	54	A = 90.7%	YAG = 13%
Steinert et al.[8]	1995	SI-18	5860	NA	12	A = 90.8% B = 35.9%	CME = 3.2% YAG = 30.2%
			500	NA	36	A = 91.4% B = 36.8%	CME = 1.4%
Irvine et al.[17]	1995	SI-30	210	NA	14	A = 95% B = 86%	
Menapace[65]	1995	SI-30	35	NA	14	bcA = 100%	
Lindstrom[12]	1995	SI-18	560	NA	12	bcA = 100% A = 96% C = 70%	CME = 0.4%
Egan et al.[66]	1996	SI-40	100	NA	12	A = 92%	
Lyle and Jin[67]	1996	Chiron 32C10/10B	50	A = 89%	3	NA	
Milazzo et al.[68]	1996	SI-18	107	NA	60	bcA = 100%	YAG = 40.6% (5y)
Hydrogel							
Percival[69]	1987	Hydrogel	50	NA	6	A = 90% B = 70%	
Condon et al.[70]	1989	Iogel 1000	20	NA	6	A = 100% B = 82%	
Menapace et al.[71]	1989	Iogel PC12	61	NA	6	A = 100% C = 86%	dec/dis = 4.2%
Tingey et al.[72]	1991	Iogel PC12	26	NA	10	mean = 20/23	dec/dis = 28%
Fishkind[73]	1993	Memory lens	500	NA	12	A = 95.4%	
Barrett[74]	1994	Iogel 2000S	67	A = 54%	18	A = 85% C = 71%	dec/dis = 1.5%
Percival[75]	1994	Iogel PC12	125	NA	<60	A = 97% B = 61%	dec/dis = 2%
Percival and Jafree[76]	1994	Iogel 2000S	20	A = 95%	6	A = 100% B = 85%	dec/dis = 10%
Pötzsch and Lösch-Pötzsch[77]	1996	Memory lens	36	NA	48	A = 91.7% B = 63.9%	YAG = 22%
Foldable acrylic							
Anderson et al.[19]	1993	AcrySof	84	NA	6	A = 94% bcA = 98.5%	
Mackool[20]	1993	ACR360 ClariFlex	74	NA	12 24	A = 97.4% A = 95.2%	
Alzner et al.[78]	1995	ACR360 ClariFlex	25	NA	3	mean = 0.7	
Oshika et al.[79]	1996	AcrySof	64	NA	24	bcA = 100%	YAG = 11.1%
Sanchez and Artaria[80]	1996	ACR360 ClariFlex	50	NA	12	A = 100% C = 83%	

A, ≤20/40; B, ≤20/20; C, ≤20/25; D, ≤20/50; bc, best cases; NA, not applicable; dec/dis, decentration/dislocation.

In summary, all foldable lens materials appear to give very satisfactory performance in both optical bench-testing and clinical evaluations. Occasional reports of untoward events are noted, but are far outweighed by the advantages of small-incision cataract surgery, possible only with foldable IOLs.

REFERENCES

1 Apple DH, Mamalis DN, Lotfield K, et al. Complications of intraocular lenses: a historical and histopathological review. *Surv Ophthalmol* 1984; **29:** 1–54.

2 Carlson KH, Cameron JD, Lindstrom RL. Assessment of the blood–aqueous barrier by fluorophotometry following poly(methylmethacrylate), silicone and hydrogel lens implantation in rabbit eyes. *J Cataract Refract Surg* 1993; **19:** 9–15.

3 Joo CK, Kim JH. Compatibility of intraocular lenses blood and connective tissue cells measured by cellular deposition and inflammatory response in vitro. *J Cataract Refract Surg* 1992; **18:** 240–6.

4 Oshika T, Yoshimura K, Miyata N. Postsurgical inflammation after phacoemulsification and extracapsular extraction with soft or conventional intraocular lens implantation. *J Cataract Refract Surg* 1992; **18:** 356–61.

5 Steinert RF, Brint SF, White SM, Fine IH. Astigmatism after small incision cataract surgery: a prospective, randomized, multicenter comparison of 4- and 6.5 mm incisions. *Ophthalmology* 1991; **98:** 417–24.

6 Brint SF, Ostrick DM, Bryan JE. Keratometric cylinder and visual performance following phacoemulsification and implantation with silicone small-incision or poly(methylmethacrylate) intraocular lenses. *J Cataract Refract Surg* 1991; **17:** 32–6.

7 Oshika T, Tsuboi S, Yaguchi S, et al. Comparative study of intraocular lens implantation through 3.2 and 5.5 mm incisions. *Ophthalmology* 1994; **101:** 1183–90.

8 Steinert RF, Bayliss B, Brint SF, et al. Long-term clinical results of AMO PhacoFlex Model SI 18 intraocular lens. *J Cataract Refract Surg* 1995; **21:** 331–8.

9 Gills JP, Sanders DR. *Small-incision Cataract Surgery: Foldable Lenses, One-stitch Surgery, Sutureless Surgery, Astigmatic Keratotomy* (Thorofare, NJ: Slack, 1990) 3–13.

10 Herzog WR, Pfeiffer RL. Comparison of the effect of poly(methylmethacrylate) and silicone intraocular lenses on rabbit corneal endothelium in vitro. *J Cataract Refract Surg* 1987; **13:** 397.

11 Burnstein NL, Ding M, Pratt MV. Intraocular lens evaluation by iris abrasion in vitro: a scanning electron microscopy study. *J Cataract Refract Surg* 1988; **14:** 520.

12 Lindstrom RL. Foldable intraocular lenses. In: Steinert RF, Fine IH, Gimbel HV, et al. *Cataract Surgery: Technique Complications and Management* (Philadelphia PA: Saunders Company, 1995) 279–94.

13 Blumenthal M, Chen V. Soft intraocular lenses. Evolution and potential. In: Percival SPB, ed. *A Color Atlas of Lens Implantation* (London: Wolfe, 1991) 122–4.

14 Uusitalo RJ, Ruusuvara P, Järvinen P, et al. Early rehabilitation after small incision cataract surgery. *Refract Corneal Surg* 1993; **9:** 67–70.

15 Shepherd JR. Small incisions and foldable intraocular lenses. *Int Ophthalmol Clin* 1994; **34:** 102–12.

16 Menapace R, Radax U, Amon M, Papapanos P. No-stitch, small-incision cataract surgery with flexible intraocular lens implantation. *J Cataract Refract Surg* 1994; **20:** 534–42.

17 Irvine S, Francis IC, Kappagoda MB, et al. Prospective study of 210 consecutive cases of endocapsular phacoemulsification using the AMO SI30 NB 3-piece foldable lens. *Aust NZ J Ophthalmol* 1995; **23:** 287–91.

18 Christ FR, Buchen SY, Deacon J, et al. Biomaterials used for intraocular lenses. In: Wise DL, Trantolo DJ, Altobelli DE, et al, eds. *Encyclopedic Handbook of Biomaterials and Bioengineering, Part B: Applications* Vol. 2 (New York: Marcel Dekker, Inc., 1995) 1261–313.

19 Anderson C, Koch DD, Green G, et al. Alcon AcrySof acrylic intraocular lens. In: Martin RG, Gills JP, Sanders DR, eds. *Foldable Intraocular Lenses* (Thorofare, NJ: Slack, 1993) 161–7.

20 Mackool RJ. IOPTEX Acrylens acrylic IOL. In: Martin RG, Gills JP, Sanders DR, eds. *Foldable Intraocular Lenses* (Thorofare, NJ: Slack, 1993) 192.

21 Lindtsrom RL, Doddi N. Ultraviolet light absorption in intraocular lenses. *J Cataract Refract Surg* 1986; **12:** 285–9.

22 Mainster MA. The spectra, classification, and rationale of ultraviolet-protective intraocular lenses. *Am J Ophthalmol* 1986; **102:** 727–32.

23 Werner JS, Spillman L. UV-absorbing intraocular lenses: safety, efficacy, and consequences for the cataract patient. *Graefe's Arch Clin Exp Ophthalmol* 1989; **227:** 248–56.

24 Christ FR, Fencil DA, Van Gent S, et al. Evaluation of the chemical, optical, and mechanical properties of elastomeric intraocular lens material and their clinical significance. *J Cataract Refract Surg* 1989; **15:** 176–84.

25 Buchen SY, Richards SC, Solomon KD, et al. Evaluation of the biocompatibility and fixation of a new silicone intraocular lens in the feline model. *J Cataract Refract Surg* 1989; **15:** 545–53.

26 DeVore DP. Long-term compatibility of intraocular lens implant materials. *J Long-Term Effects Med Implants* 1991; **1:** 205–16.

27 Chapman JM, Cheeks L, Green K. Drug interaction with intraocular lenses of different materials. *J Cataract Refract Surg* 1992; **18:** 456–9.

28 Dhaliwal DK, Mamalis N, Olson RJ, et al. Visual significance of glistenings seen in the AcrySof intraocular lens. *J Cataract Refract Surg* 1996; **22:** 452–7.

29 Grossman LW, Igel DA, Faaland RW. Survey of the optical quality of intraocular implants. *J Cataract Refract Surg* 1991; **17:** 168–74.

30 Faaland RW, Grossman LW, Igel DA. Optical quality testing of monofocal intraocular lens implants with a 3 mm and a 4 mm aperture. *J Cataract Refract Surg* 1991; **17:** 485–90.

31 Simpson MJ. Optical quality of intraocular lenses. *J Cataract Refract Surg* 1992; **18:** 86–94.

32 Portney V. Optical testing and inspection methodology for modern intraocular lenses. *J Cataract Refract Surg* 1992; **18:** 607–13.

33 Grossman LW, Faaland RW. Minimum resolution specification of intraocular lens implants using the modulation transfer function. *Appl Optics* 1993; **23:** 3497–503.

34 Norrby NES. Standardized methods for assessing the imaging quality of intraocular lenses. *Appl Optics* 1995; **34:** 7327–33.

35 Holladay JT, Ting AC, Koester CJ, et al. Intraocular lens resolution in air and in water. *J Cataract Refract Surg* 1987; **13:** 511–17.

36 Holladay JT, Ting AC, Koester CJ, et al. Silicone intraocular lens resolution in air and in water. *J Cataract Refract Surg* 1988; **14:** 657–9.

37 Kulnig W, Menapace R, Skorpik C, et al. Optical resolution of silicone and poly(methylmethacrylate) intraocular lenses. *J Cataract Refract Surg* 1987; **13:** 635–9.

38 Kulnig W, Skorpik C. Optical resolution of foldable intraocular lenses. *J Cataract Refract Surg* 1990; **16:** 211–16.

39 Knorz MC, Lang A, Hsia TC, et al. Comparison of the optical and visual quality of poly(methylmethacrylate) and silicone intraocular lenses. *J Cataract Refract Surg* 1993; **19:** 766–71.

40 Brady DG, Giamporcaro JE, Steinert RF. Effect of folding instruments on silicone intraocular lenses. *J Cataract Refract Surg* 1994; **20:** 310–15.

41 Carlson KH, Johnson DW. Cracking of acrylic intraocular lens during capsular bag insertion. *Ophthalmic Surg Lasers* 1995; **26:** 572–3.

42 Pfister DR. Stress fractures after folding an acrylic intraocular lens. *Am J Ophthalmol* 1996; **121:** 572–4.

43 Lee GA. Cracked acrylic intraocular lens requiring explanation. *Aust NZ J Ophthalmol* 1997; **25:** 71–3.

44 Kohnen T, Magdowski G, Koch DD. Scanning electron microscopic analysis of foldable acrylic and hydrogel lenses. *J Cataract Refract Surg* 1996; **22:** 1342–50.

45 Milazzo S, Turut P, Blin H. Alterations to the AcrySof intraocular lens during folding. *J Cataract Refract Surg* 1996; **22:** 1351–4.

46 Oshika T, Shiokawa Y. Effect of folding on the optical quality of soft acrylic intraocular lenses. *J Cataract Refract Surg* 1996; **22:** 1360–4.

47 Stark WJ, Worthen DM, Holladay JT, et al. The FDA report on intraocular lenses. *Ophthalmology* 1983; **90:** 311–17.

48 Skorpik C, Gnad HD, Menapace R, et al. Evaluation of 50 silicone posterior chamber lens implantations. *J Cataract Refract Surg* 1987; **13:** 640–3.

49 Neumann AC, McCarthy GR, Osher RH. Complications associated with STAAR silicone implants. *J Cataract Refract Surg* 1987; **13:** 653–6.

50 Levy JH, Pisacano AM. Initial clinical studies with silicone intraocular implants. *J Cataract Refract Surg* 1988; **14:** 294–8.

51 Shepherd JR. Induced astigmatism in small incision cataract surgery. *J Cataract Refract Surg* 1989; **15:** 85–8.

52 Neumann AC, Cobb B. Advantages and limitations of current soft intraocular lenses. *J Cataract Refract Surg* 1989; **15:** 257–63.

53 Levy JH, Pisacano AM, Anello RD. Clinical results with silicone intraocular implants. *Eur J Implant Refract Surg* 1991; **3:** 7–12.

54 Koch PD, Bradley H, Sewnson N. Visual acuity recovery rates following cataract surgery and implantation of soft intraocular lenses. *J Cataract Refract Surg* 1991; **17:** 143–7.

55 Grabow HB. Early results of 500 cases of no stitch cataract surgery. *J Cataract Refract Surg* 1991; **17:** 726–30.

56 Martin RG, Sanders DR, Van Der Karr MA, et al. Effect of small incision intraocular lens surgery on postoperative inflammation and astigmatism: a study of the AMO SI-18NB small incision lens. *J Cataract Refract Surg* 1992; **18:** 51–7.

57 Ernest PH. AMO SI-30 high refractive index three piece silicone IOL. In: Martin RG, Gills JP, Sanders DR, eds. *Foldable Intraocular Lenses* (Thorofare, NJ: Slack, 1993) 55.

58 Lindstrom RL. Post CT. AMO SI-18NB and SI-26NB three piece silicone IOLs. In: Martin RG, Gills JP, Sanders DR, eds. *Foldable Intraocular Lenses* (Thorofare, NJ: Slack, 1993) 31.

59 Steuhl KP, Schuller S, Frohn A, et al. Centration, endothelial cell count and functional results after implantation of foldable intraocular lenses. *Eur J Implant Refract Surg* 1994; **6:** 93–7.

60 Menapace R, Amon M, Papapanos P, et al. Evaluation of the first 100 consecutive PhacoFlex silicone lenses implanted in the bag through a self sealing tunnel incision using the Prodigy inserter. *J Cataract Refract Surg* 1994; **20:** 299–309.

61 Menapace R, Radax U, Vass L, Amon M, Papapanos P. In-the-bag implantation of the PhacoFlex SI-30 high refractive silicone lens through self sealing sclerocorneal and clear corneal incisions. *Eur J Implant Refract Surg* 1994; **6:** 181–2.

62 Artaria LG, Ziliotti F, Ziliotti-Mandelli A. Long-term follow-up of implantation of foldable silicone posterior lenses. *Klin Monatsbl Augenheilk* 1994; **204:** 268–70.

63 Utrata PJ, Sanders DR, De Luca M, et al. Small incision surgery with the STAAR Elastimide three-piece posterior chamber intraocular lens. *J Cataract Refract Surg* 1994; **20:** 426–31.

64 Zehetmayer M, Skorpik C, Weghaupt H, et al. Long-term results of implantation of a plate haptic silicone lens in the capsular bag. *Klin Monatsbl Augenheilk* 1994; **204:** 220–5.

65 Menapace R. Evaluation of 35 consecutive SI-30 PhacoFlex lenses with high refractive silicone optic implanted in the capsulorhexis bag. *J Cataract Refract Surg* 1995; **12:** 339–47.

66 Egan CA, Kottos PJ, Francis IC, et al. Prospective study of the SI-40NB foldable silicone intraocular lens. *J Cataract Refract Surg* 1996; **22:** 1272–6.

67 Lyle WA, Jin GJC. Prospective evaluation of early visual and refractive effects with small clear corneal incision for cataract surgery. *J Cataract Refract Surg* 1996; **22:** 1456–60.

68 Milazzo S, Turut P, Artin B, et al. Long-term follow-up of three-piece, looped, silicone intraocular lenses. *J Cataract Refract Surg* 1996; **22:** 1259–62.

69 Percival SPB. Capsular bag implantation of the hydrogel lens. *J Cataract Refract Surg* 1987; **13:** 627–9.

70 Condon PI, Barrett GD, Kinsella M. Results of the intercapsular technique with the Iogel lens. *J Cataract Refract Surg* 1989; **15:** 495–503.

71 Menapace R, Skorpik C, Juchem M, et al. Evaluation of the first 60 cases of poly-HEMA posterior chamber lenses implanted in the sulcus. *J Cataract Refract Surg* 1989; **15:** 254–71.

72 Tingey DP, Nichols BD, Jung SE, et al. Corneal endothelial response to poly(methylmethacrylate) versus hydrogel lenses after phacoemulsification. *Can J Ophthalmol* 1991; **26:** 3–6.

73 Fishkind WJ. ORC MemoryLens: a thermoplastic IOL. In: Martin RG, Gills JP, Sanders DR, eds. *Foldable Intraocular Lenses* (Thorofare, NJ: Slack, 1993) 213.

74 Barrett GD. A new hydrogel lens design. *J Cataract Refract Surg* 1994; **20:** 18–25.

75 Percival SPB. Five year follow-up of a prospective study comparing hydrogel with PMMA single piece lenses. *Eur J Implant Refract Surg* 1994; **6:** 10–13.

76 Percival SPB, Jafree AJ. Preliminary results with a new hydrogel intraocular lens. *Eye* 1994; **8:** 672–5.

77 Pötzsch D, Lösch-Pötzsch CM. Four year follow-up of the MemoryLens. *J Cataract Refract Surg* 1996; **22:** 1336–41.

78 Alzner E, Mistlberger A, Grabner G. Erste Erfahrungen mit einer neuen Generation Kleinschnittlinsen: Die weiche Acryllinse von IOPTEX (Type ACR 360). *Spektrum Augen* 1995; **9:** 27–9.

79 Oshika T, Suzuki Y, Kizaki H, et al. Two year clinical study of a soft acrylic intraocular lens. *J Cataract Refract Surg* 1996; **22:** 104–9.

80 Sanchez E, Artaria L. Evaluation of the first 50 ACR360 acrylic intraocular lens implantations. *J Cataract Refract Surg* 1996; **22:** 1373–8.

81 Oshika T, Tsuboi S. Astigmatic and refractive stabilization after cataract surgery. *Ophthalmic Surg* 1995; **26:** 309–15.

82 Pfleger T, Skorpik C, Menapace R, et al. Long-term course of induced astigmatism after clear corneal incision cataract surgery. *J Cataract Refract Surg* 1996; **22:** 72–7.

83 Afsarl A, Patel S, Woods RL, Wykes W. Visual performance in pseudophakia comparing foldable with one-piece PMMA intraocular lenses. *Invest Ophthalmol Vis Sci* 1997; **15:** S546 (abstract 2537-B227).

84 Holweger RR, Marefat B. Corneal changes after cataract surgery with 5.0 mm sutured and 3.5 mm sutureless clear corneal incisions. *J Cataract Refract Surg* 1997; **23:** 342–6.

85 Harper RA, Kirkness CM, Jay B. Colour discrimination in pseudophakia. *Eye* 1988; **2:** 382–9.

86 Marré M, Marré E, Harrer S. Farbensehen bei Katarakt, Aphakie und Pseudophakie. *Klin Monatsbl Augenheilk* 1988; **192:** 208–15.

87 Mäntyjärvi M, Tuppurainen K. Color vision in patients with a silicone intraocular lens. *J Cataract Refract Surg* 1996; **22:** 1308–12.

88 Skorpik C, Gottlob I, Weghaupt H. Comparison of contrast sensitivity between posterior chamber lenses of silicone and PMMA material. *Graefe's Arch Clin Exp Ophthalmol* 1989; **227**(5): 413–14.

89 Johansen J, Dan-Johansen M, Olsen T. Contrast sensitivity with silicone and poly(methylmethacrylate) intraocular lenses. *J Cataract Refract Surg* 1997; **23:** 1085–8.

90 Kohnen S, Ferrer A, Brauweiler P. Visual function in pseudophakic eyes with poly(methylmethacrylate), silicone and acrylic intraocular lenses. *J Cataract Refract Surg* 1996; **22:** 1303–7.

91 Milauskas AT, Kershner RM, Ziemba SL. Silicone intraocular lens implant discoloration in humans. *Arch Ophthalmol* 1991; **109:** 913–15.

92 Skorpik C, Menapace R, Scholz U, et al. Erste Erfahrungen mit Disclinsen aus Silikonmaterial. *Klin Monatsbl Augenheilk* 1993; **202:** 8–13.

93 Bucher PJ, Buchi ER, Daicker BC. Dystrophic calcification of an hydroxyethylmethacrylate intraocular lens. *Arch Ophthalmol* 1995; **113:** 1431–15.

94 Amon M, Menapace R. In vitro documentation of cellular reactions on lens-surfaces for assessing the biocompatibility of different intraocular implants. *Eye* 1994; **8:** 649–56.

95 Amon M, Menapace R, Radax U, et al. In vivo study of cell reactions on poly(methylmethacrylate) intraocular lenses with different surface properties. *J Cataract Refract Surg* 1996; **22:** 825–9.

96 Eaton AM, Jaffe GJ, McCuen II BW, et al. Condensation on the posterior surface of silicone intraocular lenses during fluid–air exchange. *Ophthalmology* 1995; **102:** 733–6.

97 Apple DJ, Federman JL, Krolicki TJ, et al. Irreversible silicone oil adhesion to silicone intraocular lenses. *Ophthalmology* 1996; **103:** 1555–62.

Chapter 24 Prevention of posterior capsule opacification after cataract surgery: theoretical and practical solutions

Okihiro Nishi

INTRODUCTION

Posterior capsule opacification (PCO) is the most frequent postoperative complication associated with decreased vision, and occurs with an incidence of up to 50% within 5 years after cataract surgery. Various mechanical, pharmaceutical and immunologic techniques have been applied in attempts to prevent PCO by removing or killing residual lens epithelial cells (LECs), but none has been confirmed to be satisfactorily practical, effective and safe for routine clinical practice.

However, there is evidence that some surgical techniques or some types of intraocular lens (IOLs) can help reduce the incidence of PCO by inhibiting the migration of LECs.[1] From a practical point of view, it is therefore of special importance to analyze how these factors affect the inhibition of migrating LECs. Herein, various methods of reducing the incidence of PCO are presented and discussed from theoretical and practical perspectives. The future direction of various pharmaceutical measures is also briefly overviewed.

CHARACTERISTICS OF POSTOPERATIVE PROLIFERATION OF LECS IN THE EMPTY CAPSULAR BAG

An understanding of the postoperative proliferation of LECs is important for efforts at PCO prevention. Residual LECs proliferate at the pre-equatorial germinative zone and migrate posteriorly onto the posterior capsule postoperatively. When the anterior capsule comes into contact with the posterior capsule, the LECs underneath the anterior capsule also migrate onto the posterior capsule abundantly, before the two capsules adhere and grow together, when collagen fibers are produced by the LECs undergoing fibrous metaplasia. The apposition of the anterior capsule on the posterior capsule can induce PCO of the fibrosis type,. because the LECs at the anterior capsular margin traumatized by capsulotomy undergo fibrous proliferation, regarded as a wound-healing process.

The IOL present in the capsular bag can inhibit migrating LECs by inducing contact inhibition. When the IOL is in the capsular bag, the IOL optic can separate both capsules, and hinder the LEC migration from the anterior capsular edge onto the posterior capsule. The inhibition of migrating LECs and the separation by the IOL optic of the capsules are the main reasons why the incidence of PCO is significantly lower in eyes with an IOL than in those without one.[2]

These effects are greater when the IOL is present in the capsular bag. The LECs also undergo fibrous proliferation when they come into contact with an IOL, causing fibrous opacification in the anterior and posterior capsules. In this event, so-called fibrous metaplasia of LECs, the LECs produce various cytokines and prostaglandin E_2,[5] which can disrupt the blood–aqueous barrier (BAB), resulting, eventually, in fibrin reactions.

Additionally, there is an age-related tendency of PCO formation:[3,4] older patients show a lower incidence of PCO indicating greater viability of youthful LECs.

METHODS AND FACTORS REDUCING THE INCIDENCE OF PCO

SURGICAL TECHNIQUES

Continuous curvilinear capsulotomy

There is no doubt that continuous curvilinear capsulotomy (CCC) can help reduce PCO by rendering the secure in-the-bag placement of an IOL. Recent reports[6,7] indicate that it is extremely important to create a well-centered CCC of the correct size for the prevention of migrating LECs. The CCC edge should be smaller than the IOL optic and cover its margin. Any decentered, oversized CCC or incomplete CCC with a radial tear will result in the apposition of both capsules. Even though the area lies in a very limited circumference, the LECs migrate from the edge of the anterior capsule onto the posterior capsule, causing PCO (Fig. 24.1).

Removal of residual LECs

LECs can easily be removed mechanically by aspiration or ultrasound aspiration.[8] Theoretically, thorough removal of residual LECs may prevent PCO. It has, however, proven to be very difficult to thoroughly remove LECs. No conclusive data are available. The technique requires additional surgical time, which can result in increased surgical trauma and, therefore, increased disruption of the BAB. Incomplete removal may rather provoke the proliferation of LECs by traumatizing them, which can also result in the increased disruption of the BAB, and poses an obstacle to atraumatic surgery that will reduce PCO. All these drawbacks preclude the routine use of the technique.

However, the fibrosis and shrinkage of the anterior capsule can be reduced or delayed by removal of LECs.[9] Therefore, the technique can be applied for eyes predisposed to anterior capsular fibrosis with shrinkage,[10–12] such as in retinitis pigmentosa and diabetic cataract.

The residual lens fiber cells that remain on the posterior capsule no longer have a cell nucleus and, therefore, are not capable of proliferation. They will be autolysed or spontaneously digested postoperatively, for which reason posterior capsule polishing was abandoned.

Atraumatic surgery and postoperative inflammation

Clinical and pathologic examinations have provided evidence that proliferation and metaplasia of residual

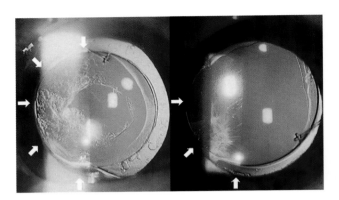

Figure 24.1. *Retroillumination slit lamp findings for the lens capsule with an AcrySof IOL. Note that the LECs have migrated from the anterior capsule positioned on the posterior capsule (arrows), forming Elschnig's pearls (left) or fibrosis (right). No LEC migration was found where the anterior capsule was positioned on the IOL optic. These figures show clearly the importance of the apposition of the CCC edge on the IOL.*

LECs are often related to the amount and duration of anterior segment inflammation intra- and postoperatively.[1,13] Atraumatic surgery, which is enhanced by small-incision surgery, is therefore of great importance. On the other hand, there is still no conclusive evidence that existing enhanced postoperative inflammation will increase the incidence of PCO. There are also some contradictory observations: out-of-the-bag fixation decreased inflammation,[14] but increased the incidence of PCO.

Non-steroidal anti-inflammatory drugs (NSAIDs) are effective in decreasing the postoperative inflammation,[15–17] particularly the form that is specifically caused by residual LECs producing various cytokines, including prostaglandin E_2.[5] NSAIDs also inhibited LEC proliferation, at least in vitro,[17] and might be efefctive in vivo as well.[18] We recommend the topical use of NSAIDs for at least 3 months postoperatively.

IOL DESIGN AND MATERIAL

Optic design

Optic surface

Many clinical and experimental studies have revealed that the posterior convexity appears to help retard LEC migration, and surgeons in general agree that a biconvex IOL should be used for the prevention of

PCO, at least for Elschnig's pearl formation.[19–22] A high rate of early fibrosis was noted with the posterior convexity.[20] This is understandable, because the posteriorly migrated LECs may be prompted or induced to undergo fibrous metaplasia by the tight contact with the posterior convex surface of the IOL. These LECs might later have formed Elschnig's pearls, had there not been tight adherence between the LECs and the IOL. On the other hand, some surgeons think that the planoconvex IOL reduces the incidence of PCO more significantly than does the biconvex IOL.[23,24] We think that the results should be interpreted less in terms of the optic surface (biconvex IOL versus planoconvex IOL) and more in regard to the optic edge, as discussed below.

Surface-modified IOLs such as heparin surface-modified IOLs[25] should reduce the PCO, but there are no conclusive data.

Optic edge and ridge

The laser ridge introduced first by Hoffer and originally conceived as hindering migrating LECs[1] is reportedly effective in the inhibition of migrating LECs,[26,27] but there are also reports indicating otherwise.[20,28] The effect of the sharp, meniscus-designed ridge of a posterior concave IOL is also controversial. Apple et al.[1] believe that the variable effects of these ridges are related to the differences in realization among the surgeons of the complete in-the-bag fixation of the IOL. The effect in retarding migrating LECs of a planoconvex IOL, as noted above and reported by Nagata[23] and Yamada,[24] is due to the sharp edge of the planoconvex IOL, which exerts compression on the posterior capsule, according to these authors. As noted, these ridge effects depend decisively on the capsular bag fixation of the IOL and on having a proper-sized, well-centered CCC. However, the anatomic particulars of the anterior segment, such as the capsular size, its position relative to the ciliary bodies and vitreous pressure, surely constitute another important factor, for the edge or ridge effect can be expected only when the posterior capsule is stretched tautly, and therefore forms a taut contact with the edge or ridge.

Haptic design

The one-piece polymethylmethacrylate (PMMA) IOL reportedly carries a lower incidence of PCO than does the three-piece IOL with polypropylene loops.[29] This difference is accounted for by the compressibility, rigidity and memory of the IOL. The polypropylene loops, with their higher compressibility and lesser rigidity and memory, are generally less likely to exert tautness or stretch on the posterior capsule, which maintains firm contact with the IOL optic, retarding LEC migration.[1] However, Davison[30] reported good results for a three-piece 12.0-mm IOL. The circular haptic IOL[31,32] reportedly reduced PCO. This type of IOL was, however, abandoned because of the technical difficulty in capsular bag placement, under conditions ensuring the preventive effect. An expansible disk lens or 'full-size IOL'[33] made of hydrogel also reportedly reduced PCO in animal studies. However, in our experience,[34,35] PCO occurred at an incidence of almost 100% even in the early postoperative period in rabbits and monkeys, even though the capsular bag was refilled tautly with silicone compounds, providing 'no space'.

The concept underlying all these IOL design-dependent factors preventing PCO for the one-piece IOL, biconvex, planoconvex, circular haptic or even full-size IOL is that they stretch the posterior capsule, which then inhibits LEC migration by direct compression, providing 'no space'. However, we think that the tautness or stretch of the posterior capsule fostered by the posterior convexity of the one-piece PMMA IOL or the sharp edge of the planoconvex IOL may help to create a firm capsular bend or angle at the optic edge rather than providing 'no space' or compression, and that this may be the factor more relevant to lowering the incidence of PCO.

Creation of discontinuous capsular bend by optic and haptic

We think, based on our recent studies, that in the inhibition of migrating LECs by these factors, an additional, but seemingly substantial, factor may be involved: inhibition of migrating LECs by discontinuous capsular bend that induces contact inhibition of LECs. We have already proposed creation of a discontinuous capsular bend or angle in the posterior capsule as a new concept for the prevention of PCO.[36] The rationale is based on our clinical and in vitro observations of LECs. On a histological section, we observed that, after an endocapsular IOL had dislocated posteriorly into the vitreous and was removed, migrating LECs were inhibited at the distinct capsular bend created by the planoconvex optic (Fig. 24.2). We also observed that LECs were inhibited on rectangular-shaped well bottoms in culture. During culture, LECs cease to proliferate due to contact inhibition when the LECs reach the rectangular well wall; this is known as 'confluent culture'.

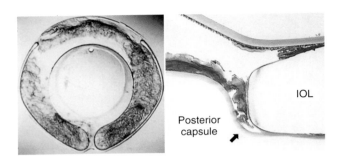

Figure 24.2. *Left: Macroscopic view of the explanted IOL that had spontaneously dislocated into the vitreous. The migrating LECs were obviously inhibited at the optic edge. Right: Histopathologic appearance of the capsular bag. LEC migration was stopped at the capsular bend created by the planoconvex optic edge (arrow). PC, posterior capsule. (Courtesy of* Journal of Cataract and Refractive Surgery *1996;* **22:** *272–5.)*

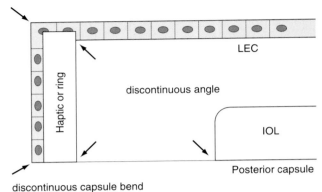

Figure 24.4. *Schematic representation of discontinuous capsular bend or angle. Migrating LECs can be inhibited there by contact inhibition.*

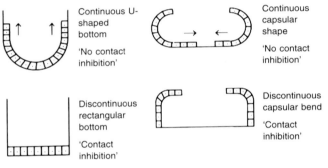

Figure 24.3. *Left: Schematic representation of the observation of migration and contact inhibition of LECs cultured in a well. Right: Migration and contact inhibition of LECs in the capsular bag which can be expected in an analogous manner as observed in the left.*

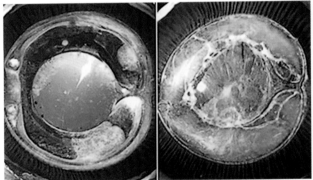

Figure 24.5. *Left: A rabbit lens capsule implanted with an IOL with a sharp-edged, band-shaped haptic like that shown in Fig. 24.4. Note that the migrating LECs are confined around the haptic. Right: Control. (By permission of* Ophthalmic Surg Lasers *1998;* **29:** *119–25.)*

However, along the wall of the U-shaped wells, LECs grew and ascended (Fig. 24.3, left). All these findings suggest that a sharp bend in the capsule can induce contact inhibition of LECs migrating on the capsule (Fig. 24.3, right). Such a bend or angle can be created by a capsule tension ring or an IOL with sharp optic edges inducing contact inhibition as illustrated in Fig. 24.4. In fact, a wide, sharp-edged, band-shaped, circular haptic of an IOL or band-shaped capsule bending ring significantly inhibited migrating LECs in rabbits (Fig. 24.5).[36]

We think that the effect of the Hoffer ridge, meniscus ridge and sharp planoconvex edge may be attributed to this concept. These ridges and edge can create a discontinuous capsular bend or angle that inhibits migrating LECs. The conflicting results obtained with this barrier edge or ridge may be caused by the different surgical techniques and the anatomy of the individual anterior segment, as discussed above. Because these IOLs were mainly used before the advent and widespread adoption of CCC, which allows secure in-the-bag fixation of an

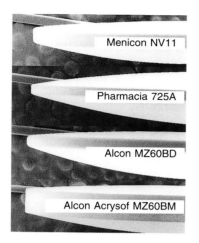
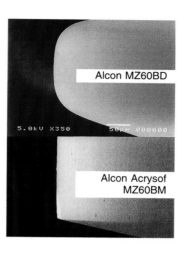

Figure 24.6. *Design of the optic edge of various IOL designs. Note the sharp, rectangular edge of the AcrySof IOL, compared to the smooth and rounded edges of the other IOL. (By permission of* Ophthalmic Surg Lasers.)

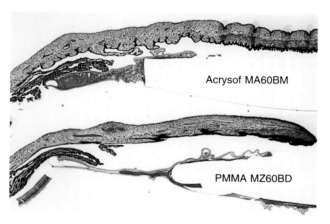
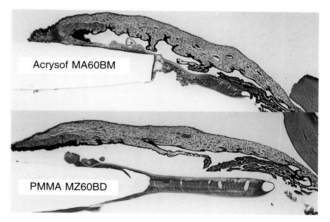

Figure 24.7. *Inhibition of migrating LECs at the sharp capsular bend created by the keen edge of an AcrySof IOL in a rabbit eye 3 weeks after surgery. These findings show clearly the reason for the lower incidence of PCO reported for this IOL. (By permission of* Ophthalmic Surg Lasers.)

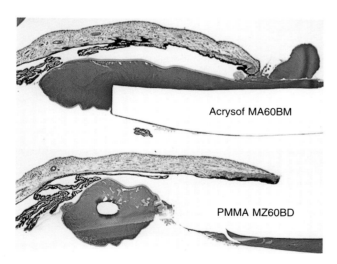
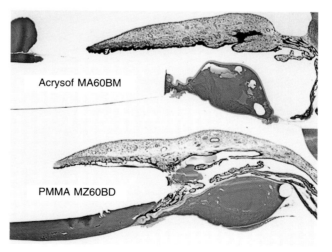

Figure 24.8. *Inhibition of migrating LECs at the sharp rectangle between the posterior capsule and the optic edge (left) and capsular bend (right) 4 weeks after surgery. (By permission of* Ophthalmic Surg Lasers.)

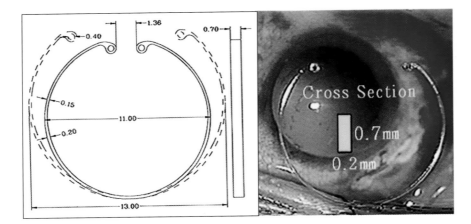

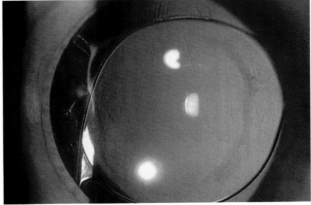

Figure 24.9. *Band-shaped capsule bending ring made from PMMA, which creates a discontinuous capsular bend. The sharp, unpolished edge is critical. (By permission of* Ophthalmic Surg Lasers.*)*

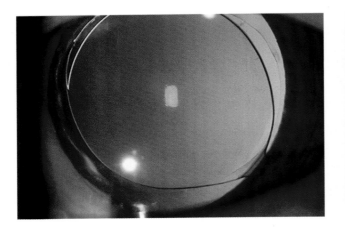

Figure 24.10. *Retroillumination findings of the lens capsule in an eye with a capsule bending ring (left) and without (right) 1 year after surgery. Note that the CCC opening is kept wide and free from fibrosis, and the posterior capsule is clear in the eye with the ring, compared to that without the ring.* (By permission of Ophthalmic Surg Lasers.)

IOL, we wonder whether these planoconvex edge or ridge IOLs might not reduce the incidence of PCO if they were reintroduced.

Creation of discontinuous capsular bend by optic edge or capsule bending ring

The AcrySof IOL reportedly has a significantly low incidence of PCO.[37,38] Our recent studies indicate that this effect may be due to the sharp and rectangular edge design of the AcrySof IOL (Fig. 24.6). The histopathologic findings for the lens capsule containing an AcrySof IOL in rabbits disclosed that the lens capsule wrapped the IOL so firmly that it conformed faithfully to the rectangular sharp optic edge of the IOL (Figs 24.7 and 24.8), and that migrating LECs were

obviously inhibited at this capsular bend or angle created by the sharp edge and posterior capsule.[39] This bend seems to have induced contact inhibition of migrating LECs. The creation of such a bend or angle requires a well-centered CCC, smaller than the IOL optic, so that the CCC edge was in apposition to the optic. On the other hand, it may be dependent not only on the rectangular edge design but also on the features of the IOL material, such as adhesiveness. Nagata[40] reported that the AcrySof IOL had triple the adhesiveness to a collagen film compared to the PMMA IOL. The adhesiveness may help to facilitate the creation of such a bend or angle. Moreover, the acrylic material itself may have effects on the inhibition of migrating LECs. It is clearly of particular importance to analyze which factor, design or material of the IOL provides inhibition of migrating LECs for the development of a new IOL designed for PCO prevention (see below), and we think that the creation of a discontinuous capsular bend is a promising design concept.

Another possibility for creating a capsular bend is the capsule bending ring (Fig. 24.9).[41] As illustrated, Menapace and we modified this ring for use in humans. The ring is 11 mm in overall length, and 0.7 mm in width. The sharp edge is critical. Menapace, Tetz and I are now conducting a multicenter clinical trial with this ring. Evaluation of the preventive effect on PCO requires a longer follow-up, but a distinctly preventive effect on the anterior capsule fibrosis was observed. Because of the band shape, the anterior capsule did not come into contact with the IOL or posterior capsule, fibrosis and constriction of the CCC opening thus being prevented (Fig. 24.10).

IOL material (foldable IOL)

The introduction of new foldable IOLs encouraged small-incision surgery, and the preference for foldable IOLs is steadily increasing. The materials used heretofore are acrylic copolymer, hydrogel and silicone. While there are no conclusive data regarding the difference between the incidence of PCO for silicone IOLs and that for PMMA IOLs, silicone IOLs cause more intense capsular fibrosis and, therefore, the constriction of the CCC.[7,42] A newly developed hydrogel IOL led to a high incidence of Elschnig's pearl formation,[43] while capsular fibrosis was very mild. The AcrySof IOL, made from acrylic material, carries a lower incidence than any other type of IOL.[37,38] It is of importance to elucidate its preventive effect on PCO and whether the effect is design-dependent, material-dependent or both, as discussed above. Ursell et al. reported[38] that the lower incidence of PCO with the AcrySof IOL may be material-dependent and is unlikely to be design-dependent in the comparative study with silicone and PMMA IOLs. However, in our recent rabbit study, migrating LECs were inhibited equally after an AcrySof IOL was implanted in one eye and a PMMA IOL with sharp rectangular optic edges similar to those of the AcrySof IOL was implanted in the fellow eye (unpublished data). This indicates that the preventive effect on PCO of an AcrySof IOL is design-dependent. However, this may be eventually corroborated by the comparative study of acrylic IOLs with sharp versus rounded edges.

It is now clear that there are three main factors to be considered that most influence the creation of a sharp bend in the capsule and the PCO incidence: design, material and a well-centered CCC apposi-

Table 24.1

Factors influencing the creation of a sharp bend in the capsule

---

Design of IOL
- sharp rectangular edges
- posterior convexity
- steep loop angle

Materials for IOL
- adhesiveness
- lesser degree of fibrosis (biocompatibility)

Surgical technique
- a well-centered CCC smaller than the IOL optic
- removal of LEC

---

tioned to the optic edge. The factors involved are listed in Table 24.1. When we carry out a study on PCO incidence as an outcome criterion, we must be aware of making these factors equivalent. In the study, the CCC edge should always lie on the IOL optic, and the IOL should be used with the same design but different material, and vice versa. This will make future studies more scientific, rendering the obtained data accurate, exact and reliable.

PHARMACEUTICAL MEASURES FOR THE PREVENTION OF PCO

There is still no pharmaceutical agent that is routinely used clinically. In this chapter, therefore, a brief overview is presented of the future potential.

Antimetabolites

Various antimetabolites, such as methotrexate, daunomycin, daunorubicin, 5-fluorouracil (5-FU), mitomycin or colchicine, are effective in inhibiting LECs in vitro. In vivo animal studies have shown, however, that whether the drugs are applied in a sustained-release fashion or as a single injection, toxic effects on the corneal endothelial cells, iris, ciliary pigment epithelial cells and retinal cells are inevitable when the antimetabolite is used at a sufficiently high concentration significantly to inhibit LECs. In an attempt to inhibit more specifically LECs but avoid side-effects on the other ocular tissues, an immunotoxin, an anti-LEC monoclonal antibody (missile) that binds specifically to LECs and carries ricin (a toxic plant protein) (bomb) was used.[44] This method is being tested in humans in a 2-year study involving 63 patients undergoing cataract surgery. A certain amount of this immunotoxin was instilled into the anterior segment at the end of surgery, and a significant reduction in lens capsule opacification was observed up to 24 months postsurgery. Behar-Cohen et al.[45] showed that the fibroblast growth factor (FGF) 2-saporin inhibited bovine LECs in vitro and reduced PCO in in vivo animal studies. A lens epithelial necrosis factor inhibited LECs in in vitro and experimental studies.[46] Further study is necessary on these methods to confirm the effect and the avoidance of the side-effects.

Other agents

Hypo-osmotic sterile water has been used to cause LEC osmolysis during surgery. Indomethacin, an NSAID, can inhibit LECs in vitro.[14] In vivo animal studies have shown that the agent can inhibit LECs when it is coated on the IOL surface and brought into direct contact with LECs.[47] However, sustained release of the agent has been confirmed to be ineffective.[48,49] The LECs may accommodate to the toxicity of the agent, and the threshold may become higher. This accommodation issue should be noted in future research when a drug is used in sustained-release preparations. Dispase, a proteolytic enzyme, or EDTA, a calcium-chelating substance used for cell dispersion, were used in in vivo animal experiments to loosen the junctional complexes of LECs with the underlying lens capsule, thus facilitating mechanical removal of the LECs.[50] Despite loosening, thorough mechanical removal of LECs having the effect of reducing the PCO incidence is still extremely difficult to perform.

Migrating LECs were significantly inhibited by sustained release of EDTA and RGD peptides (arginine–glycine–aspartic acid sequence),[51] which inhibit the expression of β-integrins on the LEC surface. The adhesion molecule integrin is involved in the migration of LECs onto the posterior capsule.[52]

PMMA lenses coated with thapsigargin, a hydrophobic inhibitor of endoplasmic reticulum Ca^{2+}-ATPase, reduced cell growth in the capsular bag in vitro. These investigations (including those with immunotoxin and FGF-saporin studies) indicate that the molecular biological approach is the future way for the pharmaceutical prevention of PCO.

As shown, all these methods are sufficiently effective in in vitro or in vivo animal studies, but clinical application of the methods is extremely difficult: the optimal concentration and sustained-release duration must be determined, and these can surely be very different individually; side-effects must be avoided; and the release method must not interfere with the optical system and surgical procedure. Toward these ends, the capsular bending ring may be an appropriate carrier.

Sustained release of a toxic substance appears to us unlikely to be clinically realized in the near future. Should a side-effect occur, the drug source must be removed surgically. A single injection might be more realistic, but the effect might be limited.

CONCLUSION

Based on this overview of the various methods of prevention of PCO, we feel, from the practical point of view, that we should now pay much more attention not to removing and killing LECs but to inhibiting the migrating LECs. The effectiveness of the surgical technique and IOL design has been a somewhat inadvertent byproduct of the process of the development of surgical procedures for effective and safe removal of a cataract and implantation of an IOL. We should now make much more intentional efforts to improve the IOL design and material specifically for the prevention of PCO. In this regard, I think creation of a sharp, rectangular capsular bend is a novel promising concept.

In conclusion, some surgical techniques and some types of IOL help reduce the incidence of PCO. There are still no conclusive data regarding the pharmaceutical measures, and the clinical application appears to be very difficult. Improving the IOL design or material appears to be a more practical means of further reducing the PCO incidence. The creation of a sharp, rectangular capsular bend appears to be a promising concept, and the creation of such a bend by improving the IOL design or material, as seen with an AcrySof IOL or obtained by utilizing a capsule bending ring, seems to be realistic. Currently, we recommend the following techniques for PCO prevention:

1) Creating a 4–4.5-mm CCC, smaller than the optic diameter, but complete and well-centered, so that the anterior capsule apposes the IOL edge.
2) Implanting a foldable AcrySof IOL, rendering the creation of a sharp, rectangular capsular bend

which induces contact inhibition of migrating LECs. The adhesiveness may help to create such a bend a provide stability and centering within the capsular bag.

3) Additionally, using an NSAID for 3 months postoperatively, in order to reduce postoperative inflammation and possibly proliferation of residual LECs.

REFERENCES

1 Apple DR, Solomon K, Tetz M, et al. Posterior capsule opacification. *Surv Ophthalmol* 1992; **37:** 73–116.

2 Nishi O. Incidence of posterior capsule opacification in eyes with and without chamber intraocular lenses. *J Cataract Refract Surg* 1986; **12:** 519–22.

3 Maltzman B, Hampt E, Notis C. Relationship between age at time of cataract extraction and time interval before capsulotomy for opacification. *Ophthalmic Surg* 1989; **20:** 321–4.

4 Oliver M, Milstein A, Pollack A. Posterior chamber lens implantation in infants and juveniles. *Eur J Implant Refract Surg* 1990; **2:** 309–14.

5 Nishi O, Nishi K, Imanishi M. Synthesis of interleukin-1 and prostaglandin E2 by lens epithelial cells of human cataracts. *Br J Ophthalmol* 1992; **76:** 338–41.

6 Ravalico G, Tognetto D, Palomba MA, Busatto P, Baccara F. Capsulorhexis size and posterior capsule opacification. *J Cataract Refract Surg* 1996; **22:** 98–103.

7 Hayashi K, Hayashi H, Nakao F, Hayashi F. Reduction in the area of the anterior capsule opening after polymethylmethacrylate, silicone, and soft acrylic intraocular lens implantation. *Am J Ophtlamol* 1997; **123:** 441–7.

8 Nishi O. Removal of lens epithelial cells by ultrasound in endocapsular cataract surgery. *Opthalmic Surg* 1987; **18:** 577–80.

9 Tasaka W, Kimura W, Kimura T, et al. Rate of reduction of anterior capsular opening following cataract surgery with removal of lens epithelial cells. *Jpn J Ophthalmol* 1997; **51:** 953–6.

10 Davison JA. Capsule contraction syndrome. *J Cataract Refract Surg* 1993; **19:** 582–9.

11 Nishi O, Nishi K. Intraocular lens encapsulation by shrinkage of the capsulorhexis opening. *J Cataract Refract Surg* 1993; **19:** 544–5.

12 Toldos JJM, Roig AA, Benabent EC. Total anterior capsule closure after silicone intraocular lens implantation. *J Cataract Refract Surg* 1996; **22:** 269–71.

13 Nishi O, Nishi K. Fibrin reaction after posterior chamber lens implantation. *Eur J Implant Refract Surg* 1992; **4:** 69–73.

14 Tsuboi S, Tsujioka M, Kusube T, Kojima S. Effect of continuous circular capsulorhexis and intraocular lens. *Arch Ophthalmol* 1992; **110:** 1124–7.

15 Jampol ML, Shelly J, Pudzisz B, et al. Nonsteroidal anti-inflammatory drugs and cataract surgery. *Arch Ophthalmol* 1994; **112:** 891–3.

16 Kraff MC, Martin RG, Neumann AC, Weinstein AJ. Efficacy of diclofenac sodium ophthalmic solution versus placebo in reducing inflammation following cataract extraction and posterior chamber lens implantation. *J Cataract Refract Surg* 1994; **20:** 138–44.

17 Nishi O, Nishi K, Fujiwara T, Shirasawa E. Effects of diclofenac sodium and indomethacin on proliferation and collagen synthesis of lens epithelial cells in vitro. *J Cataract Refract Surg* 1995; **21:** 461–5.

18 Hoshi H. Drug inhibition of lens epithelial cell proliferation. *Atarashii Ganka* 1993; **10:** 1671–7.

19 Sterling S, Wood TO. Effect of intraocular lens convexity on posterior capsules. *Am Intraocul Implant Soc J* 1986; **12:** 655–7.

20 Sellmann TR, Lindstrom RL. Effect of plano-convex posterior chamber lens on capsular opacification from Elschnig pearl formation. *J Cataract Refract Surg* 1988; **14:** 68–72.

21 Setty SS, Percival SPB. Intraocular lens design and the inhibition of epithelium. *Br J Ophthalmol* 1989; **73:** 918–21.

22 Frezotti R, Caporossi A. Pathogenesis of posterior capsular opacification. Part I. Epidemiological and clinico-statistical data. *J Cataract Refract Surg* 1990; **16:** 347–52.

23 Nagata T, Kawano T. Comparison of effects of 'pad-polished' and 'tumble-polished' intraocular lenses on posterior capsule opacification. *Jpn Soc Cataract Refract Surg* 1995; **9:** 193–6.

24 Yamada K, Nagamoto T, Yozawa H, et al. Effect of intraocular lens design on posterior capsule opacification after continuous curvilinear capsulorhexis. *J Cataract Refract Surg* 1995; **21:** 697–700.

25 Zetterstrom C. Incidence of posterior capsule opacification in eyes with exfoliation syndrome and heparin-surface-modified intraocular lenses. *J Cataract Refract Surg* 1993; **19:** 344–7.

26 Maltzman B, Hampt E, Cucci P. Effect of the laser ridge on posterior capsule opacification. *J Cataract Refract Surg* 1989; **15:** 644–6.

27 Hütz W, Küstermann R, Rösing H. Nachstar bei Intraokularlinsen mit und ohne Laserridge. In: Wenzel M, Reim M, Freyler H, Hartmann C, eds. 5. *Kongress der Deutschen Gesellschaft für Intraokularlinsen Implantation* (Berlin: Springer, 1991) 704–10.

28 Martin RG, Sanders DR, Souchek J, et al. Effect of posterior chamber IOL design and surgical placement upon post-operative outcome. *J Cataract Refract Surg* 1992; **18:** 333–41.

29 Tetz M, O'Morche D, Gwin T, et al. Posterior capsular opacification and intraocular lens decentration. Part II: Experimental findings on a prototype circular intraocular lens design. *J Cataract Refract Surg* 1988; **14:** 614–23.

30 Davison J. A short haptic diameter mod-J-loop PC-IOL for improved bag performance. *J Cataract Refract Surg* 1988; **14:** 161–6.

31 Anis A. Principles and evolution of intraocular lens implantation. *Int Ophthalmol Clin* 1982; **22:** 1–13.

32 Galand A, Delmelle M. Preliminary report on the rigid disc lens. *J Cataract Refract Surg* 1986; **12:** 394–7.

33 Apple DJ, Assia EI, Blumenthal M, Legler UFC. Verformbare Linsen. Das Konzpet den ausdehnbaren Hydrogellinse und

die Wiederhevstellung der natürlichen Kapselsackanatomie. In: Wenzel H, Reim M, Freyler H, Hartmann C, eds. *5. Kongress der Deutschsprachigen Gesellschaft für Intraokularlinsen Implantation* (Berlin: Springer Verlag, 1991) 744–53.

34 Nishi O, Nakai Y, Yamada Y, Mizumoto Y. Amplitudes of accommodation of primate lenses refilled with two types of inflatable endocapsular balloons. *Arch Ophthalmol* 1993; **111:** 1677–84.

35 Hara T, Sakka Y, Salanishi K, Yamada Y, Nakamae K, Hayashi F. Complications associated with endocapsular balloon implantation in rabbit eyes. *J Cataract Refract Surg* 1994; **20:** 507–12.

36 Nishi O, Nishi K, Mano C, Ichihara M, Honda T. Inhibition of migrating lens epithelial cells by discontinuous capsular bend created by band-shaped circular loop or capsule tension ring. *Ophthalmic Surg Lasers* 1998; **29:** 119–25.

37 Oshika T, Suzuki Y, Kizaki H, Yaguch S. Two year clinical study of a soft acrylic intraocular lens. *J Cataract Refract Surg* 1996; **22:** 104–9.

38 Ursell P, Spalton DJ, Pande MV, et al. Relationship between intraocular lens biomaterials and posterior capsule opacification. *J Cataract Refract Surg* 1998; **24:** 352–60.

39 Nishi O, Nishi K. Inhibition of migrating lens epithelial cells at the capsular bend created by the rectangular optic edge of a posterior chamber intraocular lens. *Ophthalmic Surg Lasers* 1998; in press.

40 Nagata T, Ninakata A, Watanabe I. Adhesiveness of AcrySof to a collagen film. *J Cataract Refract Surg* 1998; **24:** 367–70.

41 Nishi O, Nishi K, Menapace R. Capsule bending ring for the prevention of capsular opacification: a preliminary report. *Ophthalmic Surg Lasers* 1998; in press.

42 Auer C, Gonvers M. Silicone one piece intraocular implant and anterior capsule fibrosis. *Klin Monatsbl Augenheilk* 1995; **206:** 293–5.

43 Menapace R. Posterior capsule opacification and capsulotomy rates with taco-style hydrogel intraocular lenses. *J Cataract Refract Surg* 1996; **22:** 1318–30.

44 Clark D, Emery J, Munsell Kelleher P. Inhibition of posterior capsular opacification with an immunotoxin specific for lens epithelial cells: eighteen month results on a Phase I/II study. *J Cataract Refract Surg* 1998, in press.

45 Behar-Cohen FF, David T, D'Hermies F, et al. In vivo inhibition of lens regrowth by fibroblast growth factor 2-saporin. *Invest Ophthalmol Vis Sci* 1995; **36:** 2434–48.

46 Hunold W, Wirtz M, Kaden P, Kreiner CF. Protektiver Effect viskoelastischer Lösungen bei der Anwendung eines Nekrosefaktors zur Nachstarverhütung. In: Wenzel M, Reim M, Freyler H, Hartmann C, eds. *5. Kongress der Deutschen Gesellschaft der Intraokularlinsen Implantation* (Berlin: Springer Verlag, 1991) 711–23.

47 Nishi O, Nishi K, Yamada Y, Mizumoto Y. Effect of indomethacin-coated posterior chamber intraocular lenses on postoperative inflammation and posterior capsule opacification. *J Cataract Refract Surg* 1995; **21:** 574–8.

48 Nishi O, Nishi K, Morita T, Tada Y, Shirasawa E, Sakanishi K. Effect of intraocular sustained release of indomethacin on postoperative inflammation and posterior capsule opacification. *J Cataract Refract Surg* 1996; **22:** 806–10.

49 Tetz M, Ries MW, Lucas C, Stricker H, Völcker HE. Inhibition of posterior capsule opacification by an intraocular-lens-bound sustained drug delivery system: an experimental animal study and literature review. *J Cataract Refract Surg* 1996; **22:** 1070–8.

50 Nishi O, Nishi K, Hikida M. Removal of lens epithelial cells following loosening of the junctional complex. *J Cataract Refract Surg* 1993; **19:** 56–61.

51 Nishi O, Nishi K, Mano C, Ichihara M, Honda T, Saitoh I. Inhibition of migrating lens epithelial cells by blocking the adhesion molecule integrin: a preliminary report. *J Cataract Refract Surg* 1997; **23:** 860–5.

52 Nishi O, Nishi K, Akaishi T, Shirasawa E. Detection of cell adhesion molecules in lens epithelial cells of human cataracts. *Invest Ophthalmol Vis Sci* 1996; **38:** 579–85.

53 Duncan G, Woomstone M, Lin CSC, et al. Thapsigargin-coated intraocular lenses inhibit human lens cell growth. *Nat Med* 1997; **3:** 1026–8.

Chapter 25 Primary posterior capsulorhexis: indications, techniques and results

Albert J Galand

Posterior capsule opacification (also referred to as after-cataract) is the most important challenge to modern cataract-implant surgery, with an estimated incidence approaching 50% after 5 years.[1] Most surgeons currently rely on the Nd:YAG laser to perform posterior capsulotomy at a later stage if the capsule opacifies. There are some disadvantages to Nd:YAG laser therapy, including vision-threatening complications and increased overall cost of cataract treatment.[2]

The posterior capsule itself does not opacify. It serves as a scaffold for cellular migration. Therefore, a posterior capsulorhexis at the time of cataract surgery might prevent the central opacification that requires a postoperative Nd:YAG laser posterior capsulotomy.

In 1990, Gimbel[3] suggested a 'posterior continuous circular capsulotomy' (PCCC) in three situations: (1) to prevent the extension of an inadvertent posterior capsule tear; (2) in the presence of posterior capsule plaque; (3) in infants because they usually develop posterior capsule opacification and are often not able to have a laser capsulotomy. Blumenthal et al. also suggested the use of PCCC in special cases such as cataracts in children or dense posterior capsule plaques in adults.[4]

In August 1993, I started to perform PCCC in most adult cases of cataract implant surgery with the goal of reducing the rate of Nd:YAG laser capsulotomies. At the time of writing, I have performed 1648 PCCCs.

SURGICAL TECHNIQUE

PCCC can be done under topical, local or general anesthesia. However, due to lack of akinesia, I am reluctant to perform PCCC when the eye is under topical or even local anesthesia.

There are two prerequisites for opening the posterior capsule:

1) Visibility must be excellent; this supposes a good operative microscope, a clear cornea and sufficient mydriasis.
2) There should be no positive pressure. A 'pushy eye' is obviously an adverse condition for perforating the posterior capsule.

The timing for PCCC is after cortical clean-up and before lens implantation. To start with, some viscoelastic material is placed in the capsular bag, to flatten the posterior capsule; an equilibrium of pressure is reached on both sides of the posterior capsule. Moreover, some viscoelastic in the anterior chamber will keep it formed during the following maneuvers.

Figure 25.1 shows the four steps of the procedure.

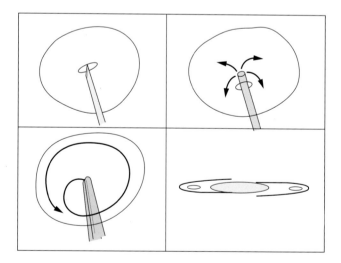

Figure 25.1. *Posterior capsulorhexis technique. (1) Perforating in front of the retrolental space of Berger. (2) Injecting viscoelastic material between the posterior capsule and the anterior vitreous. (3) Tearing with capsular forceps. (4) Position of the IOL.*

STEP 1

A 30-gauge disposable, unbent needle (Becton-Dickinson SA, Madrid, Spain) is used to perforate the central part of the posterior capsule in front of the retrolental space of Berger. Remember that the space of Berger has a diameter of ±2 mm and a depth of ±1 mm. It contains aqueous humor. Therefore, perforating the posterior capsule at this level will not disturb the anterior hyaloid membrane. Often, elderly people have an even larger space of Berger.

STEP 2

A small amount of viscoelastic material is injected into the capsular hole to fill Berger's space and to separate the posterior capsule from the anterior vitreous. This viscoelastic tamponade has to be injected gently and slowly because the cohesion of the substance may create a force sufficient to enlarge the hole in an uncontrolled manner. Regular Healon or Provisc is preferred for this maneuver. An air bubble arriving with the viscoelastic may damage the margin of the capsular hole. Should air present underneath the posterior capsule, it should be left alone.

STEP 3

A delicate capsulorhexis forceps is used to tear the posterior capsule in much the same way that one performs an anterior capsulorhexis. The posterior capsule is thinner than is the anterior capsule. However, for PCCC there are neither the nucleus nor zonular fibers which could direct the tear to the periphery. A right-handed surgeon tends to be more skilful working in a counterclockwise motion. It is important that the size of the PCCC is smaller than the size of the implant's optic. Indeed, this ensures a reconstitution of the barrier between the vitreous and the anterior chamber, particularly with early adherence of the capsulorhexis edge to the optic. In cases with a PCCC larger than the optic, there is the possibility of vitreous migration postoperatively to the pupillary space.

STEP 4

After completion of the PCCC, additional viscoelastic is injected to separate the anterior and posterior capsules, to prepare the capsular bag for implantation.

One-piece PMMA implants are the easiest to insert without intruding on the posterior capsulorhexis. It can be difficult with foldable implants. Performance of PCCC after the implantation is, in our hands, more difficult than the above-described technique.

With implants 12.0 mm in overall diameter, the PCCC may be seen to ovalize. Very soft implant loops

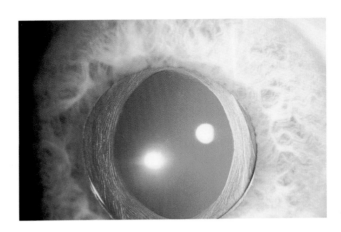

Figure 25.2. *Postoperative view of posterior capsulorhexis. The anterior capsulorhexis is underneath the iris.*

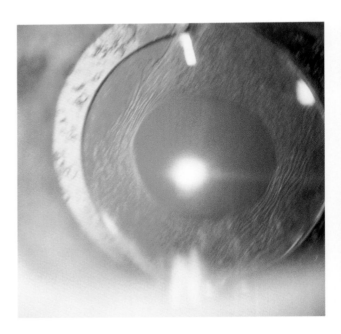

Figure 25.3. *Postoperative view of posterior capsulorhexis. The anterior capsulorhexis is approximately the size of the optic.*

are to be preferred, and an overall loop diameter of less than 11.0 mm is desirable.

At the end of the surgery, the viscoelastic is removed from the anterior chamber but no attempt is made to remove the small amount of it placed behind the posterior capsule. The postoperative view of eyes with PCCC is shown in Figs 25.2 and 25.3.

DIFFICULT CASES

- Fibrotic capsules: some degree of 'plaque' on the posterior capsule is an indication for a posterior capsulorhexis. However, in these cases the fibrous zome may misguide the tear. Sometimes, I resort partially to capsular scissors in order to avoid excessive traction with the forceps.
- If the posterior capsule is locate very deeply, it may present a problem because of the posterior limit of focus of the operative microscope.[5]
- If the corneal tunnel is too long, the capsular forceps may create striae in the cornea, resulting in poor visibility.

COMPLICATIONS

Intraoperative complications consist of poorly controlled capsular tears, resulting in an excentric or oversized capsulotomy.[6] Extension of the tearing out to the capsular fornix is less frequent than with anterior capsulorhexis. Vitreous prolapse is a rare occurrence. After a learning curve, intraoperative complications occur in less than 1% of cases, and are generally associated with difficult case types.

Postoperative complications include opacification of the PCCC window (Fig. 25.4). The major disappointment with this technique is that roughly 10% of cases present Elschnig's pearls or a fibrotic membrane in the window within a follow-up of 2 years. Diabetic retinopathy and uveitis are risk factors for closure of the PCCC.[7] Reopacification after Nd:YAG laser capsulotomy is also observed,[8] but with a much less frequent incidence, because migration of cells or material leading to opacification requires a scaffold. After Nd:YAG laser capsulotomy, the anterior hyaloid is most often destroyed. After posterior capsulorhexis, this surface is intact and may act as a support or scaffold for migration. This probably explains the higher rate of reopacification after posterior capsulorhexis than after Nd:YAG laser capsulotomy.

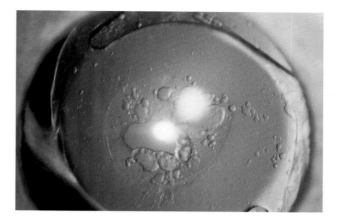

Figure 25.4. *Closure of a posterior capsulorhexis by Elschnig's pearls.*

When, in 1993, I began to perform posterior capsulorhexis on a regular basis in adult cases, the major unresolved question concerned potential risks to the retina, cystoid macular edema or retinal detachment.

With regard to cystoid macular edema (CME), I have noted an absence of clinical edema, and there has been no special rate of subnormal visual acuity. On the contrary, visual acuity after 15 days appears slightly better with a posterior capsulorhexis. In a small series, fluorescein angiography was performed at 15 days after surgery in 49 eyes with PCCC and nine eyes without PCCC. The results revealed three cases of CME in the former group and two cases in the latter, suggesting no increase in the risk of CME with a posterior capsulorhexis. Two explanations are possible. (1) Opening the capsular barrier does not trigger CME, since uveal irritation is probably necessary and no uveal irritation is induced with posterior capsulorhexis. The fact that CME does occur infrequently after Nd:YAG capsulotomy supports this explanation.[9,10] (2) A few days postoperatively, the margin of the posterior capsulorhexis apparently adheres to the implant optic. The 'barrier' is reconstituted early after surgery. Concerning retinal detachment, time seems to confirm the absence of an increased risk when a posterior capsulorhexis has been performed. Among 1579 cases of PCCC with a follow-up time from 6 to 48 months, I have observed five cases with retinal detachments (0.3%), which is less than reported after Nd:YAG capsulotomy. However, it should be noted that not all the eyes operated for cataract without posterior capsulorhexis will require a Nd:YAG capsulotomy. Interestingly enough, all five eyes with retinal detachment after PCCC had an axial length greater than 25.7 mm.

In conclusion, one can recognize that PCCC is probably safer than anticipated, and should be compared with Nd:YAG laser capsulotomy. The advantage of PCCC is to maintain the anterior hyaloid, while the Nd:YAG laser destroys it in most cases. However, leaving the anterior vitreous intact is the most likely reason for closure of the PCCC. Definitive prevention of posterior capsule opacification is not yet a reality. Nevertheless, PCCC is a valuable maneuver that cataract surgeons can apply in selected cases.

REFERENCES

1 Sterling S, Wood T. Effect of intraocular lenses convexity on posterior capsule opacification. *J Cataract Refract Surg* 1986; **12:** 655–7.

2 Steinert RF, Puliafito CA, Kumar SR, Dudak SD, Patel S. Cystoid macular edema, retinal detachment and glaucoma after Nd:YAG laser posterior capsulotomy. *Am J Ophthalmol* 1991; **112:** 373–80.

3 Gimbel HW. Posterior capsule tears using phaco-emulsification: causes, prevention and management. *Eur J Implant Refract Surg* 1990; **2:** 63–9.

4 Blumenthal M, Assia E, Neumann D. The round capsulorhexis capsulotomy and the rationale for 11.0 mm diameter IOL. *Eur J Implant Refract Surg* 1990; **2:** 15–19.

5 Van Cauwenberge F, Rakic JM, Galand A. Complicated posterior capsulorhexis: aetiology, management and outcome. *Br J Ophthalmol* 1996; **80:** 1–4.

6 Galand A, Van Cauwenberge F, Moosavi J. Posterior capsulorhexis in adult eyes with intact and clear capsules. *J Cataract Refract Surg* 1996; **22:** 458–61.

7 Tassignon MJ, De Groot V, Smets RM, Tawab B, Vervecken F. Secondary closure of posterior continuous curvilinear capsulorhexis. *J Cataract Refract Surg* 1996; **22:** 1200–5.

8 McPherson RJ, Govan JA. Posterior capsule reopacification after neodymium:YAG laser capsulotomy. *J Cataract Refract Surg* 1995; **21:** 351–2.

9 Lewis H, Singer TR, Hanscom TA, Straatsma BR. A prospective study of cystoid macular edema after neodymium:YAG laser posterior capsulotomy. *Ophthalmology* 1987; **94:** 478–82.

10 Bukelman A, Abrahami S, Oliver M, Pollack A. Cystoid macular oedema following neodymium:YAG laser capsulotomy. A prospective study. *Eye* 1992; **6:** 35–8.

Chapter 26 **Pupil stretch: techniques and results**

Luther L Fry

I would like to describe a pupil-stretching technique I have used since 1992. It is simple, very effective, and requires only two inexpensive instruments, which are probably already in your set. It involves stretching the pupil, limbus to limbus, with two Kuglin hooks.

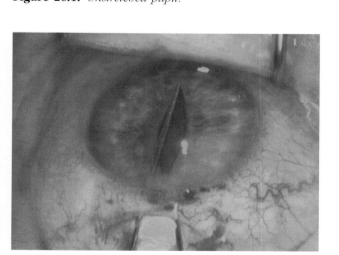

Figure 26.1. *Unstretched pupil.*

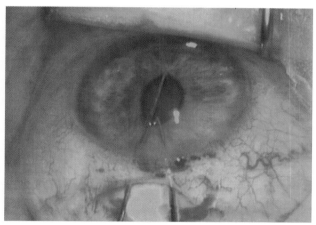

Figure 26.2. *Beginning of stretch.*

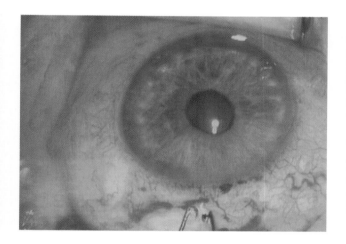

Figure 26.3. *Mid-stretch.*

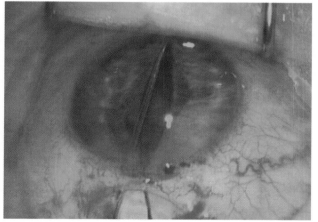

Figure 26.4. *Fully stretched.*

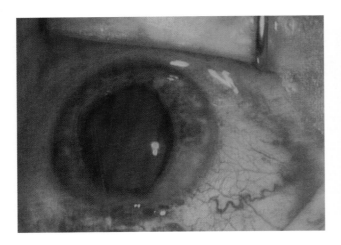

Figure 26.5. *Start of expansion with viscoelastic.*

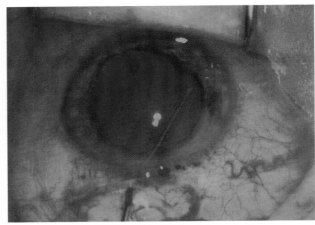

Figure 26.6. *Fully expanded.*

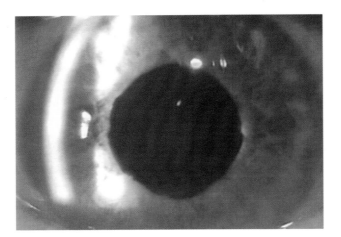

Figure 26.7. *One day after surgery.*

After stretching, the pupil is further expanded with viscoelastic. A highly retentive, non-dispersive viscoelastic, such as Healon GV, works best.

This technique yields a pupil of adequate size for easy capsulorhexis and subsequent cataract surgery in virtually all cases. In general, the smaller the pupil, the more profound the effect. I do keep a set of Grieshaber iris retractors available, but have not had to cut the iris or use the iris retractors in a single case since using the pupil stretch technique.

A few technical tips and caveats are as follows:

- With small fibrotic pupils, there may be a tendency to develop iris tears. These are usually small and

multiple. Stretching slowly (approximately 3 s) may help lessen the severity of these tears. I have not observed an iris tear large enough to cause postoperative problems, and have not noticed significant iris bleeding. Hold the stretch for a second or so at maximum stretch.

- Be sure to stretch fully out to the limbus in both directions to get maximum effect. Only one stretch is necessary. Additional stretches give little additional benefit. (Earlier, I performed a second stretch through the side-port, but eliminated this practice when it seemed to give little additional effect. Additional stretches also seem to make the iris more 'floppy' and likely to catch in the phaco tip.

- The pupil may remain permanently larger, particularly with small fibrotic pupils and iris atrophy; these cases tend to develop iris tears. These are rarely large, and may really be something of a benefit, especially in glaucoma cases, allowing postoperative fundus examination.

- In cases with an induced large pupil, particularly if there are noticeable sphincter tears, a 6.0-mm or larger optic should be used (I prefer 7.0 mm); 5.0 mm or 5.5 mm might risk incomplete pupillary coverage.

- It is easy to concentrate on only the distal Kuglin hook and forget the proximal, allowing the proximal hook to be retracted out of the wound, drawing iris with it. If one keeps this in mind, it is unlikely to happen. It is rare, and has not been associated with serious damage to the iris.

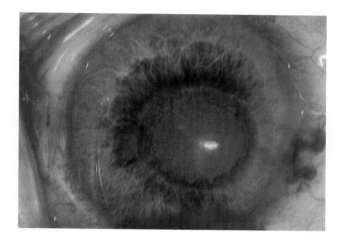

Figure 26.8. *Atrophic iris.*

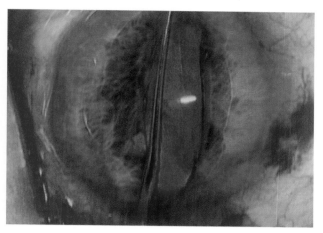

Figure 26.9. *Stretch with sphincter tear.*

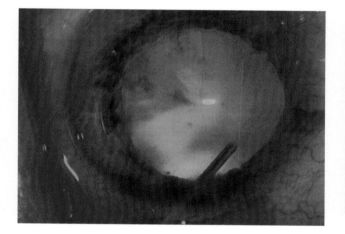

Figure 26.10. *After expansion with viscoelastic.*

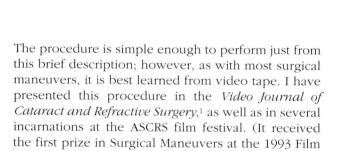

Figure 26.11. *One day after surgery.*

The procedure is simple enough to perform just from this brief description; however, as with most surgical maneuvers, it is best learned from video tape. I have presented this procedure in the *Video Journal of Cataract and Refractive Surgery*,[1] as well as in several incarnations at the ASCRS film festival. (It received the first prize in Surgical Maneuvers at the 1993 Film Festival.)

I have employed this technique since 1992, in approximately 10% of all cases; this represents roughly 600 eyes. Any surgical procedure, of course, carries a risk of complications, but I have yet to encounter my first significant complication with the pupil-stretching procedure.

I make no claim to be the originator of this procedure. I first saw Gerald Keener of Indianapolis do a similar procedure on a video tape in 1992, which gave me the idea. Subsequently, I spoke with him at a meeting, and he informed me that he learned the trick from someone else.

I would highly recommend this procedure to those of you who have not used it. I think you will find it simple, safe, effective, and inexpensive.

REFERENCE

1 Fry LL. Pupil stretching. *Video J Cataract Refract Surg* 1995; **XI**(1).

Chapter 27 Phacoemulsification and the small pupil

Bradford J Shingleton

INTRODUCTION

The miotic pupil is a common finding in the surgical practice of the comprehensive ophthalmologist. There are multiple reasons for this finding. The incidence of both cataracts and glaucoma increases with time and it is not uncommon to find patients with cataracts who have been on miotic agents for a long time. Older patients, in general, often do not dilate as well despite preoperative dilation programs. Pseudoexfoliation is also a common finding in the aging population, and the pupils in these patients do not dilate as well. Excessive intraocular iris manipulation may lead to a reduction in pupillary size during the surgical procedure, and patients who have not received satisfactory dilating drops preoperatively may also be predisposed to intraoperative miosis. Regardless of the cause, all cataract surgeons must be prepared to deal with the miotic pupil.

The miotic pupil also places significant demands on the surgical technique of the ophthalmic surgeon. A small pupil can marginalize visualization. All steps involving intraocular manipulation therefore become more difficult: capsulorhexis, phacoemulsification and intraocular lens implantation. A two-hand instrument technique is helpful for intraoperative management of the small pupil, but this requires bimanual dexterity. Because of the small pupil, skill in endocapsular phacoemulsification techniques is advantageous and surgeons must also be prepared to deal with iris suturing if sphincterotomies and iridectomies are utilized.

The goals of management of the small pupil in phacoemulsification are threefold. First, the surgeon must achieve adequate pupillary size to perform phacoemulsification. Second, preservation of pupillary activity is advantageous. Third, preservation of normal pupillary contour is desired.

TECHNIQUES FOR MANAGEMENT OF THE MIOTIC PUPIL

PREOPERATIVE CONSIDERATIONS

It is helpful to stop miotics at least 1 week preoperatively. If pupilloplasty will be required intraoperatively, one may consider adding topical steroids or NSAID agents to the preoperative regimen prior to the day of surgery. On the day of surgery, I favor dilation with tropicamide 1% and phenylephrine 2.5%. Each drop is used every 5 min by four doses preoperatively. Topical prostaglandin inhibitors may also be considered preoperatively to minimize intraoperative constriction of the pupil. Topical anesthesia with or without intracameral supplementation is not contraindicated if pupillary enlargement techniques are required intraoperatively.[1]

PUPIL-ENLARGEMENT TECHNIQUES

In all cases, it is advantageous to avoid excessive iris manipulation. Significant manipulation is required for stretching and iridectomy maneuvers but the manipulation should be kept to the minimum required for the desired result. Epinephrine 1 : 1000 (intracardiac), when added to the balanced salt solution used for coaxial irrigation, helps to maintain intraoperative dilation of the pupil. I favor 0.3 ml in 500 ml of balanced salt solution. It is very common to encounter posterior synechiae, so it is appropriate to sweep and release synechiae with viscoelastic maintenance of the anterior chamber. Some patients who have been on miotics for an extended time will have thin, veneer-like membranes that will stick the pupillary margin to the anterior capsule surface. It is appropriate to strip this membrane off and remove it from the eye if it exists. Simple sweeping and releasing of synechiae

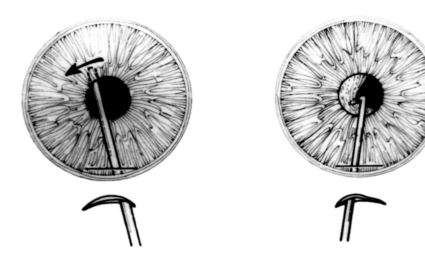

Figure 27.1. *Sweeping posterior synechiae and stripping pupillary membranes to enhance pupil size.*

followed by viscoelastic pupil expansion may be enough to achieve adequate pupillary size in many patients for phacoemulsification[2] (Fig. 27.1).

Bimanual iris stretch without scissors

Bimanual iris stretch often eliminates the need for scissors sphincterotomies.[3] This technique is best accomplished by a slow, steady bimanual stretch of the pupil to the limbal area (Fig. 27.2). I perform the technique with instruments that are often utilized in standard phacoemulsification and intraocular lens implantation, such as an angled Y-hook and Kuglen hook. Any iris hook will suffice. I initiate the slow, steady stretch in the 12-6 meridian and then follow this with extension in the 9-3 meridian. It is important to appreciate that bimanual pupillary stretch is actually a 'micro' sphincterotomy technique. The slow, steady stretch is required to avoid precipitous

iris tears, which are more common in lighter-colored irides. This technique results in excellent preservation of pupillary function and contour as well as achieving satisfactory pupillary size for phacoemulsification.

Pupillary stretch can be extended to a trimanual or quadrimanual mode. Brown has described placing a single iris retractor and coupling this with bimanual stretch to achieve triangular pupillary expansion. Beehler has developed an instrument for mechanical pupillary dilation that uses a quadrimanual approach. Both these techniques are simple to use and are effective for pupillary dilation.

Self-retaining iris retractors

Flexible[4-6] and titanium[7] iris retractors may be used to dilate pupils (Fig. 27.3). Each technique utilizes four separate paracentesis incisions. The orientation of the incisions is important in order to achieve proper dilation

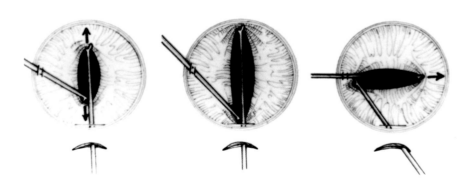

Figure 27.2. *Bimanual pupil stretch: slow, steady stretch with two instruments in two meridians.*

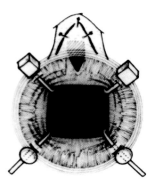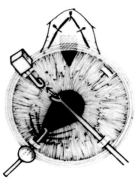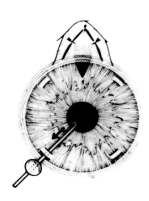

Figure 27.3. *Self-retaining iris retractors: flexible and rigid iris retractors demonstrating pupil expansion via four paracentesis incisions.*

and pupillary contour. The paracentesis incision should be directed at an angle that is the one desired for eventual positioning of the iris hook. If the paracentesis incision is parallel to the iris, the hook will tend to lift the iris off the anterior capsule and exacerbate iris chafing during the phacoemulsification procedure. If the paracentesis incision is too perpendicular, the hook will have a tendency to release the iris from its retracted position. As with bimanual iris stretch, sequential gradual hook retraction minimizes sphincter tears. If four hooks are utilized, a generous rectangular-shaped pupil is achieved. It may be appropriate to relax tension on the superior hooks prior to phacoemulsification in order to decrease iris contact with the emulsification instrument.[8] The nylon retractors utilize a silicone cinch for adjusting the iris position, and both reusable and non-reusable nylon iris retractors are available. The titanium iris retractors are sterilizable.

Self-retaining pupil expanders

Graether[9] has developed a silicone expander which achieves broad circular pupillary dilation (Fig. 27.4). This technique is initiated by placement of a small sleeve to retract the subincisional iris towards the area of the anterior chamber entry site. The expander is seated onto the iris pupillary border and released from its injector sleeve. It is then seated into an appropriate position on the pupillary margin. Phacoemulsification and intraocular lens implantation is performed and then the ring is removed by cutting the silicone interconnector between the ring-like attachments of the Graether expander.

Siepser has described the use of an expansile hydrogel ring, and Arpa, Peyman and Updegraff have described the use of an elastomeric ring.

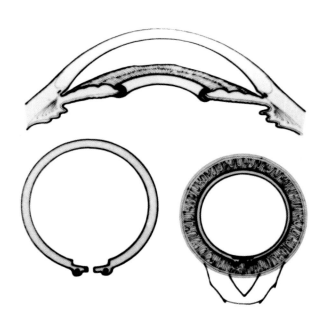

Figure 27.4. *Self-retaining pupil expander: Graether pupil expander.*

Sphincterotomies

Traditionally, a few (1–3) short or long sphincterotomies have been used to achieve pupillary size. This is extremely effective for enhancing inferior exposure. A sphincterotomy in one quadrant yields an oval-shaped pupil, and in two quadrants a 'hammock'-shaped pupil. When this technique is coupled with a superior sphincterectomy, excellent inferior and superior exposure is obtained. With long sphincterotomies, it is important to beware of iris tags that can have a remarkable tendency to be attracted to the phacoemulsification tip.

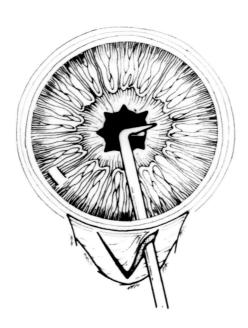

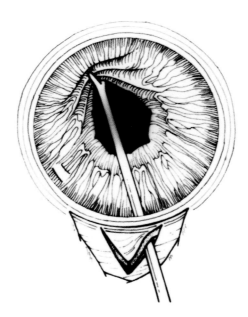

Figure 27.5.
Multiple mini-sphincterotomies coupled with pupil stretch.

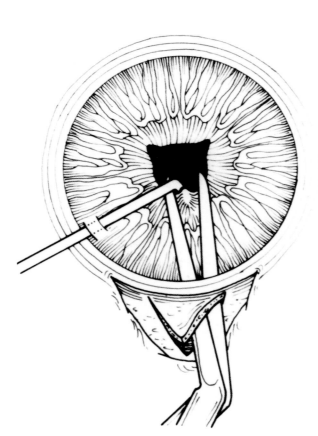

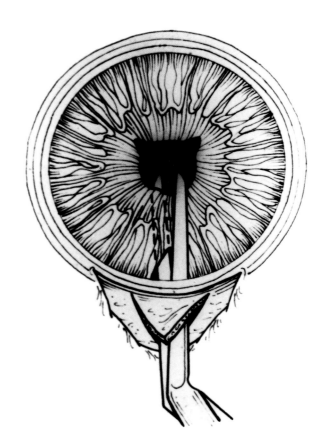

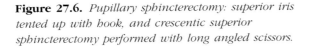

Figure 27.6. *Pupillary sphincterectomy: superior iris tented up with hook, and crescentic superior sphincterectomy performed with long angled scissors.*

Figure 27.7. *Keyhole/sector iridectomy: iridectomy extended via peripheral iridectomy to complete full opening to the pupillary margin.*

Fine,[10,11] has described the use of multiple mini-sphincterotomies (eight or more). With short cuts through part of the iris sphincter muscle, relaxation of the pupillary ring is established (Fig. 27.5). Small scissors are available that can be used to perform this technique through the phacoemulsification incision or through a paracentesis site. It may also be appropriate to stretch the iris in the area of the sphincterotomies to break fibrotic adhesions. This technique also preserves excellent pupillary function and contour.

Superior sphincterectomy

A superior sphincterectomy greatly aids superior exposure (Fig. 27.6). This is a two instrument technique that involves a hook and long, angled scissors. The hook is placed via a paracentesis incision and the superior iris is tented up. The scissors are then used to create a crescentic sphincterectomy superiorly. The arcuate configuration results in excellent exposure superiorly with preservation of near-normal reactivity and contour.

Keyhole/sector iridectomy

It may be appropriate in some patients to create and maintain a sector iridectomy. This is most likely in diabetic patients or those with significant retinal disease. The goal in these patients is to minimize manipulation and subsequent inflammation and to maximize posterior segment viewing. I favor a keyhole/sector iridectomy technique, which involves performing a superior peripheral iridectomy and then cutting the iris sphincter via the iridectomy. In certain cases, it may be appropriate to suture the sector iridectomy or sphincterotomies. 10-0 polypropylene is favored, although 10-0 nylon can be utilized. The sutures can be pre-placed or post-placed and they are subsequently tied after intraocular lens implantation.[12] It is easiest to utilize a paracentesis to enhance needle passage. All needle passages and suturing of the iris are performed with viscoelastic maintenance of the anterior chamber. A host of needles are available and many techniques have been described (Fig. 27.8a,b). The goal of iris suturing is to facilitate the restoration of a taut iris diaphragm and a more normal iris configuration.

Pharmacologic manipulation

Serpin has described the use of a mydria sponge. He and others have advocated depot release from a

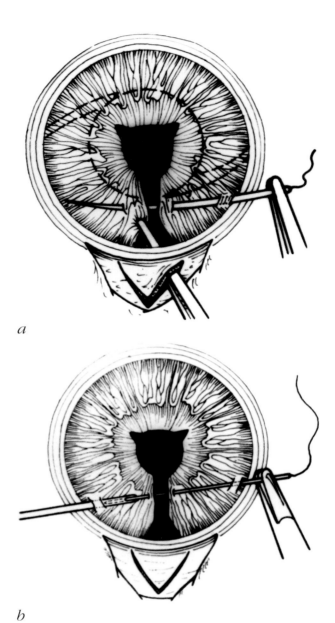

a

b

Figure 27.8. *(a) Iris suturing utilizing a long, curved needle with placement via paracentesis incisions. (b) Iris suturing utilizing a straight needle with guidance of exit via a hub needle.*

mydriatic-soaked material in the inferior fornix. Topical epinephrine (1 : 1000) and intracameral epinephrine 1 : 10 000 may also be utilized. In eyes that have significant anterior chamber inflammation and inflammatory membranes, tissue plasminogen activator (tPA) may be utilized. Generally, 5–25 µg is all that is required, and the effect is seen within 10–30 min.

SECOND INSTRUMENT

A second instrument or hook to move the iris and facilitate exposure for capsulorhexis and phacoemulsification is appropriate. This can be utilized with all the techniques noted above and will minimize iridoemulsification. Johnstone has also described an iris tuck maneuver with retraction of the iris to the wound to facilitate exposure.[13]

MICROSCOPE POSITIONING

Appropriate operating microscope tilt may enhance visualization and increase the visible diameter of the lens.

CAPSULORHEXIS

An intact capsulorhexis is important to keep the phacoemulsification tip away from the iris in endocapsular procedures. It also facilitates separation of the intraocular lens (IOL) from the iris to reduce pupillary capture of the intraocular lens and posterior migration of the iris. Small capsulorhexis openings do not preclude large optic implantation, and the anterior capsulorhexis can be enlarged after the IOL implantation if necessary to avoid anterior capsular contraction.

PHACOEMULSIFICATION

I favor a two-instrument technique for small-pupil phacoemulsification. Effective hydrodissection and hydrodelineation achieves good control of the nucleus within the capsular bag. Free rotation within the bag greatly facilitates performance of effective phacoemulsification. Many divide and conquer techniques have been described. I favor a groove, crack and chop technique that utilizes variation in vacuum, flow and power. One may consider a central groove at low vacuum with low flow and linear power. The phaco chop and nucleus aspiration can then be performed under high vacuum with moderate flow and linear power. This allows the phacoemulsification to be performed within the pupillary zone, and little manipulation is required in the capsular fornix. The epinucleus is then removed under moderate vacuum with higher flow.

To sculpt a deep central groove it is appropriate to approach steeply with the phacoemulsification tip to initiate the groove rather than parallel to the iris. One can also extend peripherally by working under the protection of the epinucleus and capsule to minimize the risk of iridoemulsification. A complete crack is needed and can be assured with deep central sculpting.

IOL IMPLANTATION

Implants of any size are possible with small-pupil phacoemulsification. Foldable IOLs allow the maximal reduction of incision size. Acrylic and silicone lenses have both been implanted with success. There may be a slightly higher incidence of pigment deposits on silicone lenses. If one is going to maintain a non-sutured large pupil or sector iridectomy, it is appropriate to use a large-diameter IOL. A posterior chamber lens in the capsular bag is the implant of choice, as this reduces pigment dispersion, which is accentuated by use of pupil-enlargement techniques. If complications with the capsule and vitreous develop during phacoemulsification in the setting of a small pupil, current-generation tripod and quadripod anterior chamber lenses may be satisfactorily implanted if the angle status is not compromised by PAS, recession or clefts. It is appropriate to avoid anterior chamber IOLs in such circumstances. A sutured posterior chamber lens with sulcus fixation should be considered in cases of inadequate capsule support and anatomic angle compromise.

PUPILLARY ASSESSMENT AFTER IOL IMPLANTATION

After the completion of IOL implantation, it is important to assess the position of the pupil. Intraoperative miotics such as acetylcholine or carbachol may be utilized. If sphincterotomies are performed, it is appropriate to stroke the iris back over the IOL to minimize synechiae to the peripheral capsule. The iris is sutured at the same time if appropriate. After iris positioning and suturing, it is best to remove residual viscoelastic and aspirate any blood or pigment that may be in the anterior chamber. This will help to reduce postoperative inflammation and synechiae formation.

POSTOPERATIVE CARE

Topical steroids are routinely used after small-pupil phacoemulsification. The frequency of administration may be increased if significant manipulation is required intraoperatively. The frequency is modified by the amount of postoperative inflammation encountered.

SUMMARY

A host of pupil-enlargement techniques are available to the ophthalmic surgeon to permit satisfactory phacoemulsification. All the techniques described in this chapter are appropriate for employment in the surgeon's armamentarium. Certain cases may be better approached by one technique rather than another and it is important for the surgeon to be comfortable with a range of techniques.

REFERENCES

1 Gills JP, Chercio M, Raanan MG. Unpreserved lidocaine to control discomfort during cataract surgery using topical anesthesia. *J Cataract Refract Surg* 1997; **23:** 545–50.

2 Joseph J, Wang HS. Phacoemulsification with poorly dilated pupils. *J Cataract Refract Surg* 1993; **19:** 551–6.

3 Shephard DM. The pupil stretch technique for miotic pupils in cataract surgery. *Ophthalmic Surg* 1994; **24:** 851–2.

4 De Juan E Jr, Hickingbotham D. Flexible iris retractors. *Am J Ophthalmol* 1991; **111:** 776–7.

5 Nichamin LD. Enlarging the pupil for cataract extraction using flexible nylon iris retractors. *J Cataract Refract Surg* 1993; **19:** 793–6.

6 Novak J. Flexible iris hooks for phacoemulsification. *J Cataract Refract Surg* 1997; **23:** 828–31.

7 Mackool RJ. Small pupil enlargement during cataract extraction: a new method. *J Cataract Refract Surg* 1992; **18:** 523–6.

8 Masket S. Avoiding complications associated with iris retractor use in small pupil cataract extraction. *J Cataract Refract Surg* 1996; **22:** 168–71.

9 Graether JM. Graether pupil expander for managing the small pupil during surgery. *J Cataract Refract Surg* 1996; **22:** 530–5.

10 Fine IH. Iridectomy technique to improve cosmesis and preserve function after cataract surgery. *Ocul Surg News* 1989; **4:** 28.

11 Fine IH. Pupilloplasty for small pupil phacoemulsification. *J Cataract Refract Surg* 1994; **20:** 192–6.

12 Masket S. Preplaced inferior iris suture method for small pupil phacoemulsification. *J Cataract Refract Surg* 1992; **18:** 518–22.

13 Johnstone MA. The iris tucking maneuver in cataract surgery for glaucoma patient with miotic pupils. *Am J Ophthalmol* 1992; **113:** 586–7.

Chapter 28 Postvitrectomy phacoemulsification

Kevin M Miller

INTRODUCTION

Cataract development is one of the most common complications of pars plana vitrectomy (PPV).[1–14] Between 12.5% and 80% of eyes develop cataracts after vitrectomy, depending on the series referenced.[2,3,5–7,9,10,13,14] Risk factors for the development and progression of cataract include older age,[9,12,14,15] degree of preoperative nuclear sclerosis,[6] intraoperative lens touch, diabetic retinopathy,[8] silicone oil injection,[16–22] and the length of follow-up.[6–13] The indications for surgery and the number of patients undergoing PPV are increasing each year as the results of surgery improve. Consequently, the number of patients requiring subsequent cataract extraction is increasing.

Advancements in posterior segment surgery have improved the visual outcomes of patients undergoing PPV. Better operating microscopes and optical subsystems, better vitrectomy instruments, a variety of intraocular gases and oils, and new pharmaceutical agents, are all responsible, in part, for the increasing volume of surgery being performed around the world. Specialists with posterior segment surgical training are readily accessible in many locations. As a result, timely access to care, which is critical to good outcomes in many conditions affecting the retina, is better than ever before.

It has been reported that patients undergoing extracapsular cataract extraction after PPV have favorable visual outcomes,[23–25] but phacoemulsification has replaced manual extraction of the lens nucleus as the current procedure of choice for a variety of reasons.[26] These include smaller incision size, less induced astigmatism, quicker visual rehabilitation, and a lower complication rate.[27–30] This chapter discusses phacoemulsification and lens implantation in patients who have had a PPV and who subsequently develop cataract. Because of anatomic changes in postvitrectomy eyes, several problems not encountered routinely in eyes with typical cataracts need to be considered.

It should be noted that cataract often obscures the retina specialist's view of the posterior segment. In such cases phacoemulsification may precede PPV by several days, weeks, or months, or it may be performed at the same time. Much has been written on simultaneous surgery, but this is not the subject of the present chapter.[24,31–33]

THE POSTVITRECTOMY EYE

Postvitrectomy eyes are anatomically different from eyes that have not had previous surgery. Theoretically, eyes that have undergone PPV are at greater risk for complications during and after phacoemulsification because they lack a formed vitreous gel, have denser cataracts, harbor the sequelae of previous surgical trauma and inflammation, and have underlying comorbidities. Scarring of the conjunctiva and Tenon's capsule may make scleral incisions more difficult to fashion. The lack of vitreous support during phacoemulsification may lead to deep anterior chambers, fluctuations of anterior chamber depth with movement of the lens–iris diaphragm, and flaccidity of the posterior capsule. Pupils may not dilate well because of posterior synechiae. Inadvertent damage to the posterior capsule or zonules during the PPV may lead to occult capsule rupture or lens subluxation. The accelerated nuclear sclerosis that has been documented in postvitrectomy eyes may make it more difficult to emulsify the lens.[1–7,9,10]

LITERATURE REVIEW

Not much has been published on postvitrectomy phacoemulsification. McDermott et al. found 22 eyes

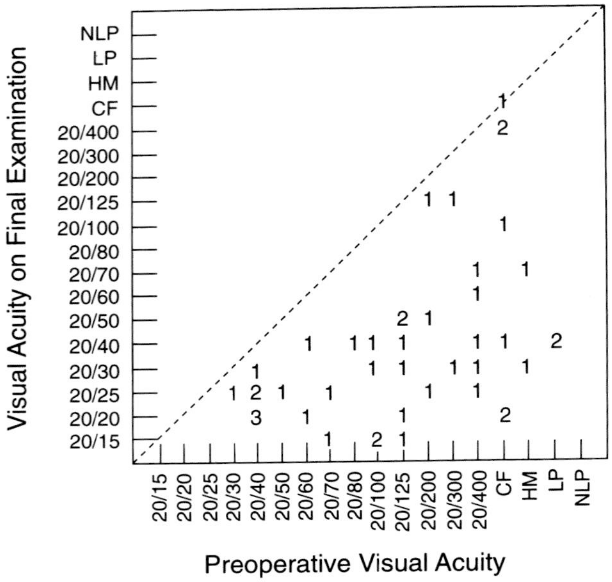

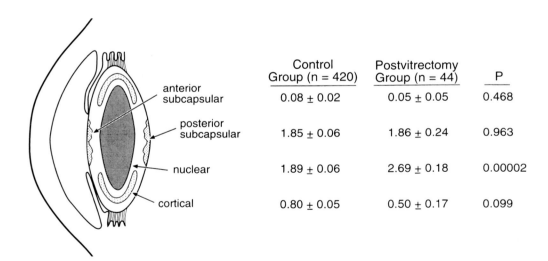

Figure 28.1. *Scattergram of best-corrected visual acuity before Kelman phacoemulsification and intraocular lens implantation versus best-corrected visual acuity at the final follow-up examination. A patient whose visual acuity improved from CF to 20/70 at the 6-week examination dropped back to CF because of a disciform macular scar. All others experienced an improvement. CF, counting fingers; HM, hand motions; LP, light perception; NLP, no light perception. From Grusha YO, Masket S, Miller KM. Phacoemulsification and lens implantation after pars plana vitrectomy.* Ophthalmology *1998; **105**: 287–94. Courtesy of* Ophthalmology.

that had previous PPV in a retrospective review of 1039 consecutive phacoemulsification cataract extractions.[34] The most common indication for vitrectomy was proliferative diabetic retinopathy, accounting for 14 eyes. Visual acuity improved postoperatively in 91% of patients. The authors observed a tendency for advanced nuclear sclerosis. They also observed deep anterior chambers, large excursions of the lens–iris diaphragm, and pupil size fluctuations during phacoemulsification. They found that many of the

	Control Group (n = 420)	Postvitrectomy Group (n = 44)	P
anterior subcapsular	0.08 ± 0.02	0.05 ± 0.05	0.468
posterior subcapsular	1.85 ± 0.06	1.86 ± 0.24	0.963
nuclear	1.89 ± 0.06	2.69 ± 0.18	0.00002
cortical	0.80 ± 0.05	0.50 ± 0.17	0.099

Figure 28.2. *Average cataract severity in a reference population of consecutive patients (420 eyes) undergoing Kelman phacoemulsification versus average cataract severity in the postvitrectomy group (44 eyes). Cataract severity was graded at the slit lamp on a 0–4 scale preoperatively as described in the text. Nuclear sclerosis was significantly more advanced in the postvitrectomy group (P = 0.00002). From Grusha YO, Masket S, Miller KM. Phacoemulsification and lens implantation after pars plana vitrectomy.* Ophthalmology *1998; **105**: 287–94. Courtesy of* Ophthalmology.

posterior capsules in their series were excessively mobile and flaccid during cortex removal. No posterior capsules tore, but some patients had posterior capsule plaques that could not be removed.

Grusha et al. identified 44 eyes of 43 patients who had phacoemulsification after PPV.[35] In their series, median visual acuity improved from 20/125 before cataract surgery to 20/30 on final examination (Fig. 28.1). Final visual acuity of 20/40 or better was achieved by 72.7% of eyes at the final examination. One eye in their series failed to improve, and it had a disciform macular scar preoperatively. They found more advanced nuclear sclerosis in the postvitrectomy eyes than in a comparison group of eyes with typical cataracts (Fig. 28.2). The most common intraoperative problem in their series was posterior capsule plaques. In two cases, surgery was made difficult by unusual fluctuations of anterior chamber depth and zonular instability. The most common early postoperative complication was corneal edema. The most common late complication was posterior capsule opacification and the need for laser capsulotomy. Inadvertent posterior capsule rupture occurred in one case, and an unplanned posterior capsulorhexis was performed in an additional three cases.

Unplanned intraoperative events and complications, early postoperative complications, and late postoperative complications from the Grusha et al. study, are detailed in Tables 28.1–28.3.

CLINICAL EXAMPLES

A few clinical examples will illustrate the types of problem encountered in postvitrectomy eyes. The first case is routine and represents 90% or more of postvitrectomy eyes. The following three cases are more complicated and illustrate problems that may occasionally be encountered.

CASE 1: A MODERATE NUCLEAR CATARACT FOLLOWING EPIRETINAL MEMBRANE DISSECTION

A 71-year-old woman underwent PPV (right eye), with epiretinal membrane dissection for macular pucker in July 1997. An inadvertent superior macular tear was

Table 28.1
Unplanned intraoperative events and complications.

Location	Pathology	N	(%)
Cornea	Peripheral corneal injury	1	(2.3)
	Stripped Descemet's membrane	1	(2.3)
Anterior chamber	Notable fluctuations in chamber depth	2	(4.5)
Iris	Prolapse	0	(0)
	Miotic pupil	0	(0)
Lens	Tears in the anterior capsulorhexis	2	(4.5)
	Marked zonular laxity or dehiscence	2	(4.5)
	Posterior capsule plaque	10	(22.7)
	Unplanned posterior capsulorhexis	3	(6.8)
	Posterior capsule rupture	1	(2.3)
	Unplanned anterior chamber intraocular lens	1	(2.3)
Posterior segment	Dropped nucleus or lens fragment	1	(2.3)
	Posterior vitreous pressure	0	(0)
	Suprachoroidal hemorrhage	0	(0)
	Vitreous loss	4	(9.1)
Other	Conversion from topical to injection anesthesia	1	(2.3)

Total eyes = 44.

From Grusha YO, Masket S, Miller KM. Phacoemulsification and lens implantation after pars plana vitrectomy. *Ophthalmology* 1998; **105:** 287–94. Courtesy of *Ophthalmology*.

Table 28.2
Early postoperative complications (complications occurring within 1 week of surgery).

Location	Pathology	N	(%)
Lids	Blepharoptosis	3	(6.8)
Cornea	Moderate to severe corneal edema	9	(20.5)
Anterior chamber	Intraocular pressure spike	0	(0)
	Wound leak	1	(2.3)
Iris	Moderate to severe postoperative iritis	1	(2.3)
	Peaked pupil with vitreous to the wound	1	(2.3)
	Prolapse	0	(0)
Lens	Incorrect intraocular lens power	0	(0)
	Intraocular lens decentration or dislocation	0	(0)
Posterior segment	Endophthalmitis	0	(0)
	Macular phototoxicity	0	(0)
	Retinal detachment	0	(0)
	Vitreous hemorrhage	0	(0)

Total eyes = 44.

From Grusha YO, Masket S, Miller KM. Phacoemulsification and lens implantation after pars plana vitrectomy. *Ophthalmology* 1998; **105:** 287–94. Courtesy of *Ophthalmology.*

Table 28.3
Late postoperative complications (complications occurring more than 1 week after surgery).

Location	Pathology	N	(%)
Lids	Blepharoptosis	1	(2.3)
Cornea	Moderate to severe corneal edema	0	(0)
	Pseudophakic bullous keratopathy	0	(0)
Iris	Chronic postoperative iritis	0	(0)
	Irregular pupil	0	(0)
	Rubeosis iridis	0	(0)
Lens	Capsulorhexis contraction	2	(4.5)
	Intraocular lens decentration	2	(4.5)
	Posterior capsular opacification	14	(31.8)
Posterior segment	New or persistent macular edema	6	(13.6)
	Persistent or recurrent choroidal neovascularization	2	(4.5)
	Proliferative diabetic retinopathy	0	(0)
	Reopened macular hole	1	(2.3)
	Retinal detachment	0	(0)
	Visually significant epiretinal membrane	7	(15.9)
	Vitreous hemorrhage	2	(4.5)

Total eyes = 44.

Complications listed in this table are not necessarily the result of cataract surgery. They may be associated with comorbidities. From Grusha YO, Masket S, Miller KM. Phacoemulsification and lens implantation after pars plana vitrectomy. *Ophthalmology* 1998; **105:** 287–94. Courtesy of *Ophthalmology.*

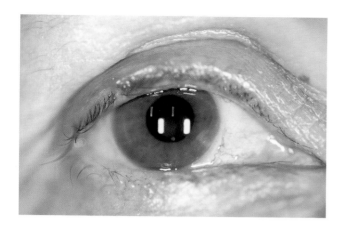

Figure 28.3. *From case 1. The postoperative day 1 appearance of a postvitrectomy eye with a moderately dense nuclear cataract that underwent phacoemulsification through a temporal corneal incision.*

created during the peel and was surrounded intra-operatively by laser retinopexy. At the time of cataract extraction she had 3+ nuclear sclerosis and a 2–3+ oil droplet posterior cortical cataract. She dilated well. Phacoemulsification and implantation of a Staar AA4207VF foldable plate haptic lens was performed under topical anesthesia in March 1998. On the first postoperative day she had mild corneal edema at the site of the temporal incision and trace endothelial stipple (Fig. 28.3). Her uncorrected visual acuity was 20/25–3. Two weeks postoperatively her best-corrected visual acuity was 20/25+1, but she complained of an inferior paracentral scotoma corresponding to the site of the retinal tear created during the vitrectomy.

CASE 2: A MATURE WHITE CORTICAL CATARACT WITH AN OCCULT POSTERIOR CAPSULE TEAR FOLLOWING REPAIR OF A CYTOMEGALOVIRUS DETACHMENT USING SILICONE OIL

A 47-year-old man with the acquired immunodeficiency syndrome developed a cytomegalovirus-related retinal detachment of his left eye from numerous atrophic retinal breaks. He underwent PPV and silicone oil injection in April 1996. At the time of cataract extraction he had a mature white cortical cataract limiting his visual acuity to light perception with projection. During surgery his pupil dilated only to 3.5 mm and a stretch pupilloplasty was performed.[36] The capsule was

membranous and the zonules were loose. The capsule was punctured a few times with a 30-gauge cystotome and further cut with the phacoemulsification probe. It was not possible to tear a circular capsulorhexis because of the membranous nature of the capsule.

After some of the anterior cortical material was removed, silicone oil began to percolate through the anterior capsule, indicating an occult posterior tear. The nucleus was sculpted cautiously and little to no posterior pressure was applied. About half the nucleus was removed successfully before the remaining large fragment dropped posteriorly. At this point silicone oil began to flow freely through the rent in the capsule and was evacuated from the eye. A dense fibrous plaque on the undersurface of the anterior capsule was cut with a combination of Westcott scissors and vitrectomy instruments. After the central anterior and posterior capsules were fully opened, a single-piece Alcon MC50BD all-polymethylmethacrylate posterior chamber lens was implanted in the ciliary sulcus. On the following day, the patient's visual acuity was counting fingers at 1 ft. His macula had been involved by the cytomegalovirus retinitis. He was sent back to his vitreoretinal surgeon for evacuation of the remaining lens fragments. The subsequent procedure was successful and his cytomegalovirus retinitis remained inactive. Unfortunately, his best-corrected visual acuity improved only to 20/80 because of macular involvement by the retinitis.

CASE 3: AN ADVANCED BRUNESCENT CATARACT AND MIOTIC PUPIL FOLLOWING EVACUATION OF A SUBMACULAR HEMORRHAGE

A 77-year-old man developed a submacular hemorrhage in the setting of macular degeneration. He underwent PPV and evacuation of the clot in March 1991. Subsequently, he developed ghost-cell glaucoma. A second PPV was performed to remove the ghost cells. Several subsequent paracenteses were performed to control intraocular pressure. At the time of cataract extraction in February 1998 he had a 3-mm non-dilating pupil and a 4+ brunescent cataract with very weak zonules (Fig. 28.4). The capsulorhexis was uneventful. Phacoemulsification time exceeded 45 min at a high-energy setting. A Staar AA4203VF foldable one-piece silicone posterior chamber intraocular lens was implanted successfully in the capsular bag. On the day after surgery, he had 3+ endothelial stria and 4+ superficial punctate keratopathy. Visual acuity was hand motions. By the second postoperative week his

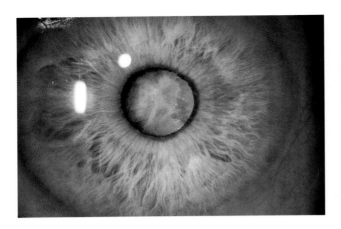

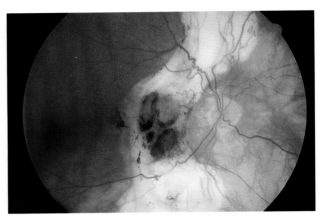

Figure 28.4. *From case 3. An eye with a brunescent cataract and miotic pupil 7 years after PPV. During the operation, the zonules were found to be weak.*

Figure 28.5. *From case 3. Macular pathology such as this disciform scar often limits the visual acuity improvement of postvitrectomy eyes after cataract extraction.*

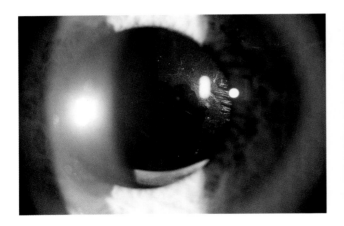

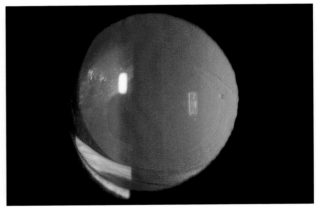

Figure 28.6. *From case 4. A primary posterior capsulorhexis was established in this eye to eliminate a dense posterior capsule plaque. The direct-illumination slit lamp view is shown on the left and a retroillumination view is shown on the right.*

visual acuity had improved to counting fingers at 1 ft eccentrically, which was his retinal potential (Fig. 28.5). By then his corneal edema had almost completely resolved. The intraocular lens was centered and the posterior capsule was clear.

CASE 4: AN ADVANCED POSTERIOR SUBCAPSULAR CATARACT WITH A DENSE POSTERIOR CAPSULE PLAQUE FOLLOWING REPAIR OF A GIANT RETINAL TEAR

A 34-year-old man underwent PPV and closed external cryotherapy for repair of a giant retinal tear in

November 1990. He had a significant inferior visual field defect and a shallow detachment of his macula at the time of vitrectomy. Gas was injected intracamerally to facilitate the repair. At the time of cataract extraction, the slit lamp biomicroscope grading of his lens was 1+ nuclear sclerosis, 2+ anterior subcapsular cataract, and 4+ posterior subcapsular cataract. He was found to have a dense central posterior capsule plaque which could not be removed intraoperatively by polishing the capsule. A small central posterior capsulorhexis was torn around the plaque and it was removed primarily (Fig. 28.6). The remaining lens capsule was clear. A Chiron 32C10XX foldable one-piece silicone posterior chamber intraocular lens was implanted in the capsular bag. His uncorrected visual acuity was 20/30+2 on the day after surgery, up from counting fingers at 1 ft prior to surgery. At the 6-week postoperative visit his best-corrected visual acuity was 20/20+.

SURGICAL APPROACH TO THE POSTVITRECTOMY CATARACT

As the previous examples illustrate, it is prudent for the surgeon to anticipate the possibility of occasional surgical problems when working with postvitrectomy cataracts, and be able to handle them. In most cases these procedures can be approached without modification of technique.

Many patients who have undergone PPV have significant posterior segment comorbidity. These patients must not be given false expectations for visual improvement with cataract surgery. If they have significant macular pathology, they should be advised that they may experience little or no improvement in central visual acuity. The benefit for some patients may only be improved color perception and peripheral vision, or a better view of the ocular fundus for the ophthalmologist. Patients should be warned that they may be more bothered by diplopia, central scotomas, metamorphopsia, and anisometropia. If they have ever had intracameral silicone oil, they may experience paradoxical aniseikonia, with a smaller image in the silicone oil-filled eye. The aniseikonia may occur in the absence of a significant anisometropia and may persist after silicone oil removal. Barring surgical complications, the improvement in visual acuity that follows cataract extraction is determined by the patient's preoperative retinal potential.

Postvitrectomy cataracts are denser, on average, than typical cataracts. More time will be spent emulsifying the lens. Care must be taken not to cause a thermal injury to the cornea and not to apply excessive force on the lens while emulsifying it. A divide and conquer or chopping technique may be indicated, depending on the surgeon's preference. In some cases, particularly in myopic eyes, the surgeon will encounter noticeable fluctuations of anterior chamber depth. If the PPV spares the anterior cortical gel (Fig. 28.7), the fluctuations may be minimal or imperceptible. If the anterior cortical gel has been removed in its entirety, as often occurs in the setting of multiple intraocular procedures, chamber fluctuations may be more significant (Fig. 28.8). Excessive

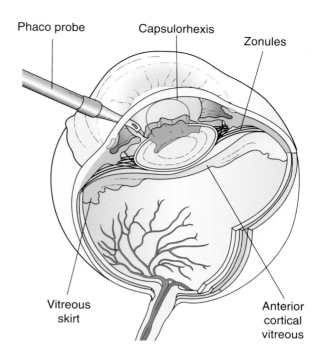

Figure 28.7. *A cushion of anterior cortical vitreous gel dampens the movement of the lens–iris diaphragm and reduces posterior capsule flaccidity.*

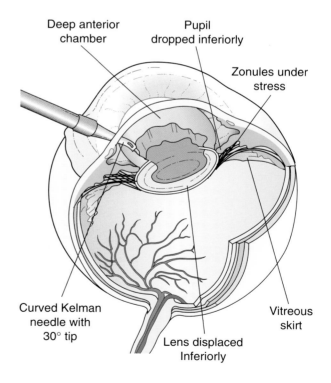

Figure 28.8. *In the absence of anterior cortical vitreous, the lens is more mobile and the posterior capsule more flaccid.*

anterior chamber depth can be reduced by keeping the irrigating bottle, and thereby the intraocular pressure, low. Movement of the lens–iris diaphragm can be reduced by maintaining constant intraocular pressure. Irrigation should be maintained whenever the phacoemulsification or irrigation–aspiration probes are in the eye. Wound leak should be minimized. The surgeon must be aware that anterior chamber depth fluctuations are uncomfortable to patients undergoing topical anesthesia surgery. If the topical approach is taken, the surgeon should consider injecting an anesthetic agent intracamerally to reduce the proprioceptive sense of the ciliary muscle. It should be mentioned that there are anecdotal reports of retinal anesthesia with intracameral injection, and that patients may experience transient blindness.

Eyes that develop mature white cortical cataracts immediately after PPV are suspect for occult posterior capsule tears. In such eyes the surgeon should consider avoiding subcapsular hydrodissection and perform a limited hydrodelineation, removing the nucleus by gentle sculpting without manual rotation. It may also be prudent to have a retina specialist available should the nucleus drop.

If intraoperative miosis is a problem, a long-acting cycloplegic agent such as cyclopentolate or atropine can be instilled. A highly retentive viscoelastic substance can be injected to force the pupil open. Additionally, the surgeon can stretch the pupil with two iris push–pull hooks.[36]

Because conjunctiva and Tenon's capsule are scarred after PPV, it is usually best to perform cataract surgery on postvitrectomy eyes through corneal incisions rather than through scleral incisions. Foldable lenses are available in most of the dioptric powers needed in clinical practice. If the surgeon must implant a non-folding anterior chamber lens, this can be performed safely through a corneal incision, but the incision should be closed with sutures.

If a dense posterior capsule plaque is encountered, the surgeon should consider incorporating the plaque in a posterior capsulorhexis. Because retina specialists usually spare the anterior cortical vitreous gel when performing a PPV, it will usually be necessary to perform a limited anterior vitrectomy as well. A larger anterior vitrectomy, however, is unnecessary. The risk of cystoid macular edema in non-diabetics who receive a primary posterior capsulorhexis is probably low. It may be preferable to open the posterior capsule primarily rather than leave patients with poor vision for several months and perform a laser capsulotomy later with the attendant risk of creating a large vitreous floater.

SPECIAL CONSIDERATIONS

INTRAOCULAR LENS CHOICE FOR EYES WITH SILICONE OIL

Silicone oil adheres to silicone intraocular lenses and interferes with vision.[37,38] The adherence problem is only slightly better with acrylic lenses. The intraocular lens material of choice at this time for eyes that must retain silicone oil is polymethylmethacrylate. Lenses that are heparin surface-modified may be preferred in the future.

Axial length measurements are best obtained after silicone oil is removed from the eye. If a retina specialist anticipates that silicone oil will be left in indefinitely, it would be wise to obtain axial length measurements before vitrectomy. It is only a matter of time before patients with silicone oil develop cataracts. Sound travels more slowly in eyes with silicone oil (1555 m/s in the normal phakic eye versus about 1000 m/s in the eye filled with silicone oil) and this alters the length calculation. If a silicone bubble does not completely fill the eye, it may move around and produce shifting echoes.

The index of refraction of silicone oil (1.405) is higher than that of the vitreous gel (1.336) which it replaces. As a result, standard theoretical and regression lens power formulas calculate a lens power which is less than that needed to achieve emmetropia, resulting in a hyperopic refractive error. The more curvature or power incorporated on the posterior surface of the lens, the greater the postoperative error. If silicone oil is in the vitreous cavity at the time of lens implantation, the surgeon should add 3–8 diopters to the calculated lens power, depending on lens shape, to achieve emmetropia. If the oil is removed after intraocular lens implantation, the patient should be forewarned that there will be a myopic shift in refraction. The shift will be greater in the presence of a biconvex lens than in the presence of a planoconvex lens, with the plano surface facing posteriorly.[39] Eyes with positive meniscus intraocular lenses (such lenses were designed to provide a laser ridge to facilitate laser posterior capsulotomy) experience the smallest change in refraction.

Additionally, eyes with good macular vision and silicone oil may experience a paradoxical aniseikonia.

Patients with silicone oil will report smaller images in their spectacle-corrected silicone oil eyes, even if they are hyperopic. The reason for this problem is not fully understood, but it is not optical. It is possible that the macular photoreceptors are spread apart by the surface tension of the silicone bubble. Interestingly, the paradoxical aniseikonia persists for some patients even after the silicone oil is removed.

INTRACAMERAL INJECTION

Pharmaceutical agents placed in the anterior chamber diffuse more easily to the retina of a postvitrectomy eye than to the back of a normal eye. The same holds true of pharmaceutical agents placed in the infusion bottle. As mentioned before, there are anecdotal reports of transient blindness resulting from intracameral injection of anesthetic agents. It might be wise to avoid putting aminoglycosides such as gentamicin and tobramycin, which have well-documented retinal toxicities, into the infusion bottle in postvitrectomy cases.[40] The surgeon should weigh

the benefit of any intracameral injection or infusion against the known and any potential unknown side-effects.

CONCLUSION

Phacoemulsification and intraocular lens implantation can be performed safely after PPV. Patients should not be given false expectations for visual recovery from cataract surgery, particularly in the setting of coexisting macular pathology. Published studies document that most patients, even those with macular disease, experience an improvement in visual acuity. To achieve consistently good results, the surgeon must anticipate the occasional problems that can occur intraoperatively and postoperatively, as with any procedure, and learn to manage them. Most patients benefit from cataract surgery when it is appropriately planned and skillfully performed.

REFERENCES

1 Novack MA, Rice TA, Michels RG, Auer C. The crystalline lens after vitrectomy for diabetic retinopathy. *Ophthalmology* 1984; **91**: 1480–4.

2 Blankenship GW, Machemer R. Long-term diabetic vitrectomy results. Report of 10 year follow-up. *Ophthalmology* 1985; **92**: 503–6.

3 Margherio RR, Cox MS, Trese MT, Murphy PL, Johnson J, Minor LA. Removal of epimacular membranes. *Ophthalmology* 1985; **92**: 1075–83.

4 McDonald HR, Verre WP, Aaberg TM. Surgical management of idiopathic epiretinal membranes. *Ophthalmology* 1986; **93**: 978–83.

5 Hutton WL, Pesicka GA, Fuller DG. Cataract extraction in the diabetic eye after vitrectomy. *Am J Ophthalmol* 1987; **104**: 1–4.

6 de Bustros S, Thompson JT, Michels RG, Enger C, Rice TA, Glaser BM. Nuclear sclerosis after vitrectomy for idiopathic epiretinal membranes. *Am J Ophthalmol* 1988; **105**: 160–4.

7 Poliner LS, Olk RJ, Grand MG, Escoffery RF, Okun E, Boniuk I. Surgical management of premacular fibroplasia. *Arch Ophthalmol* 1988; **106**: 761–4.

8 Grewing R, Mester U. Linsentrubungen nach pars-plana-vitrektomie bei diabetischer vitreoretinopathie und macular pucker. *Fortschr Ophthalmol* 1990; **87**: 440–2.

9 Cherfan GM, Michels RG, de Bustros S, Enger C, Glaser BM. Nuclear sclerotic cataract after vitrectomy for idiopathic epiretinal membranes causing macular pucker. *Am J Ophthalmol* 1991; **111**: 434–8.

10 Pesin SR, Olk RJ, Grand MG, et al. Vitrectomy for premacular fibroplasia. Prognostic factors, long-term follow-up, and time course of visual improvement. *Ophthalmology* 1991; **98**: 1109–14.

11 Nakazawa M, Kimizuka Y, Watabe T, et al. Visual outcome after vitrectomy for diabetic retinopathy. A five-year follow-up. *Acta Ophthalmol Copenh* 1993; **71**: 219–23.

12 Ogura Y, Kitagawa K, Ogino N. Prospective longitudinal studies on lens changes after vitrectomy—quantitative assessment by fluorophotometry and refractometry. *Nippon Ganka Gakkai Zasshi* 1993; **97**: 627–31.

13 Thompson JT, Glaser BM, Sjaarda RN, Murphy RP. Progression of nuclear sclerosis and long-term visual results of vitrectomy with transforming growth factor beta-2 for macular holes. *Am J Ophthalmol* 1995; **119**: 48–54.

14 Melberg NS, Thomas MA. Nuclear sclerotic cataract after vitrectomy in patients younger than 50 years of age. *Ophthalmology* 1995; **102**: 1466–71.

15 Ogura Y, Takanashi T, Ishigooka H, Ogino N. Quantitative analysis of lens changes after vitrectomy by fluorophotometry. *Am J Ophthalmol* 1991; **111**: 179–83.

16 Roussat B, Ruellan YM. Traitement du decollement de retine par vitrectomie et injection d'huile silicone. Resultats a long terme et complications dans 105 cas. *J Fr Ophthalmol* 1984; **7**: 11–18.

17 Pang MP, Peyman GA, Kao GW. Early anterior segment complications after silicone oil injection. *Can J Ophthalmol* 1986; **21**: 271–5.

18 Lucke KH, Foerster MH, Laqua H. Long-term results of vitrectomy and silicone oil in 500 cases of complicated retinal detachments. *Am J Ophthalmol* 1987; **104:** 624–33.

19 Casswell AG, Gregor ZJ. Silicone oil removal. I. The effect on the complications of silicone oil. *Br J Ophthalmol* 1987; **17:** 893–7.

20 Federman JJ, Schubert HD. Complications associated with the use of silicone oil in 150 eyes after retina-vitreous surgery. *Ophthalmology* 1988; **95:** 870–6.

21 Borislav D. Cataract after silicone oil implantation. *Doc Ophthalmol* 1993; **83:** 79–82.

22 Fisk MJ, Cairns JD. Silicone oil insertion. A review of 127 consecutive cases. *Aust NZ J Ophthalmol* 1995; **23:** 25–32.

23 Smiddy WE, Stark WJ, Michels RG, Maumenee AE, Terry AC, Glaser BM. Cataract extraction after vitrectomy. *Ophthalmology* 1987; **94:** 483–7.

24 Senn P, Schipper I, Perren B. Combined pars plana vitrectomy, phacoemulsification, and intraocular lens implantation in the capsular bag: a comparison of vitrectomy and subsequent cataract surgery as a two-step procedure. *Ophthalmic Surg Lasers* 1995; **26:** 420–8.

25 Saunders DC, Brown A, Jones NP. Extracapsular cataract extraction after vitrectomy. *J Cataract Refract Surg* 1995; **22:** 218–21.

26 Leaming DV. Practice styles and preferences of ASCRS members—1996 survey. *J Cataract Refract Surg* 1997; **23:** 527–35.

27 Watson A, Sunderraj P. Comparison of small-incision phacoemulsification with standard extracapsular cataract surgery: postoperative astigmatism and visual recovery. *Eye* 1992; **6:** 626–9.

28 Uusitalo RJ, Ruusuvaara P, Jarvinen E, Raivio I, Krootila K. Early rehabilitation after small incision cataract surgery. *Refract Corneal Surg* 1993; **9:** 67–70.

29 Feil SH, Crandall AS, Olson RJ. Astigmatic decay following small incision, self-sealing cataract surgery: one-year follow-up. *J Cataract Refract Surg* 1995; **21:** 433–6.

30 Gross RH, Miller KM. Corneal astigmatism after phacoemulsification and lens implantation through unsutured scleral and corneal tunnel incisions. *Am J Ophthalmol* 1996; **121:** 57–64.

31 Koenig SB, Han DP, Mieler WF, Abrams GW, Jaffe GJ, Burton TC. Combined phacoemulsification and pars plana vitrectomy. *Arch Ophthalmol* 1990; **108:** 362–4.

32 Mamalis N, Teske MP, Kreisler KR, Zimmerman PL, Crandall AS, Olson RJ. Phacoemulsification combined with pars plana vitrectomy. *Ophthalmic Surg* 1991; **22:** 194–8.

33 Koenig SB, Mieler WF, Han DP, Abrams GW. Combined phacoemulsification, pars plana vitrectomy, and posterior chamber intraocular lens insertion. *Arch Ophthalmol* 1992; **110:** 1101–4.

34 McDermott ML, Puklin JE, Abrams GW, Eliott D. Phacoemulsification for cataract following pars plana vitrectomy. *Ophthalmic Surg Lasers* 1997; **28:** 558–64.

35 Grusha YO, Masket S, Miller KM. Phacoemulsification and lens implantation after pars plana vitrectomy. *Ophthalmology* 1998; **105:** 287–94.

36 Miller KM, Keener Jr GT. Stretch pupilloplasty for small pupil phacoemulsification. *Am J Ophthalmol* 1994; **117:** 107–8.

37 Kusaka S, Kodama T, Ohashi Y. Condensation of silicone oil on the posterior surface of a silicone intraocular lens during vitrectomy. *Am J Ophthalmol* 1996; **121:** 574–5.

38 Apple DJ, Federman JL, Krolicki TJ, et al. Irreversible silicone oil adhesion to silicone intraocular lenses. *Ophthalmology* 1996; **103:** 1555–62.

39 McCartney DL, Miller KM, Stark WJ, Guyton DL, Michels RG. Intraocular lens style and refraction in eyes treated with silicone oil. *Arch Ophthalmol* 1987; **105:** 1385–7.

40 Miller KM. Gentamicin in ocular irrigating solutions. *J Cataract Refract Surg* 1994; **20:** 671–2.

Chapter 29 Challenging phacoemulsification procedures

Robert J Cionni

SMALL PUPILS

The presence of a small pupil during intraocular surgery increases the risk for complications. A poorly dilated pupil will decrease visualization, making surgery more dangerous, with posterior capsule rupture, iris trauma, residual cortex and malpositioned implants occurring more frequently. The ability to successfully complete phacoemulsification (phaco) and intraocular lens (IOL) implantation without a pupil-enlarging technique depends on the experience of the surgeon. Fashioning a capsulorhexis large enough to allow for nucleus manipulation and prevent capsule retraction syndrome postoperatively may require allowing the continuous tear to proceed peripheral to the pupil margin. A second dull instrument placed through the side-port can be used to retract the iris during capsulorhexis to allow direct observation of the progression of the tear. Thorough hydrodissection and hydrodelineation will be helpful for nucleus manipulation and cortical aspiration. The use of smaller phaco tips along with divide or chop techniques allows manipulation of the nucleus more easily within the confines of a smaller pupil. To be certain that all cortex is removed, a dull instrument can be used to retract the iris for direct visualization. Subincisional cortex can be removed using a 24–27-gauge J-shaped cannula after deepening the anterior chamber with viscoelastic. Direct inspection of the capsulozonular anatomy by retraction of the iris prior to IOL implantation will prevent IOL complications due to an unseen zonular dialysis or peripheral posterior capsule tear. After placement of the IOL, it is best to retract the iris and rotate the IOL to make certain the haptics are both within the capsular bag.

If the surgeon is not comfortable with a miotic pupil, it becomes necessary to enlarge the pupil for better visualization. The decision to enlarge the pupil depends on the pupil size, density of the nucleus, anterior chamber depth and health of the corneal endothelium. In a patient with a low endothelial cell count, shallow anterior chamber and brunescent nucleus, a 4-mm pupil should probably be enlarged. If only moderate nuclear sclerosis is present and the chamber is deep, a 4-mm pupil may be adequate depending on the surgeon's level of skill.

Multiple posterior synechiae can be lysed with the viscoelastic cannula. Combining a space-occupying viscoelastic with synechiolysis may enlarge the pupil significantly. If dilation is still inadequate, a ring of scar tissue incorporating the pupil can often be found. This synechial ring can be peeled free from the iris sphincter by grasping it with capsulorhexis forceps and pulling it in a tangential motion[1] (Fig. 29.1). It may be necessary to provide countertraction for the iris with a second instrument.

When synechiae are not present or when lysis of synechiae does not adequately increase pupil size, pupil stretching is often effective. Pupil stretching is accomplished by placing two dull iris retractors 180°

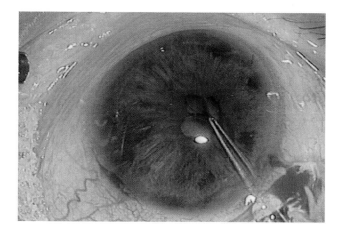

Figure 29.1. *Peeling a synechial ring with the use of capsulorhexis forceps in a patient with a history of iritis.*

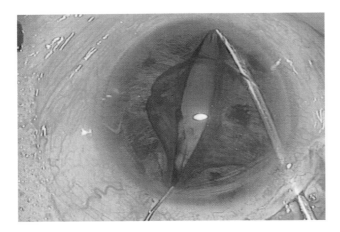

Figure 29.2. *Pupil stretch performed using an Osher iris retractor and an Osher nucleus manipulator.*

apart and slowly stretching the pupil until the retractors reach the anterior chamber angle[2] (Fig. 29.2). It is not necessary to stretch both horizontally and vertically, as the second maneuver does not usually give any increase in pupil diameter. The pupil stretch technique works quite well in most cases and usually results in a relatively normal-appearing pupil postoperatively. The use of a highly viscous and retentive viscoelastic after stretching will help to further dilate the pupil and will help to maintain dilation during capsulorhexis.

There are several alternatives to the pupil stretch technique. Multiple small incisions can be made in the iris sphincter using Vanass and reverse-style scissors. The iris is then gently stretched open further by pushing the iris tissue peripherally with a dull instrument in each direction for 360°.[3] A single large incision can be placed through the inferior iris sphincter and tissue using Vanass scissors. The sphincterotomy can be closed at the end of the case with a 10.0 proline suture using the McCannel technique. Preplacement of the suture will allow for a more reliably round and normal-appearing pupil postoperatively.[4,5] Temporary use of iris retractors will hold the pupil open during surgery; this can be done if the above techniques are inadequate or may be the preferred initial choice.[6] It is necessary to place at least three and usually four retractors to effect adequate dilation. Place the stab incisions as far posterior on the cornea as possible, to avoid elevation of the iris.[7] If the iris tents far forward, chafing may result during phaco, possibly resulting in pupil distortion and increased inflammation postoperatively. Iris retractors are available in reusable metal or disposable monofilament.

All of the above pupil-enlarging techniques can cause immediate intraocular bleeding. Use of highly retentive viscoelastic as soon as bleeding begins will usually tamponade bleeding and provide central visualization. If significant bleeding continues, one can remove all instruments and increase the intraocular pressure (IOP) by instillation of buffered saline solution (BSS) or viscoelastic via the side-port incision, provided the initial incision was fashioned to be self-sealing. Several minutes elevated IOP will often allow for hemostasis. If bleeding continues, a needle point cautery applied directly to the bleeding iris vessels under the protection of viscoelastic will effect hemostasis.

Whenever the pupil is enlarged with synechiolysis, stretching, or incisional technique, the iris will become more flaccid. Therefore, iris trauma during phaco is much more likely, as the iris tends to more easily follow viscoelastic and BSS into the phacoaspiration port. Staying alert to this possibility and resisting higher vacuum and aspiration rates will decrease the risk. It may be necessary to restrain the iris with a second dull instrument during phaco.

INTUMESCENT CATARACT

Successful phaco of the intumescent cataract remains one of the toughest challenges for the cataract surgeon today. The difficulty arises from a combination of poor visibility and increased intralenticular pressure. Successful completion of a continuous anterior capsulorhexis is jeopardized due to poor visibility resulting from the lack of a red reflex and the floating lenticular debris that escapes once the capsule is punctured. High intralenticular pressure will often cause the initial anterior capsular puncture to run peripherally into the zonules. The adult nucleus is often extremely dense despite the soft, hydrated epinucleus and cortex, making posterior capsular rupture more likely, especially if a continuous-tear capsulorhexis is not obtained. The following helpful hints are aimed at increasing the rate of successful capsulorhexis in such cases.

Use a generous amount of a highly retentive viscoelastic to deepen the anterior chamber and tamponade liquid lenticular debris. The initial anterior capsular puncture should be made just peripheral to the

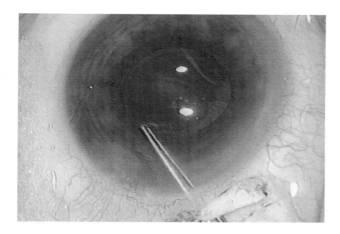

Figure 29.3. *Enlargement of the capsulorhexis after IOL placement using capsulorhexis forceps.*

central axis, so that if it does begin to run peripherally it may still be salvageable. After the initial puncture, carefully place a 27-gauge cannula through the side-port incision, through the puncture and into the hydrated lens to aspirate as much liquefied debris as possible.[8] This will decrease the intralenticular pressure, remove debris that might otherwise obscure your view, and, if enough can be aspirated, perhaps deliver some degree of a red reflex. Be careful not to move the cannula while it is inside the capsular bag, since it can easily force the initial tear peripherally. Once you have removed as much debris as possible, refill the anterior chamber with viscoelastic and continue the capsulo-rhexis. It may be easier to use capsulorhexis forceps than a bent needle, since the capsular bag may now be relatively underinflated. Strive to make the capsulo-rhexis small (4.5–5.0 mm), to avoid accidentally allow-ing the tear to run peripherally due to poor visualiza-tion. The opening can always be enlarged at a later stage of the procedure by making a small nick in the edge of the capsular rim and directing the new tear circularly around the previous edge, using forceps (Fig. 29.3). A variety of techniques, including diathermy, hemocoloration, sidelight transillumination or two-step can-opener to capsulorhexis conversion, can also be used.[9] Use high magnification to aid in visualization. Proceed slowly during capsulorhexis, and if debris begins to obscure the view, stop, aspirate the debris, and reinflate with viscoelastic. Viscoelastic can be injected directly into the capsular bag. However, over-inflating the bag can radialize the tear. If the tear encounters zonules and will not easily redirect, it is best

to convert to a can-opener technique for the remainder of the capsulorhexis. Phaco must then be performed very gently to avoid extension of the can-opener tears. Likewise, lens-cracking techniques should not be used without a successful capsulorhexis. It may, however, be safe to chop the nucleus if done carefully.

Whether continuous-tear capsulotomy is successful or not, it is not necessary to hydrodissect, since the cortex is already hydrated. If the capsulotomy is small, it is easy to damage inadvertently the capsulorhexis edge with the phaco tip. It is helpful to use a micro-Kelman-style tip to emulsify the nucleus in this situa-tion. Divide and chop techniques are well suited for most of the harder nuclei, as these techniques will allow the surgeon to see the thickness of the nucleus and develop a red reflex early on during phaco. Softer nuclei can be aspirated with little to no phaco power and relatively low vacuum levels. The dense brunes-cent nuclei are more challenging and will be discussed later in this chapter.

Despite all of the above suggestions, the intumes-cent cataract remains one of the most challenging procedures for cataract surgeons. Hopefully, new innovative approaches will develop in the future to facilitate such procedures.

BRUNESCENT CATARACT

Dense, brunescent cataracts present a greater threat for intraoperative and postoperative complications. Zonular dialysis, posterior capsule rupture, vitreous loss and posteriorly dislocated lens fragments are more likely. Prolonged phaco times at higher power levels can lead to scleral or corneal burns and corneal decompensation due to higher endothelial cell loss. Modification of standard phaco techniques may help to decrease the risk of these complications.

A more highly retentive viscoelastic with 'staying power' should be used to deepen the anterior chamber for capsulorhexis and protect the corneal endothelium during phaco. The capsulorhexis should be made large enough to allow for generous groov-ing and sculpting of the nucleus (6.0–6.5 mm). The larger capsulotomy also makes makes nucleus manipulation easier, with less likelihood of 'nicking' the anterior capsule edge with the phaco tip or a second instrument. Hydrodissection and hydrodelin-eation should be attempted; however, a large, dense nucleus and compacted cortex are often encoun-tered. If hydrodelineation is successful, manipulation of the smaller fetal portion of the nucleus will be far easier than manipulation of the entire nucleus.

A curved phaco tip will deliver power more directly to the hard nucleus. Exposure of more of the titanium tip by retraction of the silicone sleeve back further than normal will also increase the cutting efficiency of the tip. The use of higher vacuum levels will increase phacoefficiency and hold nuclear chips more firmly. However, higher vacuum levels lead to more volatile anterior chambers with higher risks for complications. High-vacuum tubing and Mackool-style phaco systems designed to minimize chamber volatility work well to decrease these risks, allowing the surgeon to utilize higher vacuum levels and more efficiently emulsify the hard nucleus.[10,11]

My preferred method for emulsification of the brunescent nucleus is a divide and debulk technique. The initial groove needs to be made two to three phaco tips wide to allow the tip to reach the hard posterior plate of the nucleus without the silicone sleeve 'hanging up' on the edges of the groove. It is often necessary to rotate the nucleus 180° to gain access to the superior portion of the nucleus. A shallow groove is made in the posterior plate at the center of the larger groove prior to cracking. A second instrument is placed deep into the groove just on top of the posterior plate, and gentle opposing forces are applied at the posterior aspect of the groove to split the nucleus (Fig. 29.4). Attempts to crack the nucleus more anteriorly are usually to no avail and require much more displacement. At this point, the surgeon can generously debulk the nucleus, leaving a thin, divided bowl of nuclear rim. Debulking is best accomplished without occlusion of the phaco tip. If the phaco tip does become occluded and embedded, care should be taken to free it with a second instrument to avoid displacement of the entire nucleus and possible zonular damage. Each half of the remaining hard bowl can then be manipulated, using a second instrument or the vacuum power of the phaco tip, into the central pupillary space for final emulsification. A second alternative is to rotate the divided nucleus 90° to groove and divide it into quadrants. These quadrants tend to prolapse anteriorly before complete debulking is accomplished, leading to more emulsification nearer the corneal endothelium. However, the use of higher vacuum levels may provide efficient enough phaco to negate the potential risk of corneal endothelial damage. While emulsifying the smaller nuclear chips, keep the phaco power low to avoid having the chips 'chatter' away from the grasp of the phaco tip. The use of short bursts of ultrasound will lessen the likelihood of a sudden occlusion break leading to ultrasound contact with the posterior capsule.

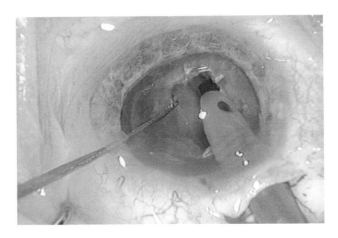

Figure 29.4. *An Osher nucleus manipulator and the phaco tip are used to divide the nucleus deep within the groove.*

Lowering of the bottle height to the minimum level required to maintain the anterior chamber will minimize the fluid irrigated through the chamber during these longer cases and decrease the amount of early corneal edema. A snug incision also decreases fluid yet too tight an incision may lead to corneal or scleral burns with long phaco times.

ZONULAR DIALYSIS

The presence of significant zonular dialysis or weakened zonules in one or more quadrants increases the difficulty of surgery tremendously, leading to a higher risk of intraoperative and postoperative complications. Each step of the procedure is compromised because of the lack of zonular integrity. Vitreous loss is common, as is the possibility of posterior nucleus dislocation. Despite successful cataract removal, adequate support for a posterior chamber IOL may be lacking. Adherence to certain principles designed to decrease zonular stress and take advantage of remaining healthy zonules will increase the likelihood of success in these patients.

A careful and detailed preoperative assessment is essential for the successful outcome of a loose cataract. Characterize the zonular defect in terms of degrees of loss, location of the defect, and presence or absence of vitreous prolapse and phacodonesis. Gonioscopy should be performed to assess for angle

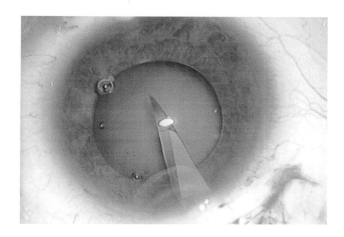

Figure 29.5. *A 15° blade is used to begin the capsulorhexis in a patient with very loose zonules due to Marfan's syndrome.*

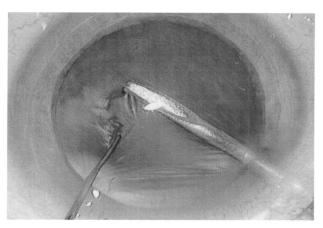

Figure 29.6. *The Osher nucleus manipulator is used to provide countertraction for capsulorhexis in a patient with loose zonules.*

recession or synechiae so that anterior chamber IOL placement can be considered should capsular bag support become insufficient.

If possible, plan to make your incision distant from the area of weakness but do not compromise your ability to perform intraocular maneuvers. Proper incision placement will help to reduce stress on the remaining zonules during the entire procedure. Maintenance of a deep, non-collapsing anterior chamber with a highly retentive and cohesive viscoelastic will help to prevent or limit forward vitreous movement. Therefore, enlarge the incision only as wide as is needed for each successive step of the procedure, to avoid egress of fluid or viscoelastic. Place a generous amount of the viscoelastic over the area of zonular dialysis for vitreous tamponade.

Begin the capsulorhexis in an area remote from the dialysis and with forces that use the countertraction of remaining, strong zonules. In more severe cases with extensive zonular loss or with significant generalized weakness, it may be necessary to begin the tear by cutting the anterior capsule with a sharp-tipped 15° blade or diamond (Fig. 29.5). The cut edge can then be grasped and directed gently to create a 5.0–6.0-mm circular opening. The capsulotomy should be large enough to allow for easy nucleus manipulation. It may be necessary to provide counteraction during capsulorhexis with a second instrument (Fig. 29.6). Hydrodissection should be performed carefully, yet thoroughly, to decrease zonular stress during nucleus rotation and cortical aspiration.

Phaco should be performed using low vacuum and aspiration rates so that the bottle height can be kept to a minimum. High bottle height leads to high IOP, which in turn forces fluid through the zonular weakness and hydrates the vitreous. The inevitable result is development of positive pressure and vitreous prolapse. However, the bottle height should not be so low as to allow chamber collapse, as such collapses also lead to vitreous prolapse. Divide and chop techniques work well in eyes with zonular dialysis as long as the surgeon is careful to apply equal forces in opposing directions so as not to displace the nucleus. It may become necessary to viscodissect nuclear quadrants free from the epinucleus or cortex, especially in the area of zonular weakness. Cortical viscodissection prior to aspiration will also limit the stress on remaining zonules and allow for cortical removal in the weakened area.[12] (Fig. 29.7). It may be best to aspirate the cortex manually using a 24–27-gauge cannula within a viscoelastic-deepened anterior chamber rather than use an automated irrigation/aspiration device.[13]

If vitreous presents at any time during the procedure, it should be removed completely from the anterior chamber. If the amount of vitreous prolapse is small, 'dry' vitrectomy can be performed, maintaining the anterior chamber with viscoelastic.[14] If there is significant prolapse, a two-handed vitrectomy should be performed, using a side-port incision for irrigation with a 27- or 25-gauge cannula. The vitrectomy handpiece can be inserted through the main incision or through a pars plana sclerotomy.[15]

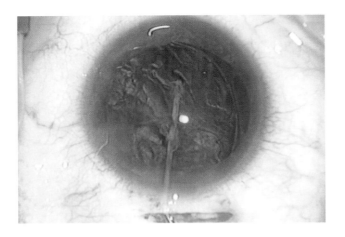

Figure 29.7. *Viscodissection of epinucleus and cortex in a patient with traumatic zonular dialysis.*

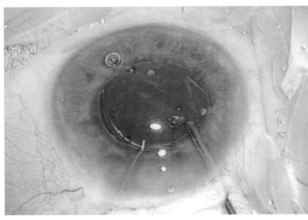

Figure 29.8. *Bending the superior haptic for in-the-bag placement using a two-handed technique to avoid stress on the zonules. (Courtesy of Robert Osher MD.)*

IOL implantation can be challenging in the face of significant zonular loss or weakness. I would recommend the use of a 6.0-mm optic or larger, just in case a small degree of lens decentration occurs postoperatively. Haptic configurations designed to allow broad contact with the peripheral capsular bag are preferred for long-term centration, but are more difficult to insert. If the dialysis is opposite the incision site, it is easy to place the inferior haptic into the bag and then use a two-handed technique to drop the superior haptic into the bag (Fig. 29.8). If the dialysis is situated at the incision site, lens placement is more difficult. Place the entire IOL into the anterior chamber first. Then, place the superior haptic into the capsular bag with a two-handed technique, prior to similarly placing the inferior haptic. Plate haptic-style silicone IOLs are a poor choice in patients with zonular dialysis or significant zonular weakness, because of the risk of postoperative decentration and capsular contraction. Foldable silicone, hydrogel or acrylic lenses are easier to place within the bag, especially if an injector is used. If you are not using an injector, insert the IOL with a technique allowing both haptics to unfold into the bag without having to 'dial in' the trailing haptic (Fig. 29.9). Placement of the haptics in the axis of the dialysis helps to expand the bag into a more natural state, decreases 'ovalization' of the bag, and usually provides adequate support and centration for the IOL. However, the IOL then relies on zonular support for only one haptic. Orienting the haptics perpendicular to the axis of the dialysis provides better zonular support but will induce 'ovalization' of the bag and perhaps a greater chance for decentration.

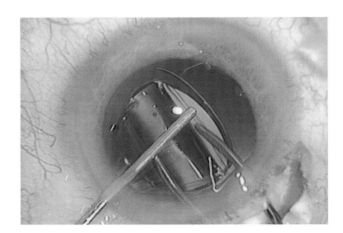

Figure 29.9. *Implantation of an AcrySof MA60 IOL using the 'mustache fold'. (Courtesy of Gary A Varley MD.)*

Use of an expanding capsular tension ring eliminates this dilemma and will be discussed later in this chapter. However, capsular tension rings cannot be used if the capsulorhexis is not intact. In that instance, place the IOL into the bag and gently rotate the IOL into the axis that provides the best centration. Once the IOL is safely within the capsular bag, viscoelastic should be removed manually to prevent further risk of vitreous prolapse. This is accomplished through the side-port incision by exchanging BSS for viscoelastic in small aliquots via a 27-gauge cannula on a 3-ml syringe.

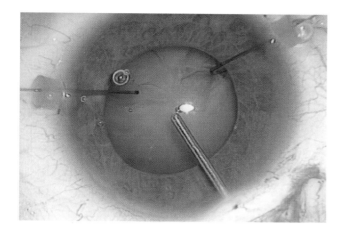

Figure 29.10. *The use of iris hooks to support a loose lens after capsulorhexis. The hooks capture the capsulorhexis edge to support the lens. (Courtesy of Robert Osher MD.)*

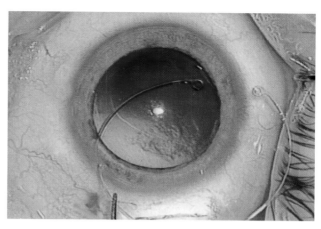

Figure 29.11. *Endocapsular ring manufactured by Morcher GmbH, Stuttgart, Germany*

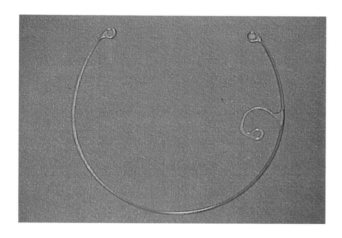

Figure 29.12. *Modified endocapsular ring as designed by Robert J Cionni. Manufactured by Morcher GmbH, Stuttgart, Germany*

Several recent advances in the management of the patient with zonular dialysis have helped to make these cases more manageable. Iris retractors can be used to engage the capsulorhexis edge at the site of a zonular dialysis.[16] The silicone stop on the hook is adjusted to hold the capsulorhexis edge to the scleral wall, thus temporarily supporting the dialysis for safer phaco and IOL placement (Fig. 29.10). This technique is especially helpful when the dialysis is at the axis of the incision.

Recently, the Morcher Company introduced the endocapsular ring (Fig. 29.11). The ring can be placed into the capsular bag at any point after successful capsulorhexis to expand and stabilize the bag.[17] Implantation can be accomplished using dull forceps or a shooter designed specifically for this ring (Hans Geuder GmbH, Heidelberg, Germany). The effect is a dramatic expansion and stabilization of a zonular dialysis or a generalized zonular weakness. The ring is left in place after IOL placement for permanent support. Removal of peripheral cortex trapped under the ring can be difficult and requires a tangential stripping action. However, the support offered by the endocapsular ring far outweighs this nuisance. At the time of this writing, the endocapsular ring is undergoing a USFDA study. It is not yet approved for use in the USA but is available in Europe.

Occasionally, despite adequate endocapsular ring expansion, the bag may remain decentered or the expanded bag may remain loose with pseudophacodonesis after IOL implantation. Additionally, long-term centration in patients with progressive generalized zonular weakness, such as that caused by pseudoexfoliation, is uncertain.[18,19] Several techniques have been devised to secure the ring and/or the bag to the scleral wall.[20] A promising technique involves a modified endocapsular ring that contains an angled hook extending off of the ring with an eyelet that provides for scleral wall suturing without violating capsular bag integrity (Fig. 29.12). A double-armed suture is passed through the eyelet of the hook (Fig. 29.13). The needles are then placed through the incision and pupil, behind the iris and

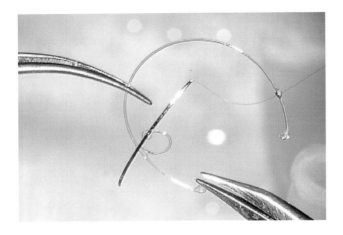

Figure 29.13. *Placement of a 10.0 proline suture through the eyelet on the 'hook' of the modified endocapsular ring prior to implantation*

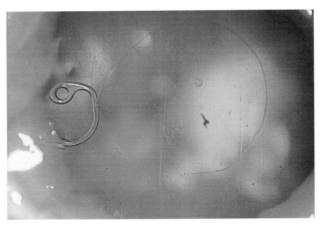

Figure 29.14. *Hook of the modified endocapsular ring being captured anterior to the capsulorhexis edge in a cadaver eye. The cornea and iris have been removed for visualization.*

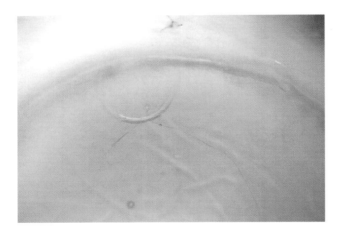

Figure 29.15. *Hook secured to the scleral wall with 10.0 prolene suture in a cadaver eye. The iris has been removed for visualization.*

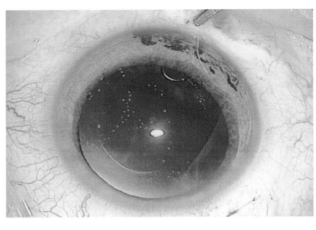

Figure 29.16. *The ring is secured into position by tying the 10.0 proline suture and burying the knot in a patient with Marfan's syndrome.*

through the scleral wall at the area of greatest zonular weakness, prior to implanting the ring. The ring is then inserted into the capsular bag. The hook is usually captured anterior to the capsulorhexis and can be used to dial the ring so that the hook orients to the site of suture placement (Fig. 29.14). The suture is secured and the knot is rotated and buried (Figs 29.15 and 29.16). Securing the ring in this fashion provides unparalleled long-term support and centration.[21] This modified ring can also be used without initial suturing. If decentration occurs

at any time postoperatively, a suture can be passed through the hook's eyelet to secure the capsular bag to the scleral wall, thereby recentering the IOL. An additional modification may soon become available with two hooks placed 180° apart for even more secure support.

The use of all endocapsular ring models is contraindicated if a complete continuous capsulorhexis is not attained. In that situation, and if there are more than 45° of zonular dialysis, it may be best to secure the IOL with sutures to the scleral wall. The entire capsular bag can be removed to prevent future opacification, or the IOL sutures can be passed through the capsular bag to stretch it and provide support.[20] Alternatively, an anterior chamber-style IOL can be used.

POSTERIOR POLAR CATARACT

Patients with posterior polar cataracts are at very high risk for posterior capsule rupture and vitreous loss.[22] These cataracts can be recognized by their characteristic 'onion-ring' appearance at the posterior pole of the lens (Fig. 29.17). A high percentage of these lenses will already have defects in the posterior capsule or thinning of the posterior capsule. The presence of satellite opacities around the axial cataract is said to be an indication of a posterior capsule opening (Daljit Singh sign). Several precautions should be taken when removing posterior polar cataracts.

The capsulorhexis should be made large enough to allow for easy manipulation of the cataract, thereby decreasing stress on the posterior capsule. Hydrodissection and/or hydrodelineation should be limited or deferred to avoid pressurizing the bag and rupturing the weak posterior capsule or extending a previous defect.

Phaco is best performed using low aspiration, low flow and low bottle height settings. High bottle height leads to higher anterior chamber pressure, especially with smaller, tighter incisions. High pressure in the anterior chamber will cause excessive deepening of the anterior chamber and stress on the posterior capsule. By the use of low vacuum and aspiration settings, chamber volatility is minimized and therefore the bottle height can be lowered. Low settings also allow phaco to occur more slowly with better control of the intraocular environment.[23]

Do not attempt divide techniques, as the stretching of the bag will challenge the decreased strength of the posterior capsule. Chop techniques can be used carefully as long as posterior forces as kept to a minimum. I prefer to sculpt maximally the nucleus to leave a nuclear and epinuclear bowl. The nuclear bowl can then be viscodissected forward for emulsification. The epinuclear bowl can then be viscodissected and emulsified in a similar fashion.

If a posterior capsule defect is not present after phaco, automated irrigation/aspiration can be

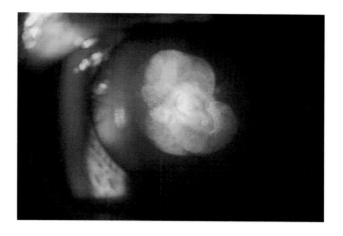

Figure 29.17. *Typical 'onion-skin' appearance of a posterior polar cataract. (Courtesy of Robert Osher MD.)*

performed. However, if a defect is detected, several steps should be altered to allow successful completion of cortex removal and IOL implantation.[13] Tamponade the posterior capsular opening with a highly retentive viscoelastic. If the defect is small, it can be converted to a posterior continuous capsulorhexis with the use of capsulorhexis forceps.[24] If the defect is already large, more care needs to be taken to avoid further enlargement of the opening during cortex aspiration, vitreous removal, if needed, and IOL placement. In the face of a posterior capsule opening, cortex is best removed manually under the protection of viscoelastic using a 25- or 27-gauge cannula. The cortex is stripped from the periphery towards the opening while the chamber is redeepened intermittently with viscoelastic. If vitreous presents, it should be removed as described previously in this chapter, taking care not to extend the posterior capsular opening.

IOL placement can proceed more easily if a defect is not present or if posterior capsulorhexis is successful. If a large opening is present, it may be best to place the IOL in the ciliary sulcus. I recommend sulcus-placed lenses with 6-mm or larger optics and overall lengths of at least 12.5 mm for more certain centration. The IOL power is decreased by 0.5 diopters from the 'in-the-bag' calculation.[25] If an opening is present in the posterior capsule, manually remove viscoelastic at the end of the procedure through the side-port incision as described earlier in this chapter.

POSITIVE PRESSURE

Phaco in the presence of positive pressure remains one of the most challenging situations facing the cataract surgeon today. Each step of the procedure becomes more challenging, with a greater likelihood of complications. Iris prolapse and trauma can occur more easily, especially if the surgeon enters the anterior chamber too near the limbus. Anterior chamber shallowing can promote unwanted peripheral extension during capsulorhexis. It may be necessary to perform phaco in the anterior chamber nearer the cornea, due to prolapse of the nucleus, causing loss of corneal endothelial cells. Complete removal of cortex can be extremely difficult because of posterior capsular bowing causing tight apposition of the anterior capsular rim to the posterior capsule. Posterior capsule rupture is more likely during any intraocular maneuvering and, if it occurs, vitreous loss is inevitable.

Positive pressure can often be prevented or corrected through an understanding of its cause. Whenever the pressure posterior to the posterior capsule is greater than the pressure within the anterior segment, positive pressure will develop. Unless an incision is self-sealing or occluded with a tightly fitted instrument, the pressure in the anterior segment is close to zero. Any pressure within the posterior segment will lead to positive pressure under this condition. Therefore, a poorly constructed clear corneal or scleral tunnel incision will increase the risk of positive pressure, while a properly fashioned incision will help to prevent its occurrence. If positive pressure develops from other causes, a self-sealing incision will aid the surgeon in managing the positive pressure as well. At each step of the procedure, the incision should be no larger than needed to allow the intended instrument to slide through the incision without displacing the globe significantly. I therefore prefer to perform capsulorhexis with a 22-gauge needle through a very small opening. The larger opening needed for use of the capsulorhexis forceps allows viscoelastic to escape and the chamber to shallow, making capsulorhexis much more difficult.

If significant positive pressure occurs during capsulorhexis and the incision is self-sealing, the surgeon may remove the forceps and perform the remainder of the capsulorhexis through a side-port incision with a 22-gauge bent needle. After deepening of the anterior chamber with a highly retentive viscoelastic agent, a clear corneal stab just to the posterior portion of the cornea is made without

actually entering. Use the tip of the needle to pierce through Descemet's membrane and complete the capsulotomy. This technique should prevent further shallowing and allow successful capsulorhexis.

It may also be necessary to perform hydrodissection through the side-port incision to prevent sudden chamber shallowing and loss of viscoelastic material. The incision can be enlarged to allow for passage of the phaco tip after capsulorhexis and hydrodissection have been completed. Sudden chamber collapse can cause forward prolapse of the IOL during final viscoelastic removal if the incision had been enlarged to allow for passage of a polymethylmethacrylate (PMMA) implant. Manual viscoelastic aspiration through the side-port incision using a 27-gauge cannula may be necessary. If at any point during the procedure the wound is too large, a 10.0 suture can be placed to decrease leakage.

Infusion rates that do not keep up with the fluid loss of aspiration and incisional leakage will lead to positive pressure and chamber shallowing. The surgeon needs to be familiar with the phaco system, to be certain that bottle height is adequate for the vacuum and aspiration settings. If the bottle height appears adequate but inflow is too slow, a kink in the irrigation tubing may be present or the irrigation bottle may not be completely 'spiked'. Occasionally, the incision may be too tight, constricting the irrigation sleeve and thereby decreasing infusion. If poor flow still exists after the above investigation, change the phaco tubing, cassette and irrigation bottle. Finally, lowering the aspiration rate may also be helpful.

Increased posterior pressure can be caused by external forces compressing the globe and transmitting the pressure through the sceral wall to the vitreous or by factors within the posterior segment itself. Identification of the etiology can often lead to a resolution of the positive pressure.

A large volume of retrobulbar or peribulbar anesthetic in a small, tight orbit can lead to significant positive pressure. Always use the smallest volume of anesthetic necessary to achieve the desired effect. If the orbit is taut after anesthetic injection, patient application of orbital massage and allowing a longer softening time with a Honan balloon or mercury bag can decrease the orbital pressure sufficiently.

Retrobulbar hemorrhage can dramatically increase orbital pressure and may necessitate the cancellation of surgery. If retrobulbar hemorrhage occurs, application of immediate pressure over closed lids and maintenance of intermittent pressure for 5–10 min should limit the orbital pressure. If, then, the globe is easy to retropulse, the lids are relatively loose, and

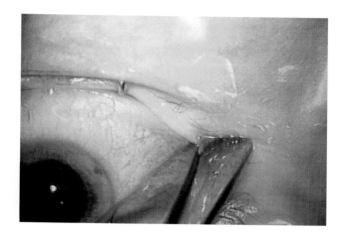

Figure 29.18. *Lysis of the lateral canthus to relieve tight lids*

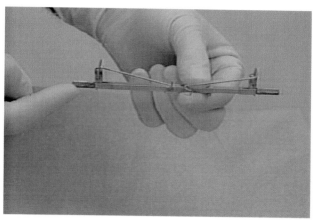

Figure 29.19. *Osher–Cionni speculum with rotating arms designed to lift the lids off the globe (Storz St Louis, Missouri).*

there is not too much proptosis, the surgeon can proceed with a small, self-sealing type of phaco procedure.[26]

Topical anesthesia eliminates the risk of positive pressure due to placement of orbital anesthetic. However, if the patient moves the eye significantly or squeezes the lids tightly during intraocular maneuvers, sudden positive pressure will develop. To avoid this possibility, determine the likelihood of poor cooperation during the preoperative examination. Simple observation of the patient's tolerance during indirect ophthalmoscopy will indicate the patient's ability to undergo topical anesthesia safely.

The anatomic finding of tight lids can compress the globe and induce positive pressure. Clamping of the lateral canthus with a hemostat for several minutes to discourage bleeding and then using scissors to perform a lateral canthotomy will decrease the pressure effect of the lids (Fig. 29.18). Extensive adipose tissue prolapse and proptosis can induce significant posterior pressure. Additional orbital softening time will sometimes prevent the development of positive pressure.

If a superior rectus suture is used, it can induce traction, which is transmitted to the scleral wall, and thereby lead to positive pressure. Superior rectus sutures should only be used when absolutely necessary.

Some speculum designs do not prevent the lids from compressing the globe adequately and their use can promote positive pressure. Utilization of a speculum which lifts the lids off the globe can help to prevent positive pressure (Fig. 29.19).

When an obese patient is placed with the feet elevated higher than the head, venous engorgement occurs within the orbit, increasing the orbital pressure and causing globe compression. Placement of the patient in a Trendeleburg position will decrease orbital pressure and thereby reduce the likelihood of positive pressure.

Several intraocular conditions can induce positive pressure during surgery. Any event that leads to hydration of the vitreous can generate considerable positive pressure. It is important to be certain of cannula placement behind the anterior capsulorhexis edge during hydrodissection. Sudden infusion of fluid into the ciliary sulcus can quickly hydrate the vitreous and even lead to a pupillary block.[27]

A high irrigation fluid bottle height increases the 'water pressure' within the anterior segment and can force fluid through the zonules and into the vitreous. This effect is more likely to occur in patients with compromised zonules or during prolonged phaco. The effect of high 'water pressure' can be seen most dramatically in younger patients with more elastic scleral walls. A high bottle height in these patients will lead to profound deepening of the anterior chamber and possible weakening of the zonules. Additionally, a higher potential energy is stored within the scleral wall and an occlusion break may cause an abrupt anterior chamber collapse.

Continued 'scleral depression' by the handpiece during phaco and cortical aspiration can also force fluid through the zonules and into the posterior segment, causing positive pressure. Intravenous mannitol may decrease the pressure caused by a hydrated vitreous, but it may also cause a paradoxical chamber shallowing if the scleral walls collapse. If positive pressure due to vitreous hydration becomes extensive, a pars plana vitreous aspiration may be indicated.[28] It is necessary, however, to confirm that a choroidal effusion or hemorrhage is not present prior to vitreous aspiration. A 25-gauge needle can be placed into the vitreous cavity through the pars plana and visualized through the pupil. Liquefied vitreous can then be aspirated, relieving the pressure. Alternatively, a small amount of vitreous can be removed with the vitrectomy cutter without the irrigation sleeve through a sclerotomy.

Choroidal hemorrhage or effusion can quickly lead to extensive positive pressure, and saving the eyes becomes the surgeon's singular mission. A dark shadow developing across the red reflex can accompany the onset of positive pressure. Use of a self-sealing incision, removal of all intraocular instruments and filling of the anterior chamber with BSS or viscoelastic will help to tamponade the hemorrhage and to limit the damage that it causes. Surgery can be completed at a later time.

If positive pressure develops, all possible causes should be examined and corrected if possible. If positive pressure persists, several techniques may allow for successful completion of the case. A prolapsed iris can prevent insertion of the phaco tip. The iris can be gently repositioned through the side-port incision with a small amount of highly retentive viscoelastic. Insertion of the phaco tip in position zero without irrigation, then advancement of the tip beyond the iris, is quite often successful.

Occasionally, it may be necessary to make a peripheral iridectomy in the prolapsed tissue to equalize the pressure on both sides of the iris. Rarely, it may be necessary to perform phaco through the peripheral iridectomy.

Phaco should be performed with low levels of aspiration and vacuum in the presence of significant positive pressure to avoid aggravation of the tendency towards chamber collapse. Short bursts of ultrasound instead of continuous phaco power may also help to decrease chamber shallowing. Raising the bottle may deepen the anterior chamber but can worsen the situation if vitreous overhydration is the culprit responsible for the pressure.

Removal of cortex can become extremely difficult and may require a manual technique. Deepening the anterior chamber and opening the capsular bag as much as possible with a highly retentive viscoelastic may allow the surgeon to use a 25- or 27-gauge cannula through the side-port incision to aspirate as much cortex as possible. A 'J'-shaped cannula introduced through the main incision may be needed to remove subincisional cortex.

IOL implantation may require special maneuvers. After expansion of the capsular bag and deepening of the anterior chamber with viscoelastic, the lens is placed into the anterior chamber. If positive pressure prevents haptic placement directly into the capsular bag, the wound is made watertight and the haptics can be dialed into the capsular bag through a side-port incision. This technique will work with both foldable and PMMA lenses.

Viscoelastic removal at the procedure's conclusion may become challenging as well, resulting in dramatic chamber collapse and anterior dislocation of the IOL. Though more time-consuming, it is best to manually exchange viscoelastic for BSS in eyes with significant positive pressure as previously described.

REFERENCES

1 Osher R. Peripupillary membranectomy. *Video J Cataract Refract Surg* 1995; **11**(1).
2 Miller K, Keener Jr G. Stretch pupilloplasty for small pupil phacoemulsification. *Am J Ophthalmol* 1994; **177**: 107–8.
3 Fine H. Pupilloplasty for small pupil phacoemulsification. *J Cataract Refract Surg* 1994; **20**: 192–6.
4 McCannel M. A retrievable suture idea for anterior uveal problems. *Ophthalmic Surg* 1976; **7**: 98–103.
5 Masket S. Preplaced inferior iris suture method for small pupil phacoemulsification. *J Cataract Refract Surg* 1992; **18**: 518–22.
6 Mackool R. Small pupil enlargement during cataract extraction. A new method. *J Cataract Refract Surg* 1992; **18**: 523–6.
7 Nichamin L. Enlarging the pupil for cataract extraction using flexible nylon iris retractors. *J Cataract Refract Surg* 1993; **19**: 793–6.
8 Cionni R. The white cataract. *Video J Cataract Refract Surg* 1992; **8**(2).
9 Krag S, Cimetta D, Osher R, John M, Basti S, Greits J. The capsule. *Video J Cataract Refract Surg* 1996; **12**(1).
10 Wilbrandt H. Comparative analysis of the fluidics of the AMO Prestige, Alcon Legacy, and Storz Premiere

phacoemulsification systems. *J Cataract Refract Surg* 1997; **23**: 766–80.

11 Mackool R. The Alcon Legacy/Mackool System. Presented at the America Society of Cataract and Refractive Surgery, April 1997.

12 Cionni R, Osher R. Complications of phacoemulsifications. In: Weinstock F, ed. *Management and Care of the Cataract Patient* (Cambridge: Blackwell Scientific Publications, 1992) 198–211.

13 Osher R, Cionni R. The torn posterior capsule: its intraoperative behavior, surgical management and long-term consequences. *J Cataract Refract Surg* 1990; **16**: 157–62.

14 Cionni R, Osher R. Complications of phacoemulsification surgery. In: Steinert R, ed. *Cataract Surgery: Techniques, Complications and Management* (Philadelphia: WB Saunders Co. 1995) 327–40.

15 Eller A, Barad R. Miyake analysis of anterior vitrectomy techniques. *J Cataract Refract Surg* 1996; **22**: 213–17.

16 Novak J. Flexible iris hooks for phacoemulsification. *J Cataract Refract Surg* 1997; **23**: 828–31.

17 Cionni R, Osher R. Management of zonular dialysis with the endocapsular ring. *J Cataract Refract Surg* 1995; **21**: 245–9.

18 Fischel J, Wishart M. Spontaneous complete dislocation of the lens in pseudoexfoliation syndrome. *Eur J Implant Refract Surg* 1995; **6**: 31–3.

19 Nishi O, Nishi K, Sakanishi K, Yamada Y. Explanation of endocapsular posterior chamber lens after spontaneous posterior dislocation. *J Cataract Refract Surg* 1996; **22**: 272–5.

20 Osher R. New approach: synthetic zonules. *Video J Cataract Refract Surg* 1997; **8**(1).

21 Cionni R, Osher R. Management of profound zonular dialysis or weakness with a new endocapsular ring designed for scleral fixation. *J Cataract Refract Surg* 1998; in press.

22 Osher R, Yu B, Koch D. Posterior polar cataracts; a predisposition to intraoperative posterior capsule rupture. *J Cataract Refract Surg* 1990; **16**: 157–62.

23 Osher R. Slow-motion phacoemulsification approach. *J Cataract Refract Surg* 1993; **19**: 223–31.

24 Gimbel H. Posterior capsule tears using phacoemulsification; causes, prevention and management. *Eur J Implant Refract Surg* 1990; **2**: 63–9.

25 Osher R, Corcoran K. Modification of the IOL power; ciliary sulcus versus capsular bag. Presented at the Welsh Cataract Congress, 1986, Houston.

26 Cionni R, Osher R. Retrobulbar hemorrhage. *Ophthalmology* 1991; **98**: 1153–5.

27 Updegraff S, Peyman G, McDonald M. Pupillary block during cataract surgery. *Am J Ophthalmol* 1994; **117**: 328–32.

28 Cionni R. Review of positive pressure. *Video J Cataract Refract Surg* 1992; **8**(3).

Chapter 30

Surgical management of posterior segment complications of cataract surgery: I

Brian Leonard

INTRODUCTION

Modern cataract surgery is a very safe procedure.[1] Final visual acuity results of 20/40 or better are achieved in 90% of all eyes and in 95% of eyes without pre-existing ocular morbidity. Clinically serious complications, however, occur in nearly 2% of cases. This implies that approximately 20 000 serious complications will develop among the more than 1 million cataract extractions performed in the USA annually.

Since most of these complications have posterior segment implications, there is abundant opportunity for scholarly and clinical collaboration between cataract surgeons and their vitreoretinal colleagues.

INADVERTENT ANESTHETIC NEEDLE PERFORATION OF THE GLOBE

Administration of periocular anesthesia for ocular surgery is one of the most commonly performed ophthalmic procedures. Because it requires the blind insertion of a needle into the orbit, there is risk of direct mechanical damage to the eye and optic nerve.[2,3]

Inadvertent subarachnoid or subdural injection of anesthetic agents[4] may lead to a variety of startling central nervous system complications, including brainstem anesthesia,[5,6] cardiac arrest,[7] contralateral nerve palsies,[8] contralateral amaurosis,[9] optic neuritis,[10,11] retinal vascular occlusion,[12] subretinal air injection,[13] and a Purtscher's-type retinopathy.[14,15] Grand mal seizures may arise from intra-arterial injection,[16] and aggressive retrobulbar hemorrhage may lead to central retinal artery closure.[17,18]

Table 30.1

Risk factors for ocular anesthetic needle perforation.

Ocular factors
  High axial myopia
  Existing scleral buckle
  Tight orbit
  Enophthalmos
Technical factors
  'Up and in' direction of gaze
  Large-gauge blunt needle
  Multiple injections
  Limited patient cooperation
  Injection by non-ophthalmologist

Globe perforation by an anesthetic needle is another significant complication. In large series with 1000 patients or more, the reported incidence of iatrogenic perforation varies from zero to 0.1%.[19–24] The most commonly stated rate of 0.1% is probably accurate, allowing for variations in existing risk factors, recognition and reporting.[24]

Although prompt diagnosis, evaluation and expert treatment of anesthetic globe perforations are of prognostic importance, most authors report very discouraging final visual outcomes.[13,25–30] Prevention of this complication is therefore essential and requires a thorough understanding of the ocular and technical risk factors involved (Table 30.1).

RISK FACTORS

Refractive error

High axial myopia, particularly with scleral thinning and staphyloma, is the most commonly quoted risk factor. Eyes with an axial length of 26.00 mm or more have a perforation risk at least 30 times greater than that of the normal population.[25] Hyperopic eyes, deeply set in a tight orbit, are also at greater risk.[28]

Existing scleral buckle

A history of previous scleral buckling, especially with an encircling band, creates both an elongation and staphyloma of the globe posterior to the hardware, increasing the exposure to needle perforation.[31]

Direction of gaze

The classic 'up and in' position of the globe was advocated to allow better access to the retrobulbar cone and to protect the inferior oblique muscle.[32] CT and MRI studies confirm that this position actually enhances needle exposure to the globe and optic nerve.[2,33]

Injection technique

Peribulbar injection has been proposed as a safer technique than retrobulbar injection, with administration of one or more large-volume injections outside the muscle cone, thereby avoiding proximity to the globe, optic nerve and subarachnoid space.[34] Although the peribulbar approach may be safer, surgeons should be aware that perforation of the globe and optic nerve can still occur.[5,6,21–30,34] Multiple injections, especially into a tight orbit, also constitute a risk factor.

Needle type

The use of blunt needles does not prevent globe or optic nerve perforation. The Weber–Fechner law states that, as resistance increases, the ability to detect increased resistance diminishes.[26] The eye and optic nerve, which are held in position by a three-dimensional web of fibrous tissue,[35] cannot move away from the oncoming needle. When perforation does occur, sharp, small-gauge needles actually create smaller, cleaner, less extensive injuries.[26] Even the short needles proposed for peribulbar technique can extend back to perforate the posterior globe or optic nerve, if the needle hub is pushed firmly and aggressively into the skin.[5]

Patient cooperation

A patient who is uncooperative because of limited intelligence, communication difficulty, anxiety, undersedation or oversedation, is at greater risk for perforation.

Training and experience

Delegation of the anesthetic block to a non-ophthalmologist is a perforation risk factor.[26,36] The national trend for anesthetic personnel to give cataract blocks is reported as the principal source of the current epidemic of ocular needle perforations in the UK.[24,37]

TREATMENT OF NEEDLE GLOBE PERFORATION

Prevention

The cataract surgeon is ultimately responsible, in each case, for assessing and responding to the presence of perforation risk factors. Some patients may be better managed with topical, limbal or general anesthesia.

Recognition

A common theme among published series is that immediate recognition of the perforation is unusual, especially by non-ophthalmologists. More often, recognition is delayed until during, after or long after the surgery. Occasionally, either the injector or the patient recalls an immediate intuitive sense that the needle entered the eye. Some immediate symptoms of perforation are acute loss of vision, a swirl of vitreous floaters and severe pain. Immediate signs of perforation include increased resistance during the injection, a dark red reflex, hypotony, shallowing of the anterior chamber, wound rupture and elevation of intraocular pressure with a stony hard globe.

Assessment

A suspected perforation, before, during or after cataract surgery, requires immediate evaluation with indirect ophthalmoscopy and scleral depression. All attempts should be made to have a vitreoretinal surgeon come to the operating room or see the patient soon after surgery.

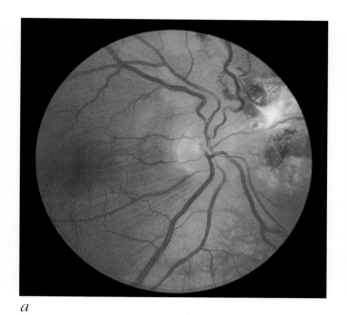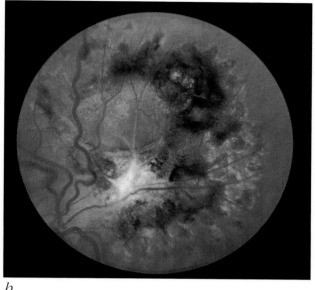

a   *b*

Figure 30.1. *Posterior anesthetic needle injury supranasal to right optic disk 2 years following vitrectomy and laser retinopexy. (a) Macula is uninvolved aside from retinal striae, and visual acuity is 20/25. (b) all vitreous was surgically delaminated and released over the injury site and this eye probably has a permanent cure.*

Needle injuries are characterized by single (penetrating) or double (perforating) transretinal punctures at the equator and posterior pole (Fig. 30.1). The posterior punctures may be elongated and multiple and are most often associated with varying amounts of progressive accumulation of choroidal, subretinal, subhyaloid and vitreous hemorrhage. Retinal detachment is a common finding, often complicated by proliferative vitreoretinopathy (Fig. 30.2).

Treatment

If the perforation is recognized at the time of injection, the cataract surgeon may occasionally consider proceeding with extraction of a very dense cataract to improve the fundus view, if adequate anesthesia and akinesia are present and if the eye is not hypotonous.[24] If the perforation is recognized intraoperatively, it is prudent to abbreviate the procedure, without lens implantation or with implantation of a 7.0-mm optic lens, without the use of miotics, and with solid wound closure, in anticipation of vitreoretinal evaluation and intervention. Posterior scleral exploration is not required, since these wounds are usually small and self-sealing. Local anesthetic agents

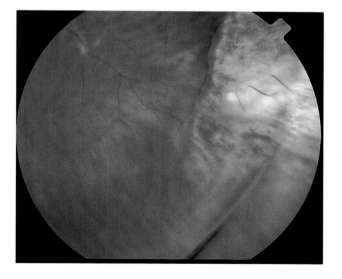

Figure 30.2. *Inferotemporal fundus of left eye with a large-gauge needle perforation following a peribulbar block delegated to a non-ophthalmologist, resulting in vitreous hemorrhage and proliferative vitreoretinopathy retinal detachment. Repair involved vitrectomy, scleral buckling, full-thickness scleral suturing and silicone oil implantation. The patient recalled an immediate intuitive sensation that the needle had entered her eye. There was no posterior perforation.*

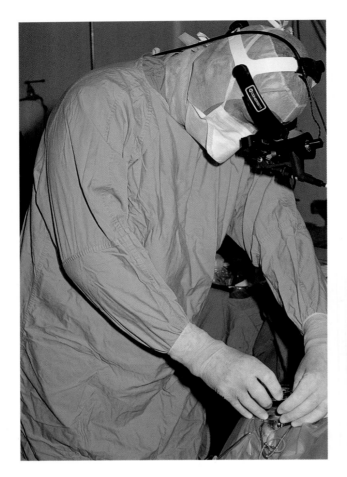

Figure 30.3. *Laser photocoagulation therapy applied around a posterior needle injury site using a laser indirect ophthalmoscope. This technique does not require intravitreal probes or slit lamp delivery systems. Far peripheral injuries can be treated with scleral depression.*

injected into the eye do not appear to be toxic to the retina[38] and do not require lavage.

The optimal treatment of retinal breaks without detachment is immediate laser indirect ophthalmoscopic retinopexy, applied before the development of retinal detachment and before clouding of the vitreous with clot break-up (Fig. 30.3).

Prompt treatment of retinal detachment with vitrectomy, internal wound debridement, retinopexy and intraocular tamponade is important to minimize the risk of proliferative vitreoretinopathy. Immediate retinotomy and surgical evacuation of extensive subretinal hemorrhage is required if the hemorrhage extends into the macula.

ZONULAR DEHISCENCE AND POSTERIOR CAPSULE RUPTURE

Intraoperative zonular dehiscence or posterior capsule rupture is a significant and common event which is estimated to occur in 3.1% of cataract operations.[1]

Opening of the posterior capsule during cataract surgery presents an opportunity for vitreous loss, posterior migration of lens material and luxation of the intraocular lens (Fig. 30.4). These events can lead

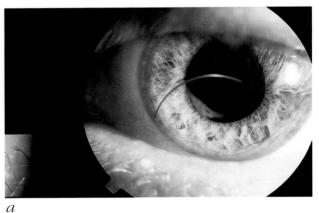

a

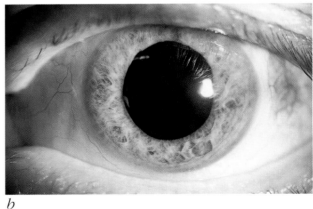

b

Figure 30.4. *(a) This intraocular lens (IOL) luxated and floated freely about the eye following intraoperative posterior capsular rupture. Vitreous presented and was adequately managed but the small linear capsular tear was not converted to a continuous capsulorhexis, allowing the tear to extend and the IOL to luxate. (b) Following vitrectomy and sulcus suture fixation of the luxated IOL.*

to a number of sight-threatening situations, including cystoid macular edema, glaucoma, retinal detachment, endophthalmitis and massive suprachoroidal hemorrhage.

Even if vitreous does not present through the capsular opening and the surgery is otherwise successfully completed, there is still some limited risk of long-term adverse effects. Pseudophakic eyes with an intact posterior capsule are less likely to develop a posterior vitreous detachment[39,40] and are less likely to develop cystoid macular edema[41,42] than eyes with primary capsulotomy.

RISK FACTORS

Any ocular or systemic disorder associated with weakened zonules creates a risk factor for capsular opening. The most significant of these are advanced age, pseudoexfoliation, previous trauma and diabetes.[43,44] Residents in training and surgeons in transition to phacoemulsification (phaco) are more likely to cause a rent in the capsule.[45] Other risk factors include an excessively hard or excessively soft nucleus, a miotic pupil, a long axial length with an awkward, deep anterior chamber, and the inability of the patient to rest quietly in a flat, supine position.

PREVENTION

The surgeon may choose to alter the choice of surgical approach or the type of anesthesia in patients at risk. Use of a capsular tension ring may be prudent (see Chapter 29).[43,46] Meticulous attention to detail in every phase of the anterior capsulotomy, hydrodissection, phaco, cortical clean-up and lens insertion is essential in high-risk eyes, with particular emphasis on protection of the posterior capsule from exposure to the sharp edges of hard nuclear fragments by judicious use of viscoelastics and thoughtful fragment manipulation.

TREATMENT

The principal goal of treatment is to complete the removal of any remaining lens material and implant an intraocular lens, without requiring vitrectomy (Table 30.2). Achieving this goal requires skill, finesse and an understanding of surgical principles.[47] Immediately upon recognizing the presence of a capsular rupture, freeze all movement of whatever

Table 30.2

Intraoperative management of posterior capsule rupture to avoid vitreous loss.

Prompt recognition and assessment of the rupture site
Freeze the handpiece in position and avoid reflex removal from the eye
Lower infusion pressure
Side-port injection of viscoelastic
Consider use of an anterior chamber maintainer
Reflux and gently remove the handpiece
Convert the linear capsular tear to a continuous curvilinear capsulorhexis
Viscodissect remaining lens material
Reinsert the handpiece and remove lens material, maintaining viscoelastic closure of the capsule rupture
Implant the intraocular lens in the bag
Constrict the pupil
Remove the viscoelastic
Hydrate or suture wounds

---

handpiece is in the eye, lower the infusion and avoid the reflex to remove the handpiece from the eye. Tamponade the capsular tear and refill the anterior chamber through a side-port incision with high-viscosity, low-cohesiveness viscoelastic (dispersive viscoelastic). Ensure that the handpiece port is free of vitreous and remove it gently from the eye. An anterior chamber maintainer may be useful at this stage.[48] If the capsule rupture is a linear tear, it should be converted at this time to a continuous posterior capsulorhexis, to avoid radial linear extension.[49] Viscodissection of remaining cortex and mobilization of any nuclear fragments to a favorable position can be done with a bent needle or probe. The lens material can then be removed with minimal infusion using manual or linear suction, taking care to maintain a viscoelastic plug over the capsular opening. Place a lens in the bag, constrict the pupil and remove the viscoelastic and any remaining cortex. Hydrate or suture the wounds as appropriate.

VITREOUS LOSS

The penalty for delayed recognition or unsuccessful management of inadvertent posterior capsular rupture is vitreous loss. This occurs in 0.8% of cataract operations and is four times more likely to occur with extracapsular technique than with phaco.[1] Presentation of vitreous into the anterior chamber interferes with completion of cataract extraction and lens implantation. Prolapsed vitreous entangled on lens capsule, iris or intraocular lens haptics or in the wound further enhances the risk of unpleasant inflammatory, infectious, proliferative and tractional posterior segment complications.[40,50]

RECOGNITION

Although vitreous can sometimes be directly observed prolapsing through an identified capsular defect, the presence of vitreous issuing through an occult defect is often telegraphed by indirect clues. A glistening string of material trailing the exit of an instrument from the eye may prompt the classic surgeon's plea, 'please let that be viscoelastic'. A perplexing plugging of the phaco or infusion/aspiration port during cortical clean-up is another clue. Lens cortex will not aspirate, even with aggressive suction levels, in the presence of vitreous.

TREATMENT

The goals of treatment are to remove all vitreous from the anterior chamber and capsular bag, and to release any vitreous wound incarceration (Table 30.3). This is best performed with closed intraocular microsurgical technique. The classic approach of methylcellulose sponge and scissors management through an open corneoscleral wound, popularized in the intracapsular era, is now considered to be dangerous and outdated. The gentle use of a methylcellulose sponge still has a limited role in inspecting wounds for residual vitreous.[51] Directional flow forces from automated vitrectomy instruments with coaxial infusion sleeves can cause dangerous capsular and posterior vitreous disruption. External vitreous wound toilet has not traditionally been a gratifying experience. This is particularly true in the phaco era. Small beveled incisions will generally only allow prolapse if vitreous is mechanically extracted by instrument exit. When vitreous incarceration does occur, however, it is much better managed with internal wound toilet by use of an automated vitrectomy instrument.

When vitreous from a visible or occult capsular break is recognized in the anterior chamber, the

Table 30.3

Management of vitreous loss.

Freeze the handpiece in position and avoid reflex removal

Lower infusion pressure

Side-port injection of viscoelastic

Viscodissect vitreous from the handpiece tip

Reflux and gently remove the handpiece

Close the wound with temporary interrupted sutures

Bimanual vitrectomy with infusion and automated vitrectomy instrument 90° from each other

Reopen the wound and inspect

Place the intraocular lens according to the availability of capsule support

Avoid methylcellulose sponge open-wound scissors vitrectomy

Avoid coaxial vitrectomy tip infusion sleeve

Consider the option of pars plana incision for bimanual vitrectomy

position of the handpiece should be frozen and not reflexively changed. Attempt a viscoelastic dissection of any vitreous adherent to or surrounding the handpiece tip with injection of a high molecular weight, low-cohesiveness viscoelastic through a side-port incision. Lower or close the infusion and gently remove the instrument from the eye. Place temporary interrupted sutures into the phaco or extracapsular corneoscleral wound to ensure a watertight closed compartment. Then perform a bimanual vitrectomy with an anterior chamber maintainer or infusion cannula and an automated vitrectomy instrument, preferably 90° apart. Either of these instruments will fit through a side-port or between interrupted wound sutures and their positions may be altered and interchanged as required to accomplish internal wound toilet, removal of vitreous and lens material from the anterior chamber and capsular bag, and posterior toilet of the capsular defect sufficient to prevent further vitreous prolapse. Internal sweeping of the iris surface is useful in detecting and releasing any residual vitreous bands. The main wound may then be reopened and an intraocular lens placed into the capsular bag, ciliary sulcus or anterior chamber, depending on the availability of capsular support. The pupil is constricted and residual viscoelastic or lens cortex removed.

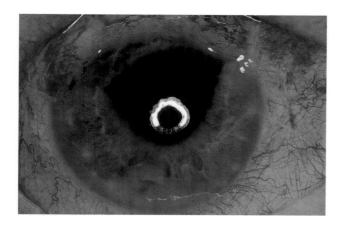

Figure 30.5. *Patient referred 2 weeks following difficult cataract surgery with superior pupillary distortion from 'wall to wall' vitreous wound incarceration. Cortical lens material is resting inferiorly in the anterior chamber. This was managed with topical anti-inflammatory medication but vitrectomy was eventually required because of chronic CME. Vitrectomy would not have been offered, despite the extensive vitreous incarceration, if visual acuity had been good and if no retinal tears had been present.*

There are some advantages to placing the vitrectomy instrument through a pars plana incision.[52] The advantages of improved internal exposure and less distorted visualization must be balanced against the surgeon's level of training and confidence.

Occasionally, vitreous loss will not be recognized until after surgery, when patients present with incarcerated strands with pupillary distortion. Most authors agree that vitrectomy surgery at this stage is not ordinarily indicated except in eyes with chronic cystoid macular edema or persisting uveitis (Fig. 30.5). Careful follow-up is important because of the risks of retinal detachment and endophthalmitis.

CYSTOID MACULAR EDEMA AFTER CATARACT SURGERY

Cystoid macular edema (CME) following cataract surgery is an intraocular inflammatory disease[53] resulting in breakdown of the blood–retina barrier with perifoveal retinal capillary leakage and outer plexiform layer fluid accumulation. Visual loss

from CME occurs after 2.1% of cataract operations.[1] CME rarely occurs within the first postoperative week,[54] but more typically develops within 4–12 weeks after surgery. In rare instances it may occur several years later.[55] Episodes of mild CME often clear spontaneously, with visual improvement, but chronic irreversible changes may occur in the form of pigment epithelial disruption, cystoid cavity rupture and subretinal fibrosis.[56]

RISK FACTORS

Any condition promoting disruption of the blood–retina barrier will favor formation of CME. These include pre-existing microvascular pathology and probably include arterial hypertension and diabetes mellitus, without detectable microvascular change.[57]

The frequency and severity of CME is directly proportional to the amount of surgical trauma. Both primary capsulotomy[41,42] and secondary Nd:YAG laser capsulotomy[58] confer some risk of triggering CME. Extracapsular technique is less likely than intracapsular technique to induce CME.[59] Phaco technique generates even less disruption of the blood–retina barrier.[60] Other risk factors include prolonged operating time, excessive intraocular manipulation, retained lens material, intraocular lens malposition and complications of vitreous presentation or incarceration.

TREATMENT

Pharmacologic therapy

No pharmacologic therapy has been established to prevent or treat clinically significant CME.[61] It seems reasonable, however, to offer topical steroid or other anti-inflammatory agents in eyes with significant inflammatory findings.[62] Many surgeons will also offer topical diclofenac, which has shown some possible effectiveness in reducing inflammation and the incidence of angiographic CME after cataract surgery.[63]

A popular 'leap of faith' approach is to offer a 6-week trial regimen of topical prednisolone 1% and a non-steroidal anti-inflammatory agent four times daily. Other less popular pharmacologic therapies with anecdotal support include sub-Tenon's repository steroid injections and oral acetazolamide.

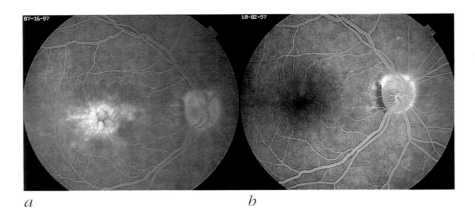

Figure 30.6. *(a) Chronic CME with vision impaired 5 months following difficult phaco-emulsification with vitreous loss and incarceration. (b) Resolution of CME 2 months after surgical management of vitreous incarceration and IOL exchange.*

a   *b*

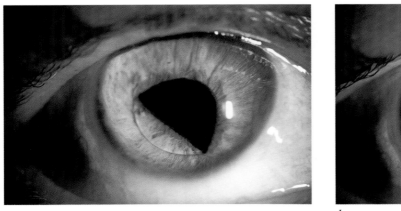 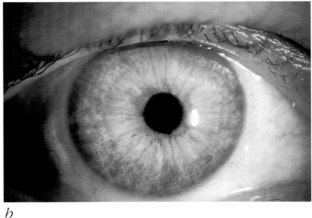

a   *b*

Figure 30.7. *(a) Pupillary capture of a sulcus-placed IOL which had been implanted backwards. Chronic iris irritation generated CME which could not be controlled with topical anti-inflammatories. (b) The CME resolved following successful management of the capture.*

Vitrectomy

Surgical correction of vitreous-generated irritative and tractional situations can reverse visual loss from CME (Fig. 30.6). The benefits of surgical release of cataract vitreous wound adhesions have been demonstrated in a prospective clinical trial.[56] CME resulting from chronic uveal irritation caused by pupillary distortion by synechiae or pupillary capture can be managed with restoration of anterior segment anatomy combined with pars plana core vitrectomy (Fig. 30.7). The more apparent the preoperative signs and symptoms of inflammation, the greater the likelihood of surgical improvement. Aside from rare cases of vitreomacular traction syndrome, there is little indication for vitreous surgery in eyes with good pupillary

mobility, intact posterior capsule and in-the-bag intraocular lens placement.

ACUTE POSTOPERATIVE INFECTIOUS ENDOPHTHALMITIS

Endophthalmitis from intraocular inoculation of microorganisms is a serious condition which occurs with an incidence of approximately 0.13%.[1,64] The modern management of endophthalmitis is strongly influenced by the findings of the Endophthalmitis Vitrectomy Study (EVS).[65] The treatment guidelines arising from this multicenter randomized controlled

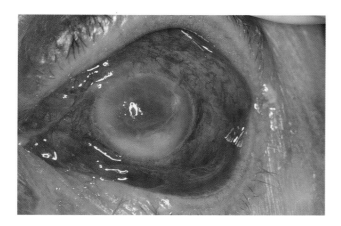

Figure 30.8. *This cataract patient presented on the sixth postoperative day with eye pain and light perception vision. The EVS guidelines suggest management with immediate three-port pars plana vitrectomy, with intravitreal, subconjunctival and topical antibiotics and subconjunctival, topical and systemic corticosteroid therapy.*

clinical trial should be familiar to all ophthalmologists (Fig. 30.8).

In addition to appropriate vitreous sampling and antimicrobial administration, the final visual outcome in cases of endophthalmitis is determined by the inherent pathogenicity of the microorganism, the size of the inoculum, and the time lapse between onset and initiation of therapy.[66]

RISK FACTORS

Although endophthalmitis is often thought of as a random event, the incidence can be favorably influenced by minimizing exposure to various ocular and systemic risk factors.

Ocular factors

The preoperative cataract surgery assessment traditionally includes screening for and treatment of ocular, eyelid and nasolacrimal infections.

Pulsed-field gel electrophoresis molecular strain typing confirms that the patient's own periocular microflora plays a significant role in causing postoperative endophthalmitis.[67] This fact emphasizes the importance of sterilizing the perioperative field,

draping out the periocular environment, keeping the periocular area sterile until the wound is tight, and operating quickly. Prolonged operating time, excessive surgical manipulation, capsular rupture and vitreous loss are some additional risk factors. Late-onset endophthalmitis risk factors include infection with low-virulence organisms, wound dehiscence, inadvertent filtering bleb, suture abscess, suture removal, and the vitreous wick syndrome.[68]

Systemic factors

Advanced age and other immunocompromising states favor infection. Diabetes is a risk factor for Gram-positive, coagulase-negative micrococcal endophthalmitis.[69]

RECOGNITION

The earliest possible diagnosis and treatment of endophthalmitis is critical to maximize the visual outcome. Since microbiological culture studies may require several days to complete, the diagnosis must usually be made on the clinical findings alone. Endophthalmitis should be suspected in any eye with greater than usual inflammatory signs or symptoms. Attentive care and patient awareness are critical elements in early diagnosis. Visual blur is the most common presenting symptom. Other classic findings are eye pain and hypopyon, but these need not be present in every case.[65] Ultrasonography may be useful in diagnosing endophthalmitis and in detecting occult posterior pathology in infected eyes with opaque media.

TREATMENT

Immediate introduction of intravitreal antibiotics to cover both Gram-positive and Gram-negative organisms is universally accepted as the principal element of treatment.

Vitreous sampling

Immediate pars plana core vitrectomy offers the most severely infected eyes the best chance of recovery,[70] possibly by debulking the infected vitreous of microorganisms and their toxins, and by clearing the ocular media. For eyes with better than light perception vision (measured by an ophthalmologist), vitrectomy does not confer any advantage over simple pars plana vitreous biopsy or vitreous tap.[65] Although vitreous is a richer source of positive cultures than aqueous, vitrectomy does not produce significantly more positive cultures than vitreous biopsy or tap, and should not be performed to improve the microbiological yield.[71]

Antimicrobial agents

The initial immediate intravitreal antibiotic administration is empirical, since it is performed at the time of vitreous sampling, prior to Gram stain or culture results. Gram-positive organisms account for the majority of infections in all types of acute endophthalmitis, but specific organisms vary according to clinical settings.[70] Although the virulence of the microorganism correlates with a history and clinical findings of an aggressive infection, this correlation is not sufficiently strong to guide the initial choice of intravitreal antibiotics.[69]

Vancomycin is currently accepted as the antibiotic of choice for Gram-positive coverage. The standard of care in endophthalmitis includes a second intravitreal antibiotic, most commonly either the cephalosporin ceftazidine or the aminoglycoside amikacin.

Adjunctive antibiotic therapy by other routes of administration does not reach the target area of the vitreous cavity as effectively as intravitreal injection. The EVS concluded that intravenous antibiotics, generally, do not improve visual outcome.[65] The role of topical and subconjunctival antibiotics, although they are widely used, has not been clarified. Some authors suggest a role for oral fluoroquinolones (ciprofloxacin or ofloxacin) as an adjunct to intravitreal therapy.[72,73]

Corticosteroids

All EVS patients received systemic, subconjunctival and topical corticosteroids. Intravitreal steroids were not used in the study and remain a subject of controversy in management.

Treatment setting

After elimination of the requirement for intravenous antibiotics, in most cases, and vitrectomy in many cases, using the EVS findings as a guide to inpatient treatment of endophthalmitis would result in an annual reduction of hospital charges in the USA of up to $40 million.[74] This cost reduction could be further enhanced by total treatment of those cases not requiring vitrectomy in an outpatient setting with daily follow-up visits. This may be feasible in eyes with an intact wound, where adequate outpatient pain control is possible, in a well-informed and compliant patient, and where daily transportation is available.

Role of the cataract surgeon

The role of the cataract surgeon in the management of endophthalmitis has been traditionally to minimize the risks of infection, to recognize or suspect endophthalmitis at the earliest possible stage and to arrange immediate referral to a vitreoretinal surgeon. A comprehensive ophthalmologist with knowledge of the unique microbiological aspects of endophthalmitis, with experience in the preoperative assessment and postoperative care of infected eyes, and who is able to offer the range of required surgical options, may choose not to refer these cases.

There is interest in managing endophthalmitis with anterior vitrectomy through a reopened cataract wound, either through a posterior capsular tear or through a posterior capsulorhexis.[75] Other authors feel that vitrectomy, vitreous biopsy or vitreous tap should only be performed through the pars plana.[76]

RETAINED LENS FRAGMENTS AFTER CATARACT SURGERY

The clinical significance of retained lens fragments varies with the amount, composition and location of the fragments. Small particles of cortex retained in the capsular bag are better tolerated than large fragments of nucleus dislocated into the posterior segment.

The incidence of posteriorly displaced lens fragments, requiring treatment, is estimated to be 0.3%. It occurs more often with phaco, since posterior capsular tears tend to be more central than with extracapsular technique. The inflammatory reaction triggered by retained lens fragments may lead to visual loss by corneal decompensation, glaucoma, CME, choroidal effusion and retinal detachment

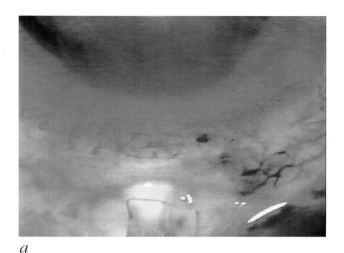
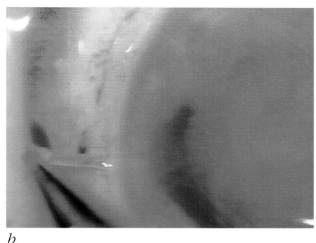

a   *b*

Figure 30.9. *Digital images retrieved from a surgical video with vitreous loss and posterior migration of lens nucleus early in the phacoemulsification phase. The surgeon is excising vitreous from the cataract wound (a) and from a side-port incision (b). Anterior segment clean-up with an automated suction cutter instrument creates less direct traction on the vitreous base and would have been the preferred approach for this situation.*

MANAGEMENT BY CATARACT SURGEON

Recognition

In cases of extreme zonular weakness, the entire lens may disappear posteriorly during anterior capsulorhexis. Usually, however, posterior migration of lens fragments occurs during the phaco phase. Although small fragments may fall back unnoticed, the migration of any significant amount of lens material is ordinarily immediately apparent to the cataract surgeon, and is often the first clue that the capsule is open.

Immediate response

Every surgeon knows, and every patient should know, that this is one of the anticipated possible side-effects of modern cataract surgery, and can occur in the hands of even the most experienced and gifted surgeon. None the less, watching a dropped, partially sculpted nucleus sail back out of sight and into the depths of the eye is a heart-stopping experience for most cataract surgeons.

The surgeon's first response should be to resist the considerable temptation to finesse the situation by attempting retrieval of the nucleus with needles,

forceps, lens loops, cryo, high-volume infusion jets or other dangerous techniques likely to create direct traction on the vitreous base (Fig. 30.9). Most patients with retained lens fragments do well if correctly managed.[77–80] The final visual outcome is probably more dependent on the extent of manipulations during the initial cataract extraction than on any other factor,[77] and the increasing tendency by surgeons to minimize surgical trauma while managing this problem probably accounts for a declining rate of associated retinal detachment.[81]

Primary toilet and closure

The cataract surgeon may attempt an anterior segment clean-up, avoiding aspiration of any vitreous gel except with an automated vitrectomy tip through the limbal wound, and retrieving only easily accessible lens fragments (Table 30.4). Placement of an intraocular lens into the capsular bag, ciliary sulcus or anterior chamber, as indicated, does not adversely affect the visual outcome.[77,79] Removal of viscoelastic and wound closure should be followed by indirect ophthalmoscopy with scleral depression, initiation of topical anti-inflammatory and intraocular pressure-lowering agents, and prompt vitreoretinal consultation.

Table 30.4
Immediate management of lost lens fragments.

Visual outcome may be good if correctly managed
Avoid blind retrieval of lost fragments by any technique
Anterior segment clean-up with automated vitrectomy
  instrument, retrieving only easily accessible fragments
Implant the intraocular lens, as indicated
Wound closure and removal of viscoelastics
Initiate topical anti-inflammatories and glaucoma therapy
Prompt vitreoretinal consultation

MANAGEMENT BY VITREORETINAL SURGEON

Observation combined with anti-inflammatory and anti-glaucoma therapy is indicated for eyes with small retained lens fragments (Fig. 30.10). Eyes with more significant amounts of lens material, especially nuclear fragments, should be considered for vitrectomy, to avoid or minimize the sight-threatening sequelae of refractory inflammation. Diagnostic ultrasonography is often useful at this stage (Fig. 30.11).

The timing of vitrectomy does not appear to influence visual acuity outcomes,[77,79,80] although preoperative medical therapy to optimize corneal clarity and intraocular pressure control is important. The preferred vitrectomy technique consists of a three-port pars plana approach, beginning with clearing of the anterior segment media, with removal of residual lens cortex and segmentation of any remaining vitreous attachment to anterior segment structures, including the intraocular lens, capsular bag and iris. A core vitrectomy, preferably with panoramic viewing technique, and truncation of the posterior vitreous base is followed by release of all vitreous attachments to lens fragments (Fig. 30.12). Once fully mobilized, the cortical fragments are usually easily removed with an automated vitrectomy tip. Nuclear material is best removed using intravitreal phaco (Fig. 30.13). Although floating the lens material with perfluorocarbon liquid protects the posterior pole from ultrasonic damage,[82] it is usually not necessary or useful except in cases with retinal detachment. Modern intravitreal phaco systems with proportional aspiration and fragmentation can safely retrieve nuclear fragments into the midvitreous cavity and fragment them safely, with low-fragmentation power settings. This technique can effectively restore visual acuity and reverse secondary glaucoma.[83] An intraocular lens may be implanted, as indicated, followed by careful peripheral fundus evaluation.

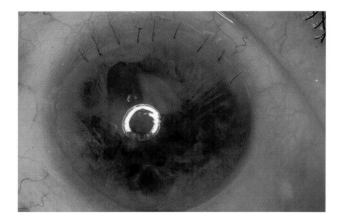

Figure 30.10. *A quiet, non-inflamed eye 4 months after difficult extracapsular cataract surgery. The cataract surgeon attempted intraoperative anterior segment clean-out with an automated vitrectomy instrument but quickly withdrew after scalloping the pupillary margin. Observation and topical anti-inflammatory therapy were not sufficient to manage the retained lens material.*

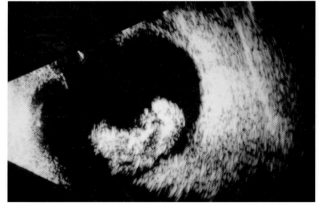

Figure 30.11. *Characteristic diagnostic echography findings of posterior luxation of a significant nuclear fragment. This is particularly useful for detecting any amount of retinal detachment or other posterior segment pathology, particularly in eyes with a significant amount of retained anterior cortical material and limited fundus visualization.*

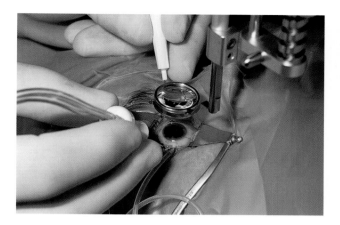

Figure 30.12. *Three-port pars plana vitrectomy with panoramic non-contact posterior imaging system. Allows a safe, controlled approach to many posterior segment complications of cataract surgery.*

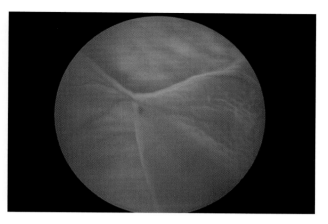

Figure 30.14. *Giant retinal tear and retinal detachment arising from excessive vitreous base manipulation during a primary attempt at blind retrieval of the nuclear fragment.*

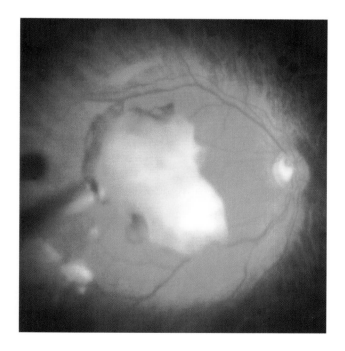

Figure 30.13. *Pars plana vitrectomy management of posterior luxation of nuclear material. The lens nucleus with attached cortex is released from all vitreous attachments and a posterior vitreous detachment is created and truncated. The nucleus is then engaged with light suction with an intravitreal phaco fragmentation probe, elevated into the midvitreous cavity and removed using proportional phacoemulsification with low power settings. This technique is associated with a good visual prognosis.*

RETINAL DETACHMENT AFTER CATARACT SURGERY

Retinal detachment is the most common globe-threatening complication of cataract surgery. The reported incidence of 0.7% with modern capsule sparing technique[1] is substantially lower than the most commonly quoted incidence of 2.2% with intracapsular technique.[84] At least 50% of retinal detachments occur within the first year after cataract surgery, and thereafter the incidence remains higher than in phakic eyes.[85] Retinal detachments occurring immediately after surgery are often due to needle perforation of the globe, vitreous wound incarceration, or vitreous base manipulation while retrieving dropped nuclear fragments (Fig. 30.14).

Non-phakic retinal detachments tend to occur more rapidly, are more extensive, and are more likely to involve the macula. Although equatorial tears may occur, non-phakic detachments arise more often from multiple, small tears along the posterior margin of the vitreous base.

RISK FACTORS

A number of independent ocular and surgical risk factors are associated with increased chances of retinal detachment following cataract surgery.[86,87]

Ocular factors

These include young age, male sex, high axial myopia and a history of retinal detachment or lattice degeneration.

Posterior capsular rupture

Intraoperative opening of the posterior capsule, even if adequately managed, cancels the protective effect associated with modern cataract surgical technique. Vitreous loss adds an additional risk factor, giving an incidence of retinal detachment as high as 20%.[85] Other high-risk factors include posterior migration of lens fragments, intraocular lens luxation or any situation associated with extra surgical manipulation.

Nd:YAG posterior capsulotomy

Laser posterior capsulotomy is associated with a four-fold excess risk of pseudophakic retinal detachment.[88] This effect appears to be due to the presence of a capsular opening rather than direct laser trauma. There is a mean latency of 6 months from capsulotomy to detachment, with 85% of detachments occurring within the first year following capsulotomy. Although the risk may be greater for some patients than others, there is a need for strong clinical justification, in every case, for performing laser capsulotomy. Surgeons should make every effort to minimize controllable factors contributing to opacification of the posterior capsule.[89]

PREVENTION

In patients with risk factors, a vitreoretinal assessment before and after cataract surgery or Nd:YAG capsulotomy may provide an opportunity to treat retinal tears, or vitreoretinal precursors of retinal tears.

REATTACHMENT SURGERY

Conventional repair

The time-honored surgical repair of a non-phakic retinal detachment has been a scleral buckling procedure. Because of the tendency for there to be multiple holes and the unique relationship between peripheral retina and vitreous base, the repair usually includes an encircling element. Adjunctive vitreous surgery may be required to manage vitreous incarceration, dropped nuclear material, a luxated intraocular lens, vitreous hemorrhage or proliferative vitreoretinopathy.

Primary vitrectomy

Repair of non-phakic retinal detachments with primary vitrectomy is being proposed as an attractive alternative to conventional scleral buckling because of better intraoperative visualization of the peripheral fundus, controlled removal of vitreous traction and the opportunity for clearing vitreous opacities. There are early claims of a superior reattachment rate and a reduced rate of proliferative vitreoretinopathy.[90]

Pneumatic retinopexy

Pneumatic retinopexy is a retinal reattachment operation performed in an office setting, combining laser or cryo retinopexy with intravitreal injection of an expanding gas bubble. Because of the limited peripheral retinal visualization, the presence of multiple small retinal tears and the unique vitreoretinal traction, the success rate of this procedure in non-phakic eyes has been disappointing, especially following posterior capsulotomy or intracapsular cataract extraction.[91] Recent data suggest that pneumatic retinopexy, when combined with a complete 360° peripheral laser retinopexy, may be an efficacious and cost-effective procedure in selected cases.[92]

MASSIVE SUPRACHOROIDAL HEMORRHAGE

Massive suprachoroidal hemorrhage is an imposing complication of cataract surgery, with a poor visual prognosis,[93] occurring with an incidence of 0.2%.[94] Rupture of a weakened long or short posterior ciliary artery is the principal event, probably precipitated by ocular hypotony,[95] and possibly preceded by serous choroidal effusion with vascular stretching.[96] A rupture may occur intraoperatively or may be delayed for hours, days, or months, especially in a soft, inflamed eye.

RISK FACTORS

Reported risk factors mostly include situations favoring ocular hypotony, posterior ciliary artery weakness or intraocular inflammation.[97]

Systemic factors

Advanced age, generalized arterial sclerosis, hypertension and diabetes probably promote rupture of engorged, stretched posterior ciliary arteries. Blood dyscrasias and coagulation disorders may be factors, despite reports promoting the safety of clear corneal incisions in anticoagulated patients.[98]

Ocular factors

Glaucoma, choroidal sclerosis, axial myopia, choroiditis, recent intraocular surgery on the same eye and a history of massive suprachoroidal hemorrhage in the fellow eye are important risk factors.

Perioperative factors

Labile intraoperative hypertension, acute arterial pressure changes due to retrobulbar infiltration of local anesthetic containing adrenaline, and the release of catecholamines during general anesthesia, may promote ciliary artery blowout. Any situation associated with prolonged intraoperative ocular hypotony is a major risk factor.

MANAGEMENT BY CATARACT SURGEON

Recognition

The extent and location of the hemorrhage is determined by the size and location of the ruptured vessel. Limited suprachoroidal hemorrhage is reported to occur in 3% of cataract operations[99] (Fig. 30.15). There is a spectrum of clinical presentations, varying from blood seeping into the angle of the anterior chamber or lens capsule, to a full-blown expulsive suprachoroidal hemorrhage with extrusion of intraocular contents through the cataract wound.

Intraoperative massive suprachoroidal hemorrhage presents with a sequence of progressive signs of positive wound pressure, shallowing of the anterior chamber, iris prolapse, vitreous loss, a stone-hard

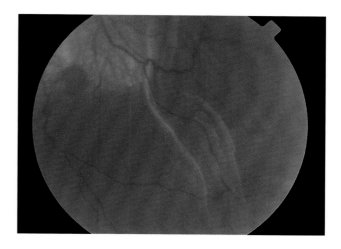

Figure 30.15. *A limited suprachoroidal hemorrhage extending 360° and not involving the macula. This is probably a common occurrence and is often of no clinical significance apart from associated pain and discomfort.*

eye, loss of red reflex and prolapse of retina and choroid. The earliest and most important finding is often severe pain, restlessness and agitation in a patient with a previously adequate block and previously adequate sedation. Under general anesthesia, the patient may begin to buck vigorously and spike a blood pressure rise, incorrectly leading the anesthesia staff to believe it was they who created the ensuing disaster.

Immediate response

The cataract wound should be immediately closed and the procedure concluded at the first sign of massive suprachoroidal hemorrhage.[97] Any hesitation, even to reposition incarcerated tissue, may result in continued expulsion of intraocular contents and loss of the eye. A Verhoeff sclerotomy[100] or other desperate transscleral drainage maneuver is rarely effective and best reserved for cases where the wound cannot be closed.[97]

MANAGEMENT BY VITREORETINAL SURGEON

Observation is recommended for non-appositional suprachoroidal hemorrhages, without retinal or uveal incarceration. Diagnostic ultrasonography is a valuable tool in assessing these eyes at this stage[101]

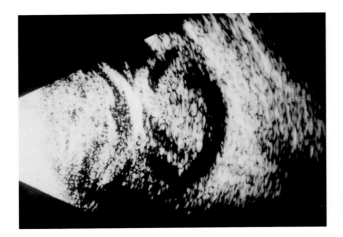

Figure 30.16. *Diagnostic echography of appositional suprachoroidal hemorrhage. This is frequently the most appropriate means of diagnosing and monitoring the extent of the condition.*

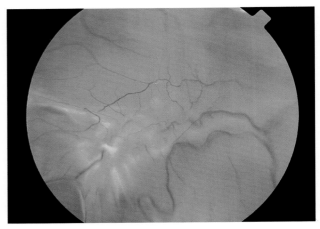

Figure 30.17. *Proliferative vitreoretinopathy retinal detachment with fixed folds and tractional tears in an inferior location. Surgical management of this condition will require some dissection under automated air–fluid exchange and will often require the use of intravitreal silicone oil, which would not be possible through a silicone IOL.*

(Fig. 30.16). Surgical drainage of appositional hemorrhages in eyes with retinal detachment or incarceration is best performed after a 7–10-day observation period to allow clot fibrinolysis.[97] Predictors of a poor visual outcome include wound incarceration, retinal detachment, poor visual acuity or afferent pupillary defect on presentation, and an apposition configuration lasting longer than 14 days.[93]

VITREORETINAL SURGERY AND SILICONE INTRAOCULAR LENSES

Adequate management of many posterior segment complications of cataract surgery may require vitreoretinal procedures with either intraocular gas or silicone oil tamponade (Fig. 30.17). In eyes with previously implanted silicone lenses there is a very significant limitation of posterior segment visualization during dissections performed under automated air–fluid exchange, because of fluid condensation on the posterior lens surface.[102] In addition, silicone oil may interact with silicone lenses, creating a thick, opaque coating on the lens surface. This coating is tenaciously adherent and cannot be dislodged intraoperatively by mechanical wiping or viscodissection.[103] Although these opacities may occur with any intraocular lens, including the human crystalline lens,[104] they are most pronounced with silicone lenses. Silicone lens implantation is therefore not recommended for patients at risk for posterior segment complications.

REFERENCES

1 Powe NR, Schein OD, Gieser SC, et al. Synthesis of the literature on visual acuity and complications following cataract extraction with intraocular implantation. Cataract Patient Outcome Research Team. *Arch Ophthalmol* 1994; **112:** 239–52. (Published erratum appears in *Arch Ophthalmol* 1994; **112:** 889. Comment in *Arch Ophthalmol* 1994; **112:** 875.)
2 Unsöld R, Stanley JA, DeGroot J. The CT-topography of retrobulbar anesthesia: anatomic–clinical correlation of complications and suggestion of a modified technique. *Graefes Arch Klin Exp Ophthalmol* 1981; **217:** 125–36.
3 Feibel RM. Current concepts in retrobulbar anesthesia. *Surv Ophthalmol* 1985; **30:** 102–10.
4 Drysdale DB. Experimental subdural retrobulbar injection of anesthetic. *Ann Ophthalmol* 1984; **16:** 716–18.
5 Edge KR, Davis A. Brainstem anesthesia following peribulbar block for eye surgery. *Anaesth Intens Care* 1995; **23:** 219–21.
6 Singer SB, Preston R, Hodge WG. Respiratory arrest following peribulbar anesthesia for cataract surgery: case report and review of literature. *Can J Ophthalmol* 1997; **32:** 450–4.

7 Albright GA. Cardiac arrest following regional anesthesia with etidocaine and bupivacaine. *Anesthesiology* 1979; **51:** 285–7.

8 Antoszyk AN, Buckley EG. Contralateral decreased visual acuity and extraocular muscle palsies following retrobulbar injection. *Ophthalmology* 1986; **93:** 462–5.

9 Friedberg HL, Kline OR Jr. Contralateral amaurosis after retrobulbar injection. *Am J Ophthalmol* 1986; **101:** 688–90.

10 Carroll FD. Optic nerve complications of cataract extraction. *Trans Am Acad Ophthalmol Otolaryngol* 1973; **77:** OP623–9.

11 Pautler SE, Grizzard WS, Thompson LN, Wing GL. Blindness from retrobulbar injection into the optic nerve. *Ophthalmic Surg* 1986; **17:** 334–7.

12 Giuffre G, Vadala M, Manfre L. Retrobulbar anesthesia complicated by combined central retinal vein and artery occlusion and massive vitreoretinal fibrosis. *Retina* 1995; **15:** 439–41.

13 Morgan CM, Schatz H, Vine AK, et al. Ocular complications associated with retrobulbar injections. *Ophthalmology* 1988; **95:** 660–5.

14 Grizzard WS. Ophthalmic anesthesia. *Ophthalmol Annu* 1989; 265–93.

15 Lemagne JM, Michiels X, Van Causenbroeck S, Snyers B. Purtscher like retinopathy after retrobulbar anesthesia. *Ophthalmology* 1990; **97:** 859–61.

16 Meyers EF, Ramirez RC, Boniuk I. Grand mal seizures after retrobulbar block. *Arch Ophthalmol* 1978; **96:** 847–52.

17 Goldsmith MO. Occlusion of the central retinal artery following retrobulbar hemorrhage. *Ophthalmologica* 1967; **153:** 191–6.

18 Kraushar MF, Seelenfreund MH, Freilich DB. Central retinal artery closure during orbital hemorrhage from retrobulbar injection. *Trans Am Acad Ophthalmol Otolaryngol* 1974; **78:** OP65–70.

19 Cibis PA. General discussion: opening remarks. In: Schepens CL, Regan CDJ, eds. *Controversial Aspects of the Management of Retinal Detachments* (Boston: Little Brown, 1965) 222.

20 Ramsay RC, Knobloch WH. Ocular perforation following retrobulbar anaesthesia for retinal detachment surgery. *Am J Ophthalmol* 1978; **86:** 61–4.

21 Kimble JA, Morris RE, Witherspoon CE, Feist RM. Globe perforation from peribulbar injection. *Arch Ophthalmol* 1987; **105:** 749.

22 Arnold PN. Prospective study of a single-injection peribulbar technique. *J Cataract Refract Surg* 1992; **18:** 157–61.

23 Davis DB, Mandel MR. Efficacy and complication rate of 16224 consecutive peribulbar blocks: a prospective multicenter study. *J Cataract Refract Surg* 1994; **20:** 327–37.

24 Gillow JT, Aggarwal RK, Kirkby GR. A survey of ocular perforation during ophthalmic local anaesthesia in the United Kingdom. *Eye* 1996; **10:** 537–8.

25 Duker JS, Belmont JB, Benson WE, et al. Inadvertent globe perforation during retrobulbar and peribulbar anaesthesia. *Ophthalmology* 1991; **98:** 519–26.

26 Grizzard WS, Kirk NM, Pavan PR, Antworth MV, Hammer ME, Roseman RL. Perforating ocular injuries caused by anesthesia personnel. *Ophthalmology* 1991; **98:** 1011–6.

27 Hay A, Flynn HW Jr, Hoffman JI, Rivera AH. Needle penetration of the globe during retrobulbar and peribulbar injections. *Ophthalmology* 1991; **98:** 1017–24.

28 Berglin L, Stenkula S, Algvere PV. Ocular perforation during retrobulbar and peribulbar injections. *Ophthalmic Surg Lasers* 1995; **26:** 429–34.

29 Polkinghorne PJ. Inadvertent perforation of the globe during regional anaesthesia. *Aust NZ J Ophthalmol* 1996; **24:** 43–5.

30 Gillow JT, Aggarwal RK, Kirkby GR. Ocular perforation during peribulbar anaesthesia. *Eye* 1996; **10:** 533–6.

31 Ramsay RC, Knobloch WH. Ocular perforation following retrobulbar anesthesia for retinal detachment surgery. *Am J Ophthalmol* 1978; **86:** 61–4.

32 Ellis PP. Retrobulbar injections. *Surv Ophthalmol* 1974; **18:** 425–30.

33 Liu C, Youl B, Moseley I. Magnetic resonance imaging of the optic nerve in extremes of gaze: implications for the positioning of the globe for retrobulbar anesthesia. *Br J Ophthalmol* 1992; **76:** 728–33.

34 Davis DB, Mandel MR. Peribulbar anesthesia. A review of technique and complications. *Ophthalmol Clin North Am* 1990; **3:** 101–10.

35 Koornneef L. *Spatial Aspects of Orbital Musculo-Fibrous Tissue in Man: New Anatomical and Histological Approach* (Amsterdam: Swets & Zeitlinger, 1977).

36 Miller-Meeks MJ, Bergstrom T, Karp KO. Prevalent attitudes regarding residency training in ocular anesthesia. *Ophthalmology* 1994; **101:** 1353–6.

37 Boase DL. Local anaesthesia revisited. *Eye* 1996; **10:** 531–2.

38 Liang C, Peymann GA, Sun G. Toxicity of intraocular lidocaine and bupivacaine. *Am J Ophthalmol* 1998; **125:** 191–6.

39 McDonnel PJ, Patel A, Green WR. Comparison of intracapsular and extracapsular cataract surgery: histopathologic study of eyes obtained postmortem. *Ophthalmology* 1985; **92:** 1208–23.

40 Green WR. Vitreoretinal juncture. In: Ryan SJ, ed. *Retina*, 2nd edn (Philadelphia: Mosby, 1994) 1869–930.

41 Kraff MC, Sanders DR, Jampol LM, Peyman GA, Lieberman HL. Effect of primary capsulotomy with extracapsular surgery on the incidence of pseudophakic cystoid macular edema. *Am J Ophthalmol* 1984; **98:** 166–70.

42 Wright PL, Wilkinson CP, Balyeat HD, Popham J, Reinke M. Angiographic cystoid macular edema after posterior chamber lens implantation. *Arch Ophthalmol* 1988; **106:** 740–4.

43 Fine IH, Hoffman RS. Phacoemulsification in the presence of pseudoexfoliation: challenges and options. *J Cataract Refract Surg* 1997; **23:** 160–5.

44 Chitkara DK, Smerdon DL. Risk factors, complications, and results in extracapsular cataract extraction. *J Cataract Refract Surg* 1997; **23:** 570–4.

45 Snyder RW, Donnenfeld ED. Teaching phacoemulsification to residents and physicians in transition. *Int Ophthalmol Clin* 1994; **34:** 191–9.

46 Gimbel HV, Sun R, Heston JP. Management of zonular dialysis in phacoemulsification and IOL implantation using the capsular tension ring. *Ophthalmic Surg Lasers* 1997; **28:** 273–81.

47 Masket S. Consultation section. How would you handle a tear in the posterior capsule, detected at the end of phacoemulsification, with the cortex intact and no vitreous loss? *J Cataract Refract Surg* 1997; **23:** 12–18.

48 Blumenthal M, Assia EI, Chen V, Avni I. Using an anterior chamber maintainer to control intraocular pressure during phacoemulsification. *J Cataract Refract Surg* 1994; **20:** 93–6.

49 Galand A, van Cauwenberge F, Moosavi J. Posterior capsulorhexis in adult eyes with intact and clear capsules. *J Cataract Refract Surg* 1996; **22:** 458–61.

50 Frost NA, Sparrow JM, Strong NP, Rosenthal AR. Vitreous loss in planned extracapsular cataract extraction does lead to a poorer visual outcome. *Eye* 1995; **9:** 446–51.

51 Smiddy WE, Chong LP. Management of vitreous loss at cataract surgery. In: Wright KW, ed. *Color Atlas of Ophthalmic Surgery* (Philadelphia: JB Lippincott, 1995) 171–8.

52 Kusak S, Tsujioka M, Mano T, Tsuboi S, Ohashi Y. Two-port vitrectomy for vitreous loss during sutureless cataract surgery. *Am J Ophthalmol* 1994; **117:** 533–4.

53 Jampol LM. Cystoid macular edema following cataract surgery. *Arch Ophthalmol* 1988; **106:** 894.

54 Klein RM, Yannuzzi L. Cystoid macular edema in the first week after cataract extraction. *Am J Ophthalmol* 1976; **81:** 614–15.

55 Mao LK, Holland PM. 'Very late onset' cystoid macular edema. *Ophthalmic Surg* 1988; **19:** 633–5.

56 Fung WE. Vitrectomy for chronic aphakic cystoid macular edema. Results of a national, collaborative, prospective, randomized investigation. *Ophthalmology* 1985; **92:** 1102–11.

57 Menchini U, Bandello F, Brancato R, Camesasca FI, Galdini M. Cystoid macular edema after extracapsular cataract extraction and intraocular lens implantation in diabetic patients without retinopathy. *Br J Ophthalmol* 1993; **77:** 208–11.

58 Steinert RF, Puliafito CA, Kumar SR, Duda SD, Patel S. Cystoid macular edema, retinal detachment and glaucoma after Nd:YAG laser posterior capsulotomy. *Am J Ophthalmol* 1991; **112:** 373–80.

59 Severin TD, Severin SL. Pseudophakic cystoid macular edema: a revised comparison of the incidence with intracapsular and extracapsular cataract extraction. *Ophthalmic Surg* 1988; **19:** 116–18.

60 Pande MV, Spalton DJ, Kerr-Muir MG, Marshall J. Postoperative inflammatory response to phacoemulsification and extracapsular cataract surgery: aqueous flare and cells. *J Cataract Refract Surg* 1996; **22**(S1): 770–4.

61 Blair NP, Kim SH. Cystoid macular edema after ocular surgery. In: Albert DM, Jakobiec FA, eds. *Principles and Practice of Ophthalmology* (Philadelphia: WB Saunders, 1994) 898–906.

62 Jampol LM. Cystoid macular edema following cataract surgery. *Arch Ophthalmol* 1989; **107:** 166.

63 Rossetti L, Bujtar E, Castoldi D, Torrazza C, Orzalesi N. Effectiveness of diclofenac eyedrops in reducing inflammation and the incidence of cystoid macular edema after cataract surgery. *J Cataract Refract Surg* 1996; **22**(S1): 794–9.

64 Javitt JC, Vitale S, Canner JK, et al. National outcomes of cataract extraction. Endophthalmitis following inpatient surgery. *Arch Ophthalmol* 1991; **109:** 1085–9.

65 Endophthalmitis Vitrectomy Study Group. Results of the endophthalmitis vitrectomy study. A randomized trial of immediate vitrectomy and of intravenous antibiotics for the treatment of postoperative bacterial endophthalmitis. *Arch Ophthalmol* 1995; **113:** 1479–96.

66 Whitcher JP. The treatment of endophthalmitis—still an exercise in frustration. *Br J Ophthalmol* 1997; **81:** 713–14.

67 Bannerman TL, Rhoden DL, McAllister SK, Miller JM, Wilson LA. The source of coagulase-negative staphylococci in Endophthalmitis Vitrectomy Study. A comparison of eyelid and intraocular isolates using pulsed-field gel electrophoresis. *Arch Ophthalmol* 1997; **115:** 357–61.

68 Han DP. Endophthalmitis. In: Freeman WR, ed. *Practical Atlas of Retinal Disease and Therapy*, 2nd edn (Philadelphia: Lippincott-Raven Publishers, 1997) 373–82.

69 Johnson MW, Doft BH, Kelsey SF, et al. The Endophthalmitis Vitrectomy Study. Relationship between clinic presentation and microbiologic spectrum. *Ophthalmology* 1997; **104:** 261–72.

70 Meredith TA. Vitrectomy for infectious endophthalmitis. In: Ryan SJ, ed. *Retina*, 2nd edn (Philadelphia: Mosby, 1994) 2525–37.

71 Barza M, Pavan PR, Doft BH, et al. Evaluation of microbiological diagnostic techniques in postoperative endophthalmitis in the Endophthalmitis Vitrectomy Study. *Arch Ophthalmol* 1997; **115:** 1142–50.

72 Okhravi N, Towler HM, Kykin P, Matheson M, Lightman S. Assessment of a standard protocol on visual outcome following presumed bacterial endophthalmitis. *Br J Ophthalmol* 1997; **18:** 719–25.

73 Donnenfeld ED, Perry HD, Snyder RW, Moadel R, Elsky M, Jones H. Intracorneal, aqueous humor, and vitreous penetration of topical and oral ofloxacin. *Arch Ophthalmol* 1997; **115:** 173–6.

74 Wisniewski SR, Hammer ME, Grizzard WS, et al. An investigation of the hospital charges related to the treatment of endophthalmitis in the Endophthalmitis Vitrectomy Study. *Ophthalmology* 1997; **104:** 739–45.

75 Gimbel HV. Endophthalmitis: immediate management using posterior capsulorhexis and anterior vitrectomy through reopened cataract surgery incision. *J Cataract Refract Surg* 1997; **23:** 27–31.

76 Masket S. Managing endophthalmitis. *J Cataract Refract Surg* 1997; **23:** 814–15.

77 Kim JE, Flynn HW Jr, Smiddy WE, et al. Retained lens fragments after phacoemulsification. *Ophthalmology* 1997; **101:** 1827–32.

78 Lambrou FH Jr, Stewart MW. Management of dislocated lens fragments during phacoemulsification. *Ophthalmology* 1992; **99:** 1260–2.

79 Borne MJ, Tasman W, Regillo C, Malecha M, Sarin L. Outcomes of vitrectomy for retained lens fragments. *Ophthalmology* 1996; **103:** 971–6.

80 Margherio RR, Margherio AR, Pendergast SD, et al. Vitrectomy for retained lens fragments after phacoemulsification. *Ophthalmology* 1997; **104:** 1426–32.

81 Smiddy WE, Flynn HW Jr, Kim JE. Retinal detachment in patients with retained lens fragments or dislocated posterior chamber intraocular lenses. *Ophthalmic Surg Lasers* 1996; **27:** 856–61.

82 Movshovich A, Berrocal M, Chang S. The protective properties of liquid perfluorocarbons in phacofragmentation of dislocated lenses. *Retina* 1994; **14:** 457–62.

83 Vilar NF, Flynn HW, Smiddy WE, et al. Removal of retained lens fragments after phacoemulsification reverses secondary glaucoma and restores visual acuity. *Ophthalmology* 1997; **104:** 787–92.

84 Scheie HG, Morse PH, Aminlari A. Incidence of retinal detachment following cataract extraction. *Arch Ophthalmol* 1973; **89:** 293–302.

85 Young LH, D'Amico DJ. Retinal detachment. In: Albert DM, Jakobiec FA, eds. *Principles and Practice of Ophthalmology* (Philadelphia: WB Saunders, 1994) 1084–92.

86 Tielsch JM, Legro MW, Cassard SD, et al. Risk factors for retinal detachment after cataract surgery. A population-based case-control study. *Ophthalmology* 1996; **103:** 1537–45.

87 Jacobi FK, Hessemer V. Pseudophakic retinal detachment in high axial myopia. *J Cataract Refract Surg* 1997; **23:** 1095–102.

88 Rickman-Barger L, Florine CW, Larson RS, Lindstrom RL. Retinal detachment after neodymium:YAG laser posterior capsulotomy. *Am J Ophthalmol* 1989; **107:** 531–6.

89 Rosen B. Retinal detachment after laser capsulotomy. *J Cataract Refract Surg* 1997; **23:** 7–8.

90 Barts-Schmidt KU, Kirchhof B, Heimann K. Primary vitrectomy for pseudophakic retinal detachment. *Br J Ophthalmol* 1996; **80:** 346–9.

91 Ambler JS, Meyers SM, Aegerra H, Paranadi L. Reoperations and visual results after failed pneumatic retinopexy. *Ophthalmology* 1990; **97:** 786–90.

92 Tornambe PE. Pneumatic retinopexy: the evolution of case selection and surgical technique. A twelve-year study of 302 eyes. *Trans Am Ophthalmol Soc* 1997; **95:** 551–78.

93 Scott IU, Flynn HW Jr, Schiffman J, Smiddy WE, Ehlies F. Visual acuity outcomes among patients with appositional suprachoroidal hemorrhage. *Ophthalmology* 1997; **104:** 2039–46.

94 Payne JW, Kameen AJ, Jensen AD, Christy NE. Expulsive hemorrhage: its incidence in cataract surgery and a report of four bilateral cases. *Trans Am Ophthalmol Soc* 1985; **83:** 181–204.

95 Wolter JR. White thrombi in massive subchoroidal hemorrhage: indicators of the site of its origin and of the mechanism of its control. *Br J Ophthalmol* 1985; **69:** 303–6.

96 Gressel MG, Parrish RK II, Heuer DK. Delayed nonexpulsive suprachoroidal hemorrhage. *Arch Ophthalmol* 1984; **102:** 1757–60.

97 Smiddy WE, Chong LP. Management of expulsive hemorrhagic choroidal detachment. In: Wright KW, ed. *Color Atlas of Ophthalmic Surgery* (Philadelphia: JB Lippincott, 1995) 103–12.

98 Roberts CW, Woods SM, Turner LS. Cataract surgery in anticoagulated patients. *J Cataract Refract Surg* 1991; **17:** 309–12.

99 Hoffman P, Pollack A, Oliver M. Limited choroidal hemorrhage associated with intracapsular cataract extraction. *Arch Ophthalmol* 1984; **102:** 1761–5.

100 Verhoeff FH. Scleral puncture for expulsive subchoroidal hemorrhage following sclerostomy: scleral puncture for postoperative separation of the choroid. *Ophthalmic Rec* 1915; **24:** 55–9.

101 Chu TG, Cano MR, Green RL, et al. Massive suprachoroidal hemorrhage with central retinal apposition. A clinical and echographic study. *Arch Ophthalmol* 1991; **109:** 1575–81.

102 Eaton AM, Jaffe GJ, McCuen BW, Mincey GJ. Condensation on the posterior surface of silicone intraocular lenses during fluid–air exchange. *Ophthalmology* 1995; **102:** 733–6.

103 Apple DJ, Federman JL, Krolicki TJ, et al. Irreversible silicone oil adhesions to silicone intraocular lenses. A clinicopathologic analysis. *Ophthalmology* 1996; **103:** 1555–62.

104 Apple DJ, Isaacs RT, Kent DG, et al. Silicone oil adhesion to intraocular lenses: an experimental study comparing various biomaterials. *J Cataract Refract Surg* 1997; **23:** 536–44.

Chapter 31 Surgical management of posterior segment complications of cataract surgery: II

Oswaldo Moura Brasil

The most frequent secondary segment complications of cataract surgery that can be treated by the vitreous and retina surgeon can be divided into four groups:

- retinal detachment
- dislocated crystalline lens, nucleus or fragments and intraocular lenses
- cystoid macular edema
- endophthalmitis.

RETINAL DETACHMENT

Retinal detachment occurs in approximately 0.005–0.01% of the population. The incidence in aphakic eyes is 1–3%, and among patients with retinal detachment, 20–40% have aphakic or pseudophakic eyes.[1–4]

This relationship is probably due to the state of the vitreous. After cataract surgery, there is a greater trend towards vitreous liquefaction, posterior vitreous detachment and collapse. Peripheral retinal tears can be formed by traction at the vitreous base. This condition, associated with a liquefied vitreous, is a risk factor for the development of retinal detachment, with fast evolution and greater extension. The aphakia can also be a risk factor for the formation of proliferative vitreous retinopathy (PVR).[5]

Posterior capsulotomy represents another risk factor for the development of retinal detachment. Both primary and secondary capsulotomies, even those with YAG laser, represent a three times greater risk of retinal detachment. If vitreous loss or vitreous incarceration occurs, the risk of retinal detachment increases by approximately 20–25%.[6–8]

Approximately 50% of the detachments following cataract surgery occur during the first year after cataract surgery. After that, the incidence is approximately 1% a year.[9,10]

Myopic patients are at substantially greater risk, due to their increased vitreous degenerative disorders.

Surgical treatment of these detachments is directly related to the patient's clinical manifestations. From our point of view, there is no specific surgical procedure for aphakic and pseudophakic eyes. When traction is significant, vitreous incarceration exists, or in the presence of PVR, vitrectomy is indicated. The retinal tears should be treated with laser or cryo and the peripheral traction can be neutralized by scleral buckle with silicone explants.[11]

DISLOCATED CRYSTALLINE LENS, NUCLEUS OR FRAGMENTS AND INTRAOCULAR LENSES

There are several conditions where the crystalline lens can be dislocated. Cataract surgery is one of them (Figs 31.1 and 31.2). Sometimes surgery is not necessary for the removal of a dislocated crystalline lens in the vitreous cavity. When there are no complications or when the crystalline lens is not in the visual axis disturbing the vision, rehabilitation is possible with contact lenses only. When inflammatory reactions, ocular hypertension, vitreous hemorrhage, retinal detachment or other complications occur, it is necessary to remove it. When just the nucleus or fragments are dislocated to the vitreous cavity, we believe that surgery is usually indicated as a matter of urgency (Figs 31.3 and 31.4). The complications are more frequent under these circumstances.[12,13]

The surgical technique consists of pars plana vitrectomy with three ports, ultrasonic fragmentation

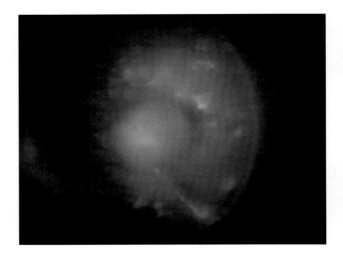

Figure 31.1. *Crystalline lens dislocated in vitreous cavity.*

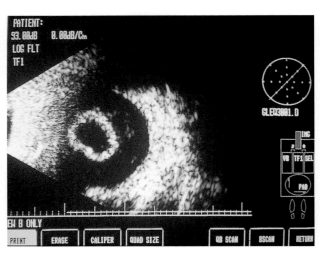

Figure 31.2. *Ultrasound image of crystalline lens dislocated in the vitreous cavity.*

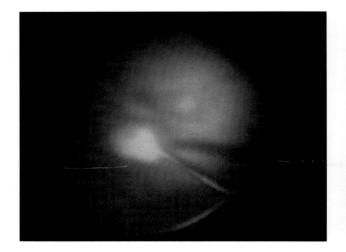

Figure 31.3. *Crystalline lens fragment dislocated in the vitreous cavity.*

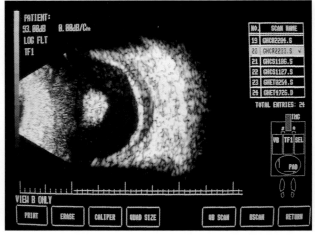

Figure 31.4. *Ultrasound image of crystalline lens fragment dislocated in the vitreous cavity.*

of the nucleus and aspiration of the cortical remnants (Fig. 31.5). When the nucleus is very hard, it is safer to bring it to the anterior chamber and remove it by limbal incision. Excessive ultrasound trauma is avoided with this procedure. We always find it convenient in these surgical procedures, after vitrectomy and before removing the crystalline lens, to protect the retina by injecting perfluoroctane (Fig. 31.6), a heavy liquid that works by moving the crystalline lens or its fragments to the center of the vitreous cavity (Fig. 31.7).[14–16]

Dislocated intraocular lens in the vitreous cavity is another surgical indication. In general, it is necessary to remove or reposition the intraocular lens. A pars plana vitrectomy should be performed, with removal of as much of the basal vitreous gel as possible, the posterior hyaloid should be removed, the retina should be protected by injecting perfluoroctane, and a choice should be made between removing or suturing the lens.[17]

When the decision is the removal of the lens, it should be driven to the anterior chamber and

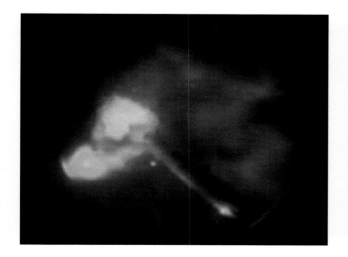

Figure 31.5. *Ultrasound fragmentation of the nucleus inside the vitreous cavity.*

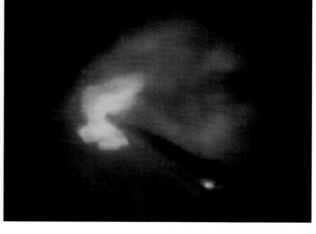

Figure 31.6. *Perfluorocarbon injected under the nucleus to protect the retina during fragmentation.*

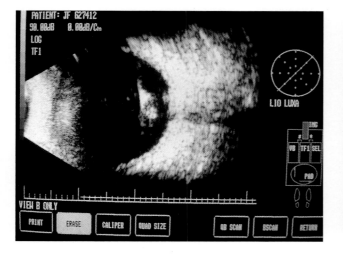

Figure 31.7. *Ultrasound image of intraocular lens dislocated in the vitreous cavity.*

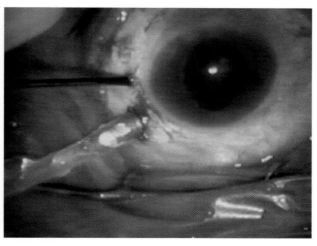

Figure 31.8. *Temporal sclerotomy.*

removed by limbal incision. In such cases, it is still possible to place a new lens in the anterior chamber or suture it in the sclera at the level of the ciliary sulcus.[18,19]

Our preference is suture of the lens without removing it from the cavity. In this case, we do a three-incision vitrectomy, placing one of them approximately 1.5 mm from the limbus at the 9 o'clock meridian on the right eye and at the 3 o'clock meridian on the left eye (Fig. 31.8). This incision is used to accomplish the vitrectomy and also to suture one of the loops with prolene 9–0 on the sclera (Figs 31.9–31.11). We still need a fourth limbal incision on the opposite side to suture the other loop of the lens. After vitrectomy and injection of perfluoroctane, we grasp the loops, one on each side, and suture them to the sclera (Brasil OM, unpublished).

If there are concurrent problems, such as retinal detachment, vitreous hemorrhage, or diabetic retinopathy (Fig. 31.12), these should be treated soon after the suture of the lens.

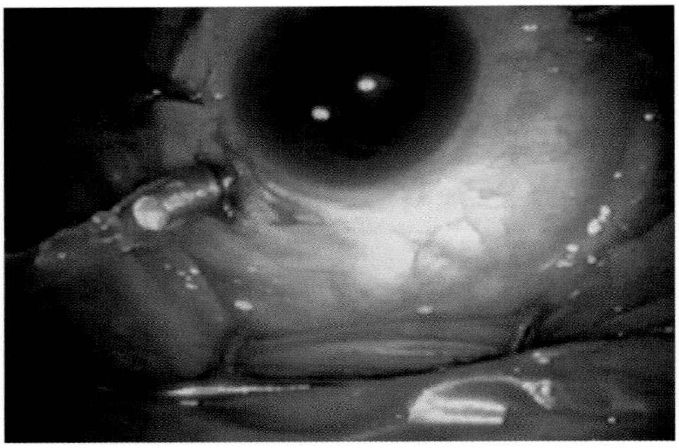

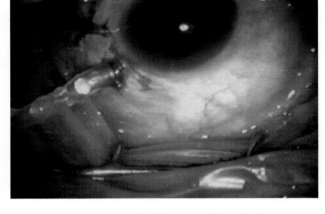

Figure 31.9. *Intraocular forceps grasping the haptic inside the vitreous cavity.*

Figure 31.10. *Intraocular forceps pulling the haptic through the sclerotomy.*

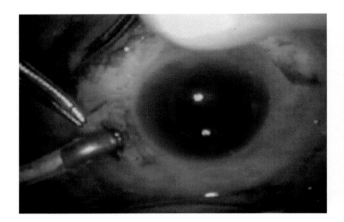

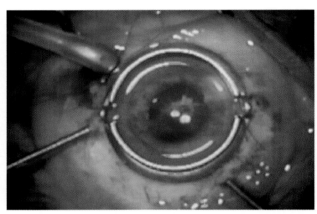

Figure 31.11. *Suture of the haptic to the sclera.*

Figure 31.12. *Pars plana capsulotomy.*

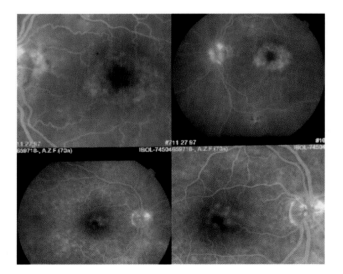

Figure 31.13. *Fluorescein angiography of cystoid macular edema.*

CYSTOID MACULAR EDEMA

Cystoid macular edema (Fig. 31.13) can be a complication of uncomplicated cataract surgery, as well as being associated with vitreous loss, vitreous incarceration in the operative wound (Fig. 31.14) or capture of the intraocular lens in the pupillary area (Figs 31.15 and 31.16).

The mechanism of cystoid macular edema development is uncertain. The chronic inflammatory reaction may be related to cataract surgery with incarceration of tissues. When clinical treatment fails to control the edema, surgical treatment with pars plana vitrectomy associated with the removal of the

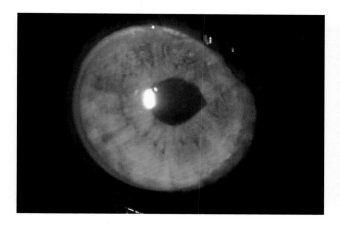

Figure 31.14. *Vitreous incarceration in the operative wound.*

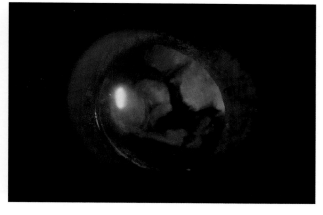

Figure 31.15. *Capture of the intraocular lens in the pupillary area and cortex fragments.*

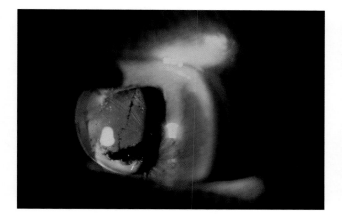

Figure 31.16. *Capture of the intraocular lens in the pupillary area.*

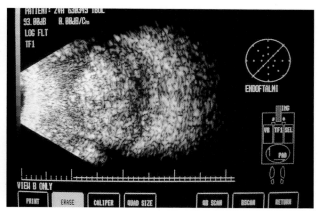

Figure 31.17. *Ultrasound image of endophthalmitis.*

posterior hyaloid shows excellent results, even when some time has elapsed without improvement.[20,21]

ENDOPHTHALMITIS

Endophthalmitis, although not a frequent complication, must, because of its severity, be approached as an emergency procedure (Fig. 31.17).

According to the results of the US National Study of Cataract Outcomes, the estimated risk of endophthalmitis in the first 12 months after cataract surgery is 0.17%.[22]

Nowadays, the treatment usually accepted for endophthalmitis is intravitreous antibiotic injections of vancomycin (1 mg/0.1 ml) and ceftazidime (2.25 mg/0.1 ml) or vancomycin and amikacin (0.4 mg/0.1 ml).[23]

To evaluate the role of immediate vitrectomy and antibiotic therapy, a multicenter, randomized clinical trial was carried out, named the US Endophthalmitis Vitrectomy Study. The conclusions of this study were that omission of systemic antibiotic treatment can reduce toxic effects, cost, and length of hospital stay. Routine immediate vitrectomy is not necessary in patients with better than light perception vision at presentation, but is of substantial benefit for those who have light perception-only vision.[24]

REFERENCES

1 Haimann WS, Burton TC, Brown CK. Epidemiology of retinal detachment. *Arch Ophthalmol* 1982; **100:** 289–92.

2 Schepens CL. Retinal detachment and aphakia. *Arch Ophthalmol* 1951; **45:** 1–17.

3 Norton EWD. Retinal detachment in aphakia. *Am J Ophthalmol* 1964; **58:** 111–14.

4 McPherson AR, O'Malley RE, Bravo J. Retinal detachment following late posterior capsulotomy. *Am J Ophthalmol* 1983; **95:** 593–7.

5 Foos RY. Posterior vitreous detachment. *Trans Am Acad Ophthalmol Otolaryngol* 1979; **76:** 480–6.

6 Winslow RL, Taylor BC. Retinal complications following YAG laser capsulotomy. *Ophthalmology* 1985; **92:** 785–9.

7 Ober RR, Wilkinson CP, Fiore JV, Maggiano JM. Rhegmatogenous retinal detachment after neodymium–YAG laser capsulotomy in phakic and pseudophakic eyes. *Am J Ophthalmol* 1986; **101:** 81–9.

8 Fastenberg DM, Schwartz PL, Lin HZ. Retinal detachment following neodymium–YAG laser capsulotomy. *Am J Ophthalmol* 1984; **97:** 288–91.

9 Meredith TA, Maumenee AE. A review of one thousand cases of intracapsular cataract extractions: I. Complications. *Ophthalmic Surg* 1979; **10:** 32–41.

10 Folk JC, Burton TC. Bilateral aphakic retinal detachment. *Retina* 1983; **3:** 32–5.

11 Brasil OM. Tratamento cirúrgico—indicações e técnicas. In: Brasil OM, ed. *Vítreo–Clínica & Cirurgia* 1st edn (Rio de Janeiro: Editora Cultura Médica, 1990) 66–77.

12 Kapusta NA, Chen JC, Lam WC. Outcomes of dropped nucleus during phacoemulsification. *Ophthalmology* 1996; **103:** 1184–7.

13 Borne MJ, Tasman W, Regillo C, Malecha M, Sarin L. Outcomes of vitrectomy for retained lens fragments. *Ophthalmology* 1996; **103:** 971–6.

14 Lewis H, Blumenkranz MS, Chang S. Treatment of dislocated crystalline lens and retinal detachment with perfluorocarbon liquids. *Retina* 1992; **12:** 299–304.

15 Liu K, Peyman GA, Chen M, Chang S. Use of high density vitreous substitute in removal of posteriorly dislocated lenses or intraocular lenses. *Ophthalmic Surg* 1991; **22:** 503–7.

16 Shapiro MJ, Resnick KI, Kim SH, Weinberg A. Management of the dislocated crystalline lens with a perfluorocarbon liquid. *Am J Ophthalmol* 1991; **112:** 401–5.

17 Lewis H, Sanchez G. The use of perfluorocarbon liquid in the repositioning of posteriorly dislocated intraocular lenses. *Ophthalmology* 1993; **100:** 1055–9.

18 Sternberg T Jr, Michels RG. Treatment of dislocated posterior chamber intraocular lenses. *Arch Ophthalmol* 1986; **104:** 1391–6.

19 Chan CK. An improved technique for management of dislocated posterior chamber implants. *Ophthalmology* 1992; **99:** 51–7.

20 Harbour JW, Smiddy WE, Rubsamen PE, Murray TG, Davis JL, Flynn HW Jr. Pars plana vitrectomy for chronic pseudophakic cystoid macular edema. *Am J Ophthalmol* 1995; **120:** 302–7.

21 Falcone PM. Vitreomacular traction syndrome confused with pseudophakic cystoid macular edema. *Ophthalmic Surg Lasers* 1996; **27:** 392–4.

22 Norregaard JC, Thoning H, Bernth-Peteren P, Anderssen TF, Javitt JC, Anderson GF. Risk of endophthalmitis after cataract extraction: results from the International Cataract Surgery Outcomes study. *Br J Ophthalmol* 1997; **81:** 102–6.

23 Roth DB, Flynn HW Jr. Antibiotic selection in the treatment of endophthalmitis: the significance of drug combinations and syngergy. *Surv Ophthalmol* 1997; **41:** 395–401.

24 Endophthalmitis Vitrectomy Study Group. Results of the Endophthalmitis Vitrectomy Study. A randomized trial of immediate vitrectomy and of intravenous antibiotics for the treatment of postoperative bacterial endophthalmitis. *Arch Ophthalmol* 1995; **113:** 1479–96.

Chapter 32 Posterior capsule management in congenital cataract surgery

Abhay Vasavada

Clarity and integrity of the posterior capsule are of paramount importance for achieving successful technical and functional outcome. Maintenance of a clear visual axis is a high priority when planning the management of cataracts in the amblyogenic age range. The posterior capsule opacifies rapidly in children (Fig. 32.1) and often defeats the purpose of preventing amblyopia.[1,2] The incidence of posterior capsule opacification approaches 100% in infants and small children.[1,2] The younger the child, the more acute the problem,. because capsular opacification is inevitable and the amblyogenic effect greater.[3,4] Integrity of the posterior capsule is essential for stable intraocular lens (IOL) implantation. However, treatment of the posterior capsule determines where and how safely the IOL can be fixated (Fig. 32.2). The way in which the posterior capsule is managed determines the ultimate case outcome to a large extent. In small children the anterior vitreous face and posterior capsule are closely interlinked. While dealing with the posterior capsule, it is also important to keep this relationship in mind.

Primary posterior capsulotomy with a needle or a vitrectomy instrument, secondary pars plana or limbal capsulotomy/vitrectomy, pars plana lensectomy and primary posterior continuous curvilinear capsulorhexis (PCCC) with and without anterior vitrectomy are some of the available options in dealing with such cases.[2–6] YAG laser capsulotomy is also possible in older and cooperative children.

POSTERIOR CAPSULOTOMY— PRIMARY VERSUS SECONDARY

Posterior capsulotomy may be performed at the time of cataract removal or secondarily.[1,2,5,6] Primary capsulotomy alone may not be adequate. The incidence of primary capsulotomy closure has been reported to be over 60% when capsulotomy was not

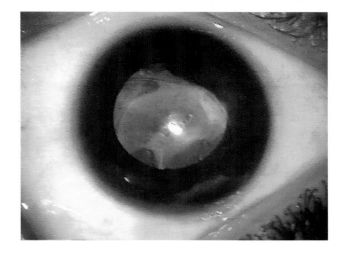

Figure 32.1. *Fibrous posterior capsule opacification in a child of 2½ years who received a polymethylmethacrylate (PMMA) IOL in the bag 1 year ago. Notice the decentration.*

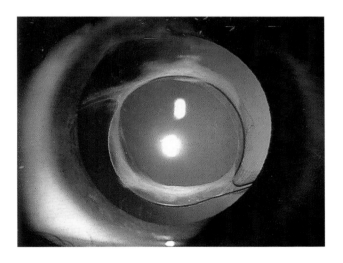

Figure 32.2. *Bag-fixed PMMA IOL in a 4-year-old child, 1 year after surgery. Anterior vitrectomy and optic capture through PCCC were performed.*

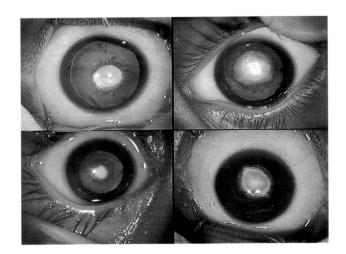

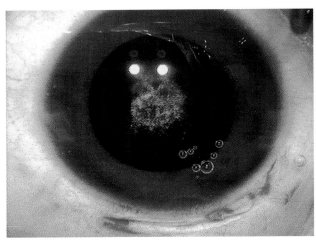

Figure 32.14. *Congenital cataract with pre-existing capsular changes. Upper and lower left had posterior capsule plaque. Upper and lower right had pre-existing posterior capsule defect.*

Figure 32.15. *Central plaque opacity is seen after the lens aspiration in a 1-year-old child.*

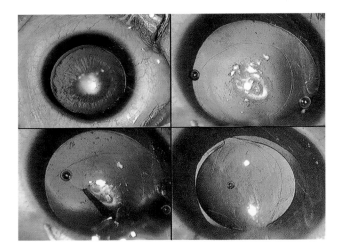

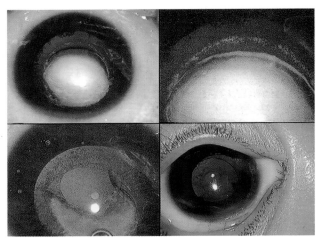

Figure 32.16. *Management of posterior capsule plaque. Upper left: Congenital cataract in a child aged 1½ years. Upper right: Dense plaque on posterior capsule. Lower left: Posterior capsulorhexis encompassing the plaque. Lower right: IOL implantation—haptic fixated in the bag, optic capture through PCCC.*

Figure 32.17. *Upper left: Pre-existing posterior capsule defect in a 7-month-old child. Upper right: Higher magnification showing white granules present in anterior vitreous. Lower left: Posterior capsule defect became apparent during lens aspiration. Lower right: 1-year follow-up of the same eye showing ciliary sulcus-fixated PMMA IOL and clear central axis. The opening in the posterior capsule has contracted.*

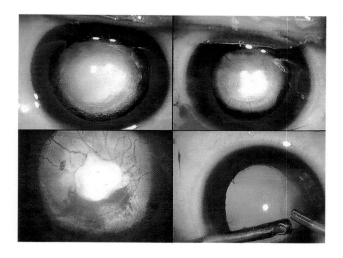

Figure 32.18. *PHPV. Upper left: 2-month-old infant with a dense white cataract in the right eye. Upper right: Fibrovascular thick tissue in place of posterior capsule seen after lens aspiration. Lower left: Intraoperative bleeding from tunica vasculosa. Lower right: Appearance after excision of the tissue with two-port anterior vitrectomy.*

PERSISTENT HYPERPLASTIC PRIMARY VITREOUS (PHPV) (FIG. 32.18)

The vascularized plaque becomes visible once the cataract is aspirated. Intralenticular hemorrhage may occur. The fibrovascular tissue may be excised with two-port vitrectomy. IOL implantation is usually not attempted in such eyes.

IMPORTANT POINTS

Management of the posterior capsule is the essence of a successful technical outcome. Primary posterior capsulorhexis should be seen as mandatory in younger children. Anterior vitrectomy (central) is essential in infants and small children. Both may be performed before IOL implantation. Optic capture gives stability and is an important element in IOL fixation.

REFERENCES

1 Parks MM, Hiles DA. Management of infantile cataracts. *Am J Ophthalmol* 1967; **63:** 10–19.
2 Basti S, Ravishankar U, Gupta S. Results of a prospective evaluation of three methods of management of pediatric cataracts. *Ophthalmology* 1996; **103:** 713–20.
3 Oliver M, Milstein A, Pollack A. Posterior chamber lens implantation in infants and juveniles. *Eur J Implant Refract Surg* 1990; **2:** 309–14.
4 Parks MM. Posterior lens capsulectomy during primary cataract surgery in children. *Ophthalmology* 1983; **90:** 344–5.
5 Gimbel HV, DeBroff BM. Posterior capsulorhexis with optic capture. Maintaining a clean visual axis after pediatric cataract surgery. *J Cataract Refract Surg* 1994; **20:** 658–64.
6 Buckley EG, Klombers LA, Seaber JH, Scalise-Gordy A, Minzter R. Management of the posterior capsule during pediatric intraocular lens implantation. *Am J Ophthalmol* 1993; **115:** 722–8.
7 Morgan KS, Karchioglu ZA. Secondary cataracts in infants after lensectomies. *J Pediatr Ophthalmol Strabismus* 1987; **24:** 45–8.
8 Nishi O. Fibrinous membrane formation on the posterior chamber lens during the early postoperative period. *J Cataract Refract Surg* 1988; **14:** 73–7.
9 Tablante RT, Lapus JV, Cruz ED, Santos AM. A new technique of congenital cataract surgery with primary posterior chamber intraocular lens implantation. *J Cataract Refract Surg* 1988; **14:** 149–57.
10 Hiles DA, Watson BA. Complication of implant surgery in children. *Am Intraocul Implant Soc J* 1979; **5:** 24–32.
11 Vasavada A, Chauhan H. Intraocular lens implantation in infants with congenital cataracts. *J Cataract Refract Surg* 1994; **20:** 592–8.
12 Vasavada A, Desai J. Primary posterior capsulorhexis with and without anterior vitrectomy in congenital cataracts. *J Cataract Refract Surg* 1997; **23:** 645–51.
13 Von Noorden GK, Crawford MLJ. The sensitive period. *Trans Ophthalmol Soc UK* 1979; **99:** 442–6.
14 Vaegan TD. Critical period for deprivation amblyopia in children. *Trans Ophthalmol Soc UK* 1979; **99:** 432–9.
15 Mackool RJ. Management of the posterior capsule during pediatric intraocular lens implantation. *Am J Ophthalmol* 1994; **117:** 121–3.
16 Zetterstrom C, Kugelberg U, Oscarson C. Cataract surgery in children with capsulorhexis of anterior and posterior capsules and heparin-surface modified intraocular lenses. *J Cataract Refract Surg* 1994; **20:** 599–601.
17 Gimbel HV, Ferensowicz M, Raanan M, DeLuca M. Implantation in children. *J Pediatr Ophthalmol Strabismus* 1993; **30:** 69–79.
18 Koch DD, Kohnen T. Retrospective comparison of techniques to prevent secondary cataract formation after posterior chamber intraocular lens implantation in infants and children. *J Cataract Refract Surg* 1997; **23:** 657–63.
19 Mcleod D. Congenital cataract surgery: a retinal surgeon's viewpoint. *Aust NZ J Ophthalmol* 1986; **14:** 79–84.
20 Mackool RJ, Chhatiawala H. Pediatric cataract surgery and intraocular lens implantation. A new technique for

preventing or excising postoperative secondary membranes. *J Cataract Refract Surg* 1991; **17:** 62–6.

21 Neuhann T, Neuhann Th. *The Rhexis Fixated Lens.* Film presented at the Symposium on Cataract, IOL and Refractive Surgery. April 1991, Boston, USA.

22 Kugelberg U, Zetterstrom C. Ocular growth in new born rabbit eyes implanted with a poly (methyl methacrylate) or silicone intraocular lens. *J Cataract Refract Surg* 1997; **23:** 629–34.

23 Kugelberg U, Zetterstrom C. After cataract and ocular growth in new born rabbit eyes implanted with a capsule tension ring. *J Cataract Refract Surg* 1997; **23:** 635–40.

24 Kloti R. Bipolar Nassfeld diathermie in der Mikrochisurgie. *Klin Monatsbl Augenheilkd* 1984; **184:** 442–4.

25 Comer RM, Abdulla N, O'Keefe M. Radiofrequency diathermy capsulorhexis of the anterior and posterior capsules in pediatric cataract surgery: preliminary results. *J Cataract Refract Surg* 1997; **23:** 641–4.

26 Scott Atkinson C, Hiles DA. Treatment of secondary posterior capsular membranes with the Nd:YAG laser in a pediatric population. *Am J Ophthalmol* 1994; **118:** 496–501.

27 Vasavada A, Diwan RP. Plaque management—needling. *Video J Cataract Refract Surg* 1996; **XII**(I).

Chapter 33 **Pediatric lens implantation: technique and results**

Joaquim Neto Murta and Maria J Quadrado

The treatment of pediatric cataracts has changed greatly in recent years but remains a challenge. Early treatment, accurate optical correction of aphakia according to the rapid change in the refractive power of the eye, mainly during the first year, prompt and careful amblyopia treatment and parental motivation are the most important factors in the visual outcome of the management of pediatric cataracts.

The timing and the surgical techniques for removing pediatric cataracts have changed considerably over the last decades.[1–3] Procedures such as discission, linear extraction, intracapsular extraction or aspiration techniques popularized by Scheie in the early 1960s were associated with significant intraoperative and postoperative complications (vitreous wicks to corneoscleral wound, secondary pupillary membrane, opacification of posterior capsule, pupillary distortion, corneal clouding, aphakic glaucoma, retinal detachment, etc.) forcing multiple surgical procedures with relatively rare surgical success.[4–7] Apart from historical interest, they should be kept in mind because many times we have to deal with eyes that have been submitted to such procedures (Figs 33.1a,b and 33.2).

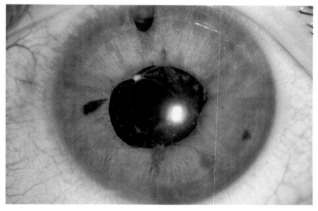

a

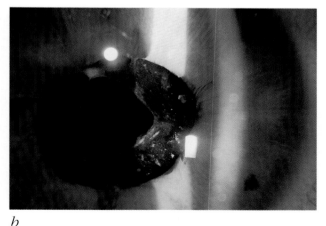

b

Figure 33.1. *a, b (high magnification).*

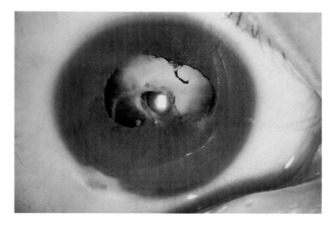

Figure 33.2. *Anterior and posterior synechiae, lens proliferation, distortion of the pupil in eyes submitted to aspiration techniques and multiple discisions in order to clear the visual axis.*

The management of pediatric cataracts involves not only the removal of the obstruction of the visual axis but also an accurate optical correction of aphakia in a crucial period when the visual system is still developing. A correct optical correction of aphakia and a prolonged amblyopic treatment, until 9 years of age, are as important as the surgical treatment of the pediatric cataract.

A variety of options are available to correct aphakia namely spectacles, contact lenses and intraocular lenses (IOLs). Epikeratoplasty is no longer used because, even with lenticules made from fresh tissues, an extended period of time was sometimes necessary for the lenticule to become transparent, with associated poor refractive predictability.[8–10] Spectacles and contact lenses have the advantage of being easily changeable, allowing an adequate refractive correction, so important in a period when rapid changes in refractive power occur. However, peripheral aberrations, constricted visual fields, weight and appearance in spectacles and intolerance in contact lenses are some of the disadvantages of these methods.[11–14] On the other hand, IOLs have the great advantage of offering a permanent aphakia correction allowing easier amblyopic rehabilitation, but are immutable and can induce large anisometropia, particularly when they are implanted in infants.[15–17]

At present, because of the rapid growth of the globe within the first months of life, causing great changes in the refractive power of the eye, two main surgical techniques are used to treat pediatric cataracts: lensectomy with anterior vitrectomy, which can be performed using either a limbal, a pars plana or a pars plicata approach, and implantation of an IOL, paying particular attention to management of the posterior lens capsule and anterior vitreous opacification and ocular inflammation.

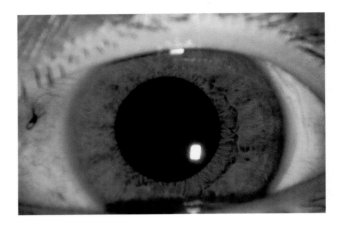

Figure 33.3. *Lensectomy and anterior vitrectomy through a pars plicata approach (3 days after surgery). Pupil is free and reactive.*

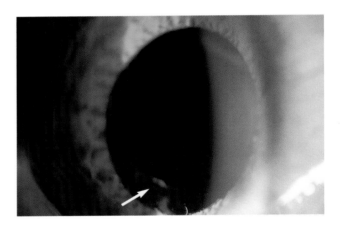

Figure 33.4. *Lensectomy and anterior vitrectomy through a pars plicata approach. Note rim of anterior and posterior capsules (white arrow).*

LENSECTOMY AND ANTERIOR VITRECTOMY

In children under 18 months of age, we, like others,[2,18–22] advocate a lensectomy and anterior vitrectomy through the pars plicata, using a closed vitrectomy system and leaving a rim of anterior and posterior capsules which fuse posteriorly, allowing a secondary posterior IOL implantation in the sulcus, with a risk comparable to that found in the adult population[23–25] (Figs 33.3 and 33.4).

The pars plicata approach allows easier removal of peripheral cortex, less iris manipulation, less damage to the corneal endothelium, and optimal visualization throughout the procedure, and minimizes, when compared to pars plana entry, the risk of damaging the peripheral retina in these small eyes, in which the pars plana is not fully developed.[21,26] This procedure allows a clear visual axis from the start, less secondary cataract formation, and an adequate and changeable optical correction until the refraction of the eye becomes more stable.

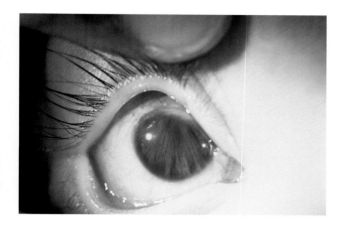

Figure 33.5. *Lensectomy and anterior vitrectomy through a limbal approach in an infant. Pupil border is adherent to the wound.*

The limbal approach is a more familiar surgical technique to most of the anterior segment pediatric surgeons, but a widely dilated pupil is most important, namely to aspirate correctly all the cortex, a condition not often possible with infants even after mydriatic medication, and is associated with more complications such as anterior synechiae, wound dehiscence, vitreous wicks to the corneoscleral wound, surgically induced astigmatism, and epithelial ingrowth (Fig. 33.5). Pupils in infants do not dilate well and intraoperative manipulation makes them even smaller.

INTRAOCULAR LENS IMPLANTATION

Implantation of IOLs in children was pioneered by Choice, Binkhorst and Hiles.[12,27,28] IOL implantation in the pediatric age group, although initially raising some criticism and controversy among pediatric ophthalmologists, has increased in recent years, becoming a common procedure to treat aphakia in children older than 18 months.[3,29–34]

Implanting an IOL before 1 year of age, however, remains a very controversial issue. The difference in size of the globe when compared to the adult eye, its rapid growth (axial length, corneal curvature, diameter of the lens and sulcus size) and the use of standard adult IOLs in these eyes, are some of the multiple factors responsible for the many associated complications.

There are important differences between the treatment of cataracts in children and in adults. Implanting an IOL in an adult eye is normally a very successful procedure with a very low rate of complications. Implanting an IOL in a child is technically more demanding compared to adult surgery and, despite remarkable advances in technology, carries a higher risk of complications. These complications can be divided into two main groups: the long-term complications such as retinal detachment, glaucoma or haptic erosion in secondary IOL implantation, which may develop later in life, and the short-term complications such as secondary cataract formation with opacification of the visual axis or formation of pseudophakic membranes, resulting from the greater inflammatory response that occurs in a child's eye after intraocular surgery.

Different surgical techniques have been then developed in order to avoid these complications and it is particularly important to pay attention to the details of each eye with its unique features and challenges.

ANTERIOR CAPSULOTOMY

Continuous curvilinear capsulorhexis, without any radial tears, should be performed in order to ensure the intercapsular placement of the IOL, which is vital to avoid its decentration or tilting and to prevent its direct contact with uveal tissue, thus reducing uveal response.[35,36]

The anterior capsule of the child's eye is more resistant to tear than that of the adult, and its increased elasticity, associated with low scleral rigidity and increased intravitreal pressure, frequently results in an inadvertent peripheral extension of the capsulotomy.[3,37]

The anterior capsulotomy should be done manually[38] or with a diathermy needle, which is particularly useful in cases of intumescent or mature cataractous lenses.[39,40] On many occasions it is advisable to start in a more central position and perform a small continuous opening in the anterior capsule which should be enlarged after the implantation of the IOL with the cystotome or with intraocular scissors, because progressive constriction of the capsulorhexis has been described.[41]

MANAGEMENT OF THE POSTERIOR CAPSULE AND ANTERIOR VITREOUS

Opacification of the posterior capsule is nearly universal in infantile eyes if the posterior capsule is

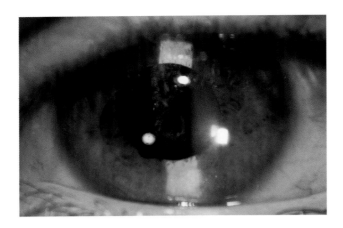

Figure 33.6. *Opacification of posterior capsule 2 months after an IOL implantation in a child 5 years of age.*

left intact and may be extremely rapid in onset[42] (Fig. 33.6). On the other hand, and mainly in children under 5 years of age, an anterior vitrectomy is mandatory. Posterior capsulotomy alone does not guarantee a permanent clear visual axis.[11,43–47] The intact hyaloid vitreous face may act as a scaffold for the migration and proliferation of lens epithelium cells, as well as exudates and cells that result from the breakdown in the blood–aqueous barrier, increasing the risk of dense secondary membrane formation.[10,37,48] These new opacities in the visual axis constitute a significant cause of amblyopia and will usually establish the need for a second surgical procedure.

Nd:YAG laser capsulotomy in intact posterior capsules in young children normally requires high amounts of laser energy and multiple treatments, usually performed under general anesthesia, to open these thickened capsules.[29,49,50]

Posterior capsulotomy with a diameter of 3–4 mm can be done with the vitreous cutting instrument, a cystotome or radiofrequency diathermy.[29,37,38,40,43,51,52] The posterior capsule is less elastic and resistant to tear than the anterior capsule. Posterior continuous curvilinear capsulorhexis is easily performed after puncture of the posterior capsule with the cystotome and introduction of a dense viscoelastic material such as Healon GV, between the posterior capsule and the anterior hyaloid.

To reduce the need for reoperations, different surgical techniques have been proposed to manage, separately or simultaneously, the posterior capsule and the anterior vitreous. Gimbel[53,54] has advocated creating a manual posterior capsulorhexis and then prolapsing the IOL optic through the posterior capsule, making unnecessary anterior vitrectomy in children above 2 years of age. There are recent reports[47] of secondary cataracts after longer follow-up periods as well as the unique complication of opacification of the anterior IOL surface after this technically demanding surgical approach. Zetterstrom et al.[55] reported only posterior capsulotomy prior to IOL implantation, with only one eye, out of 21, developing opacification of the visual axis. However, the mean age of the children was quite high (5.6 ± 4.0 years).

An increasing number of surgeons[11,44,46,47] recommend the importance of moderately aggressive anterior vitrectomy along with a posterior capsulotomy in the treatment of pediatric cataracts at least under 5 years of age, in order to prevent secondary cataract formation.

Different surgical techniques have been proposed. Dahan and Salmenson[43] advocate a posterior capsulectomy and an anterior vitrectomy with a vitreous cutting instrument followed by implantation of the IOL. Some authors[56] found the correct intercapsular fixation of the haptics quite difficult, with a higher risk of intraoperative decentration of the IOL, and proposed doing the posterior capsulectomy and anterior vitrectomy in the early postoperative period. Buckley et al.[52] advocated the implantation of the IOL followed by the posterior capsulectomy and anterior vitrectomy through a pars plana approach, which is awkward because a second entry is obligatory. Tablante et al.[57] describe a more complicated technique which involves a limbal approach to allow the implantation of the IOL in the sulcus, anterior to the cataract, and a pars plana approach to remove the cataract and the anterior vitreous, leaving a rim of capsule to support the IOL. Apart from the fact that it requires a second entry site, this technique has the great disadvantage of using in-sulcus implantation in the primary procedure. Mackool and Chhatiawala[51] proposed a retropseudophakic vitrectomy performed via a limbal approach (LARV), thus avoiding the second entry but increasing the risk of an incomplete anterior vitrectomy with establishment of vitreous wicks to the corneoscleral wound.

We advocate the double capsulorhexis with anterior vitrectomy in all pediatric cataracts in patients less than 5 years of age. In a series of 28 pediatric cataracts, in children between 18 months and 5 years, treated with this technique and with the

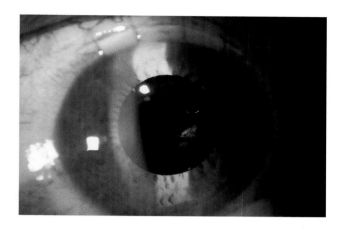

Figure 33.7. *Anterior and posterior capsulorhexis with implantation of a heparin surface-modified IOL.*

implantation of heparin surface-modified IOLs in the capsular bag, the visual axis remained clear after a minimum follow-up of 2 years (Fig. 33.7).

In children older than 5 years we do not perform anterior vitrectomy after the double capsulorhexis, because the inflammatory response is less aggressive and the need for Nd:YAG laser is unusual. When necessary, the children normally cooperate and the treatment may be similar to that given to adults.

IOL FOR PEDIATRIC IMPLANTATION (POWER, DESIGN, SIZE AND BIOMATERIAL)

The pediatric eye presents some particular features that are especially important during the first 2 years of life: (1) the rapid growth of the eye (an average increase of 2.4–3.3 mm in axial length during the first year and an additional 1.2–2.2 mm during the second year);[58,59] (2) the keratometry readings change from 52.00 ± 4.00 D to 42.00 ± 4.00 D in the first 6 months of life,[58] changing remarkably the refractive power of the eye; and (3) the increase of the capsular bag diameter (7.0 mm at birth, 9.0 mm at 2 years, 9.0–10.0 mm at 5 years and 10.0–10.5 mm at 16 years), up of 90% of the lens growth occurring in the first 24 months.[60] These characteristics of the eye during the first 2 years of life, along with an unexpected myopic shift that may occur after surgery,[16,17,61] raise serious questions regarding the safety and accuracy of IOL

implantation in very young children. The choice of the most appropriate IOL power, size and design is particularly difficult.

The myopic shift is more apparent in children who had surgery at a very young age,[62] and occurs faster and is greater in myopic than in hyperopic children of the same age,[63] and in amblyopic eyes.[16,59,64–66] We believe, like others,[62] that it is not appropriate to implant an IOL with the aim of inducing a small myopia in a child's eye, with the objective of stimulating the near vision even without the use of spectacles, because significant myopic shifts may be induced.

Different approaches have been proposed to calculate an IOL in patients of pediatric age, trying to compensate for the myopic shift. Some have advocated an implantation of standard adult IOL power in all cases,[12,55,67] others have advocated introducing an IOL aiming for emmetropia in any case, risking a large myopic shift,[29,37,61] and others have favored an intermediate mode but advocated an arbitrarily fixed undercorrection.[17,52] We think that the most advisable method of calculating the IOL power in patients of pediatric age is the one proposed by Dahan,[62] where the K-readings in newborns are ignored and replaced by an average of 44.00 D, and undercorrections of the IOL power of 20% and 10% are introduced, in babies and in toddlers respectively.

Another major concern in pediatric lens implantation is related to the size and design of the IOL. Despite the fact that iris-fixated IOLs and anterior chamber IOLs have been used for pediatric implantation, they are no longer recommended because of the high rate of complications observed.[27,28,62,68] Wilson-Holt et al.[69] described the occurrence of severe uveitis in a fellow eye of a child after iris-supported IOL implantation, suggesting sympathetic ophthalmia. Posterior chamber IOLs in the capsular bag or secondarily in the ciliary sulcus are advocated by the vast majority of surgeons.[3,32,46,47,54,55,62]

Many complications observed with implantation of IOLs in small eyes are related to the use of standard, adult-size IOLs. Wilson et al.[60] demonstrated that downsizing of IOLs is not necessary after the age of 2 with the exception of very small eyes, because lens growth is completed by this time. A flexible, open-loop, one-piece, all polymethylmethacrylate, modified C-loop capsular IOL with an overall length of 12–12.5 mm, which has a very good loop memory, would possibly be a good choice.[60] C-loops may also have the advantage of minimizing the central migration of lens epithelial cells.[42]

Again, the main problems occur within the first 24 months of life. An oversized IOL will distort the capsular bag and possibly result in erosion through the capsula, leading to excessive pressure on uveal structures. A 10 mm-diameter flexible, open-loop, one-piece, all polymethylmethacrylate, modified C-loop capsular IOL is, probably, the best choice, but may be difficult to obtain in the market.[60]

Although surgical technique is a very important issue, it is necessary to determine first if an implanted IOL will be well tolerated in a very young eye. Improvements in IOL biocompatibility are definitely necessary to reduce the postoperative sequelae. Some degree of foreign body reaction is present after IOL implantation,[70–72] but in high-risk patients such as children, where the inflammatory response is much more aggressive, this reaction, which usually does not appear until 1 or 2 days postoperatively, could be particularly severe.

Anterior uveitis is the most common complication.[29,61,68,73] Deposition of inflammatory cells and formation of fibrinous membranes in the anterior and posterior surfaces of the IOL (Figs 33.8–33.10), significant anterior and posterior synechiae, displacement of one of the IOL haptics into the anterior chamber (iris capture), and pupillary irregularities (Figs 33.11 and 33.12) can occur. Postoperative inflammation can be minimized by avoiding trauma and iris manipulation during surgery, by applying corticosteroids frequently, and by using IOL materials which induce less inflammation.

Significant reductions in the rates of cellular adhesion and inflammation have been achieved in different groups of patients receiving heparin surface-modified IOLs.[55,74,75] Heparin surface treatment may preserve the blood–aqueous barrier better than regular PMMA IOLs.

We compared the postoperative inflammation and the postoperative opacification on the visual axis after the surgical removal of 42 pediatric cataracts, older than 4 years, using double capsulorhexis, aspiration of the nucleus and cortex and implantation of heparin surface-modified IOLs (Fig. 33.13) (group I; 30 eyes) and regular PMMA IOLs (group II; 12 eyes). We observed, in group I, only two secondary membranes (6.6%), which disappeared after topical steroid treatment and in all cases the visual axis remained clear; in group II, 11 of the 12 eyes developed secondary membranes, and a second procedure to clear the visual axis (Nd:YAG laser or pars plicata anterior vitrectomy) was necessary in four cases. More deposits of inflammatory cells, on the anterior surface of the IOL, were also observed in group II when compared to group I.

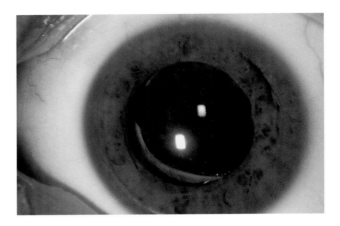

Figure 33.8. *Deposition of inflammatory cells on the anterior surface of an IOL.*

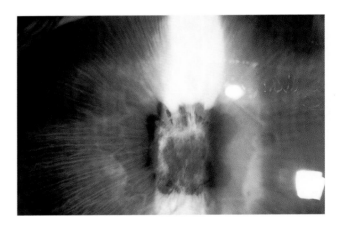

Figure 33.9. *Secondary membrane across the pupil over the anterior surface of a regular polymethylmethacrylate IOL.*

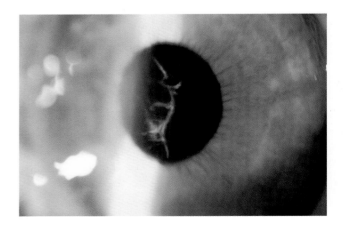

Figure 33.10. *Retropseudophakic membrane after IOL implantation in a child 7 years of age which resolved after topical corticosteroids.*

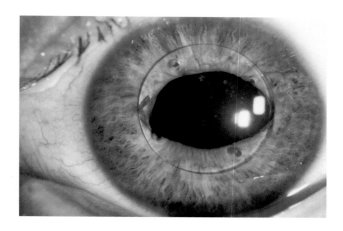

Figure 33.11. *Iris capture of a posterior chamber IOL.*

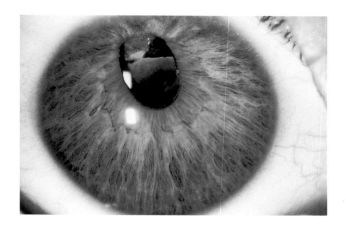

Figure 33.12. *Distortion of the pupil in a pseudophakic eye (4-year follow-up).*

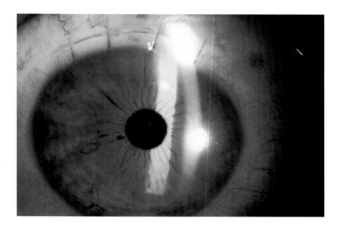

Figure 33.13. *Double capsulorhexis and heparin surface-modified IOL in an 8-year-old. Note that the eye is quiet and the visual axis is free.*

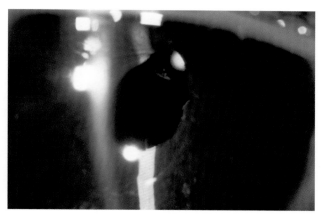

Figure 33.14. *Secondary ciliary sulcus heparin surface-modified IOL implantation in a 6-year-old child submitted to aspiration and two secondary discisions of the posterior capsule (9-month follow-up).*

Other IOL materials with reduced bioreactivity, such as acrylic foldable lenses, have been used with encouraging results (Masket S, personal communication), but longer follow-up periods are necessary for appropriate evaluation.

SECONDARY IMPLANTATION IN CHILDREN

The success of secondary IOL implantation in adults is already well established.[76–78] In children, despite initial reports indicating a high rate of complications,[3] recent reports have shown encouraging results due to the use of safer and less traumatic surgical techniques, new viscoelastics and improved IOL biomaterials. Correct surgical technique (synechiolysis with dense viscoelastic material, iris spatula or scissors) and implantation of a less reactive IOL such as a heparin surface-modified IOL, are two important factors responsible for the good results observed (Fig. 33.14). As mentioned above, iris-supported and flexible anterior chamber IOLs should never be employed.

Monocular aphakic children are the most appropriate candidates for this kind of procedure, mainly when contact lens intolerance develops and visual rehabilitation is threatened. In a series of 10 aphakic eyes, of ages between 2 and 12 years, submitted to lensectomy and anterior vitrectomy through the pars plicata (2) and aspiration technique with multiple discisions (8), we performed secondary ciliary sulcus heparin surface-modified IOL implantation. No major inflammatory responses or complications were observed.

In spite of the low rate of complications with this procedure,[24,25] the long-term safety of the sulcus fixation of these lenses in the pediatric population should be determined.

PROTOCOL FOR PEDIATRIC CATARACT SURGERY

In a child under 18 months of age we advocate a lensectomy, leaving a rim of anterior and posterior capsule, and an anterior vitrectomy with a mechanical suction-cutting instrument. Optical correction of aphakia is done with spectacles or contact lenses in bilateral cases and with contact lenses in unilateral aphakia. When the child or the parents become non-compliant with contact lenses, a secondary IOL implantation in the ciliary sulcus (heparin surface-modified IOL) should be performed.

Some surgeons encourage IOL implantation in very young children, based on the high quality of the aphakic correction of IOL. The enormous variation in size and refractive power of the eye during this period makes the choice of the size and the power of the IOL to implant extremely difficult. High anisometropias can be created, forcing an exchange of IOLs which induces serious inflammatory responses.

In children more than 18 months of age we advocate a double capsulorhexis with implantation of a heparin surface-modified IOL in the capsular bag. An anterior vitrectomy performed after the posterior capsulorhexis is mandatory in all eyes less than 5 years of age. Encouraging results with the use of other IOL materials such as acrylic foldable lenses have been presented, but longer follow-up observations are necessary in order to evaluate their safety and efficacy.

REFERENCES

1 Sheppard RW, Crawford JS. The traetment of congenital cataracts. *Surv Ophthalmol* 1973; **17:** 340–7.

2 Lloyd IC, Goss-Sampson M, Jeffrey BJ, et al. Neonatal cataract: aetiology, pathogenesis and management. *Eye* 1992; **6:** 184–96.

3 Lambert SR, Drack AV. Infantile cataracts. *Surv Ophthalmol* 1996; **40:** 427–58.

4 Cordes FC. Failure in congenital cataract surgery: a study of 56 enucleated eyes. *Am J Ophthalmol* 1957; **43:** 1–6.

5 Scheie HJ. Aspiration of congenital or soft cataracts: a new technique. *Am J Ophthalmol* 1960; **50:** 1048–56.

6 Scheie HJ, Rubenstein RA, Kent RB. Aspiration of congenital or soft cataracts: further experience. *Am J Ophthalmol* 1967; **63:** 3–8.

7 Parks MM, Hiles DA. Management of infantile cataracts. *Am J Ophthalmol* 1967; **63:** 10.

8 Arffa RC, Marvelli TL, Morgan KS. Long-term follow-up of refractive and keratometric results of pediatric epikeratophakia. *Arch Ophthalmol* 1986; **104:** 668–70.

9 Morgan KS, McDonald MB, Hiles DA, et al. The nationwide study of epikeratophakia for aphakia in children. *Am J Ophthalmol* 1987; **103:** 366–74.

10 Dutton JJ, Baker JD, Hiles DA, Morgan KS. Visual rehabilitation of aphakic children. *Surv Ophthalmol* 1990; **34:** 365–84.

11 BenEzra D, Paez JH. Congenital cataract and intraocular lenses. *Am J Ophthalmol* 1983; **96:** 311–14.

12 Hiles DA. Intraocular lens implantation in children with monocular cataracts, 1974–1983. *Ophthalmology* 1984; **91:** 1231–7.

13 Hoyt CS. The optical correction of pediatric aphakia. *Arch Ophthalmol* 1986; **104:** 651–2.

14 BenEzra D, Rose L. Intraocular versus contact lenses for the correction of aphakia in unilateral congenital and developmental cataract. *Eur J Implant Refract Surg* 1990; **2:** 303–7.

15 Dahan E. Lens implantation in microphthalmic eyes of infants, *Eur J Implant Refract Surg* 1989; **1:** 9–11.

16 Huber C. Increasing myopia in children with intraocular lenses (IOL): an experiment in form deprivation myopia? *Eur J Implant Refract Surg* 1993; **5:** 154–8.

17 Sinskey RM, Amin PA, Lingua R. Cataract extraction and intraocular lens implantation in an infant with monocular congenital cataract. *J Cataract Refract Surg* 1994; **20:** 647–51.

18 Stark WJ, Taylor HR, Michels RG, Maumenee AE. Management of congenital cataracts. *Ophthalmology* 1979; **86:** 1571–8.

19 Taylor D. Choice of surgical technique in the management of congenital cataract. *Trans Ophthalmol Soc UK* 1981; **101:** 114–17.

20 Calhoun JH. Cataracts. In: Harley RD, ed. *Pediatric Ophthalmology*, 2nd edn (Philadelphia: Saunders, 1983) 549–67.

21 Peyman GA, Raichard M, Oesterle C, et al. Pars plicata lensectomy and vitrectomy in the management of congenital cataracts. *Ophthalmology* 1981; **88:** 437–9.

22 Hiles DA, Kilty LA. Disorders of the lens. In: Isenberg SI, ed. *The Eye in Infancy* (St Louis, MI: Mosby-Year Book, Inc., 1988) 336–73.

23 Dahan E, Salmenson BD, Levin J. Ciliary sulcus reconstruction for posterior implantation in the absence of an intact posterior capsule. *Ophthalmic Surg* 1989; **20:** 776–80.

24 Sharma A, Basti S, Gupta S. Secondary capsule-supported intraocular lens implantation in children. *J Cataract Refract Surg* 1997; **23:** 675–80.

25 DeVaro JM, Buckley EG, Awner S, Seaber J. Secondary posterior chamber intraocular lens implantation in pediatric patients. *Am J Ophthalmol* 1997; **123:** 24–30.

26 Green BF, Morin JD, Brent HP. Pars plicata lensectomy/vitrectomy for development cataract extraction: surgical results. *J Pediatr Ophthalmol Strabismus* 1990; **27:** 229–32.

27 Choyce DP. Correction of uniocular aphakia by means of anterior chamber acrylic implant. *Trans Ophthalmol Soc UK* 1958; **78:** 459–70.

28 Binkhorst CD, Gobin MH. Treatment of congenital and juvenile cataract with intraocular lens implants. *Br J Ophthalmol* 1970; **54:** 759–65.

29 Gimbel HV, Ferensowicz M, Raanan M, DeLuca M. Implantation in children. *J Pediatr Ophthalmol Strabismus* 1993; **30:** 69–79.

30 Hiles DA, Atkinson SC. Intraocular lens for correction of aphakia in children. In: Cotlier E, Lambert SR, Taylor D, eds. *Congenital Cataracts* (Boca Raton, FL: RG Landes/CRC Press, 1994) 127–37.

31 Wilson ME, Bluestein EC, Wang XB. Current trends in the use of intraocular lenses in children. *J Cataract Refract Surg* 1994; **20:** 579–83.

32 Zetterstrom C. Intraocular lens implantation in the pediatric eye. *J Cataract Refract Surg* 1997; **23:** 599–600.

33 Kora Y, Inatomi M, Yoshinao F, et al. Long-term study of children with implanted intraocular lenses. *J Cataract Refract Surg* 1992; **18:** 485–8.

34 Wilson ME. Intraocular lens implantation: has it become the standard of care for children? *Ophthalmology* 1996; **103:** 1719–20.

35 Apple DJ, Mamalis N, Loftfield K, et al. Complications of intraocular lenses. A historical and histopathological review. *Surv Ophthalmol* 1984; **291:** 1–54.

36 Assia EI, Legler UF, Merrill C, et al. Clinicopathologic study of the effect of radial tears and loop fixation on intraocular lens decentration. *Ophthalmology* 1993; **100:** 153–8.

37 Vasavada A, Chauhan H. Intraocular lens implantation in infants with congenital cataracts. *J Cataract Refract Surg* 1994; **20:** 592–8.

38 Gimbel HV, Neuhann T. Development, advantages, and methods of the continuous circular capsulorhexis technique. *J Cataract Refract Surg* 1990; **16:** 31–7.

39 Delcoigne CD, Hennekes R. Circular continuous anterior capsulotomy with high frequency diathermy. *Bull Soc Belge Ophthalmol* 1993; **249:** 67–72.

40 Comer RM, Abdulla N, O'Keefe M. Radiofrequency diathermy capsulorhexis of the anterior and posterior capsules in pediatric cataract surgery: preliminary results. *J Cataract Refract Surg* 1997; **23:** 641–4.

41 Hansen SO, Crandall AS, Olson RJ. Progressive constriction of the anterior capsular opening following intact capsulorhexis. *J Cataract Refract Surg* 1993; **19:** 77–82.

42 Apple DJ, Solomon KD, Tetz MR, et al. Posterior capsule opacification. *Surv Ophthalmol* 1992; **37:** 73–116.

43 Dahan E, Salmenson BD. Pseudophakia in children: precautions, technique, and feasibility. *J Cataract Refract Surg* 1990; **16:** 75–82.

44 Dahan E, Welsh NH, Salmenson BD. Posterior chamber implants in unilateral congenital and developmental cataracts. *Eur J Implant Refract Surg* 1990; **2:** 295–302.

45 Basti S, Ravishankar U, Gupta S. Results of a prospective evaluation of three methods of management of pediatric cataracts. *Ophthalmology* 1996; **103:** 713–20.

46 Vasavada A, Desai J. Primary posterior capsulorhexis with and without anterior vitrectomy in congenital cataracts. *J Cataract Refract Surg* 1997; **23:** 645–51.

47 Koch DD, Kohnen T. Retrospective comparison of techniques to prevent secondary formation after posterior chamber intraocular lens implantation in infants and children. *J Cataract Refract Surg* 1997; **23:** 657–63.

48 Cobo LM, Ohsawa E, Chandler D, Arguello R, George G. Pathogenesis of capsular opacification after extracapsular cataract extraction. An animal model. *Ophthalmology* 1984; **91:** 857–61.

49 Atkinson CS, Hiles DA. Treatment of secondary posterior capsular membranes with the Nd:YAG laser in a pediatric population. *Am J Ophthalmol* 1994; **118:** 496–501.

50 Brady KM, Atkinson CS, Kilty LA, Hiles DA. Cataract surgery and intraocular lens implantation in children. *Am J Ophthalmol* 1995; **120:** 1–9.

51 Mackool RJ, Chhatiawala H. Pediatric cataract lens implantation: a new technique for preventing or excising postoperative secondary membranes. *J Cataract Refract Surg* 1991; **17:** 62–6.

52 Buckley EG, Klombers LA, Seaber JH, Scalise-Gordy A, Minzter R. Management of the posterior capsule during pediatric intraocular lens implantation. *Am J Ophthalmol* 1993; **115:** 722–8.

53 Gimbel HV, DeBroff BM. Posterior capsulorhexis with optic capture: maintaining a clear visual axis after pediatric cataract surgery. *J Cataract Refract Surg* 1994; **20:** 658–64.

54 Gimbel HV. Posterior continuous curvilinear capsulorhexis and optic capture of the intraocular lens to prevent secondary opacification in pediatric cataract surgery. *J Cataract Refract Surg* 1997; **23:** 652–6.

55 Zetterstrom C, Kugelberg U, Oscarson C. Cataract surgery in children with capsulorhexis of anterior and posterior capsules and heparin-surface-modified intraocular lenses. *J Cataract Refract Surg* 1994; **20:** 599–601.

56 Metge P, Cohen H, Chemila JF. Intercapsular implantation in children. *Eur J Implant Refract Surg* 1990; **2:** 319–23.

57 Tablante RT, Cruz EDG, Lapus JV, Santos AM. A new technique of congenital cataract surgery with primary posterior chamber intraocular lens implantation. *J Cataract Refract Surg* 1988; **14:** 149–57.

58 Gordon RA, Donzis PB. Refractive development of the human eye. *Arch Ophthalmol* 1985; **103:** 785–9.

59 Manzitti E, Gamio S, Damel A, Benozzi J. Eye length in congenital cataracts. In: Cotlier E, Lambert SR, Taylor D, eds. *Congenital Cataracts* (Boca Raton, FL: RG Landes/CRC Press, 1994) 251–9.

60 Wilson ME, Apple DJ, Bluestein E, Wang XH. Intraocular lenses for pediatric implantation: biomaterials, designs, and sizing. *J Cataract Refract Surg* 1994; **20:** 584–91.

61 Sinskey RM, Stoppel JO, Amin P. Long-term results of intraocular lens implantation in pediatric patients. *J Cataract Refract Surg* 1993; **19:** 405–8.

62 Dahan E, Drusedau MU. Choice of lens and dioptric power in pediatric pseudophakia. *J Cataract Refract Surg* 1997; **23:** 618–23.

63 Mantyjarvi MI. Changes in refraction in schoolchildren. *Arch Ophthalmol* 1985; **103:** 790–2.

64 Rabin J, Van Sluyters RC, Malach R. Emmetropization: a vision-dependent phenomenon. *Invest Ophthalmol Vis Sci* 1981; **20:** 561–4.

65 Yamamoto M, Hirofumi M, Shigeru H, et al. Axial length and amblyopia in pediatric aphakia. In: Cotlier E, Lambert SR, Taylor D, eds. *Congenital Cataracts*. (Boca Raton, FL: RG Landes/CRC Press, 1994) 245–50.

66 Tigges M, Tigges J, Fernandes A, et al. Postnatal axial eye elongation in normal and visually deprived rhesus monkeys. *Invest Ophthalmol Vis Sci* 1990; **31:** 1035–46.

67 BenEzra D. Cataract surgery and intraocular lens implantation in children. *Am J Ophthalmol* 1996; **121:** 224–5.

68 Hiles DA. Visual rehabilitation of aphakic children: intraocular lenses. *Surv Ophthalmol* 1990; **34:** 371–9.

69 Wilson-Holt N, Hing S, Taylor DSI. Bilateral blinding uveitis in a child after secondary intraocular lens implantation for unilateral congenital cataract. *J Pediatr Ophthalmol Strabismus* 1991; **28:** 116–18.

70 Ohara K. Biomicroscopy of surface deposits resembling foreign-body giant cells on implanted intraocular lenses. *Am J Ophthalmol* 1985; **99:** 304–11.

71 Amon M, Menapace R. In vivo documentation of cellular reactions on lens-surfaces for assessing the biocompatibility of different intraocular implants. *Eye* 1994; **8:** 649–56.

72 Shah SM, Spalton DJ, Kerr-Muir M. Specular microscopy of the anterior intraocular lens surface. *Eye* 1993; **7:** 707–10.

73 Markham RHC, Bloom PA, Chanda A, Newcomb EH. Results of intraocular lens implantation in pediatric aphakia. *Eye* 1992; **6:** 493–8.

74 Borgioli M, Coster DJ, Fan RFT, et al. Effect of heparin surface modification of polymethylmethacrylate intraocular lenses on signs of postoperative inflammation after cataract extraction: one-year results of a double-masked multicenter study. *Ophthalmology* 1992; **99:** 1248–55.

75 Shah SM, Spalton DJ. Comparison of the postoperative inflammatory response in the normal eye with heparin-surface-modified and poly(methyl methacrylate) intraocular lenses. *J Cataract Refract Surg* 1995; **21:** 579–85.

76 Kraff MC, Sanders DR, Lieberman HL, Kraff J. Secondary intraocular lens implantation. *Ophthalmology* 1983; **90:** 324–6.

77 Biro Z. Results and complications of secondary intraocular lens implantation. *J Cataract Refract Surg* 1993; **19:** 64–7.

78 MuKluskey P, Harrisberg B. Long-term results using scleral-fixated posterior chamber intraocular lenses. *J Cataract Refract Surg* 1994; **20:** 34–9.

Chapter 34 Combined trabeculectomy and phacoemulsification without antimetabolites: techniques and results

Almir Ghiaroni

The coexistence of primary open glaucoma and cataract is becoming more frequent in the aging population. The management of these coexisting conditions has long been a source of controversy. The basic surgical approaches are sequential surgery or a combined procedure.[1]

The combined procedure eliminates the extra morbidity and cost associated with two successive surgical procedures and leads to faster rehabilitation.[2] It also reduces the risk of the intraocular pressure spikes that often occur after cataract surgery, especially in glaucoma patients.[3–6]

The combination of trabeculectomy with cataract extraction and intraocular lens (IOL) implantation in one operation has proved to be relatively safe and effective in the treatment of glaucoma patients who develop cataracts.[7–13]

Foldable IOLs combined with phacoemulsification have the advantage of smaller wound size, which can be expected to minimize long-term against-the-rule meridional shift and conjunctival scarring.[14]

Parker et al. reported their results on phaco-trabeculectomy associated with foldable IOLs. Considering their results regarding visual acuity, induced astigmatism, intraocular pressure control and presence of a filtering bleb, we can observe that the best aspects of small-incision cataract surgery and filtration surgery performed under a scleral flap have been retained.[15]

Other advantages of small-incision methods for combined glaucoma and cataract surgery, besides rapid visual rehabilitation with an early, stable postoperative refraction, include a large area of undisturbed tissue in the conjunctiva and at the limbus for future glaucoma surgery or revisions as necessary, little inflammation and limited bleb fibrosis.[16–17]

In the present report, I analyzed the results of a series of patients who had undergone phacoemulsification with implantation of foldable IOLs associated with trabeculectomy but without antimetabolites.

SUBJECTS AND METHODS

Eighty-one eyes of 72 patients who had phaco-trabeculectomy combined with implantation of foldable IOLs were evaluated. The age of the patients ranged from 45 to 87 years (average: 70.1 years), and the postoperative follow-up ranged from 12 to 54 months (average: 28.3 months). The indication for surgery was the presence of visually compromising cataracts in patients who required use of anti-glaucomatous medication for elevated intraocular pressure. Anterior chamber angles were open in all eyes and were classified as Grade III–IV by gonioscopy. No patients had a history of previous argon laser trabeculoplasty or other ocular surgical intervention. The number of topical medications used by the patients preoperatively ranged from one to three (average: 1.4 medications). Preoperative corrected visual acuity ranged from 20/40 to 20/400 (average: 20/80). Preoperative intraocular pressure ranged from 13 to 26 mmHg (average: 19.29 mmHg).

The surgical technique consisted basically of:

- A fornix-based conjunctival flap located between 11:00 and 1:00.
- Cauterization of superficial episcleral vessels with a bipolar cautery.
- A half-thickness scleral flap 4 mm in length beginning approximately 2.5 mm posterior to the limbus.

- A clear corneal side-port incision 1 mm in length performed with a 15° straight blade.
- A corneal incision 3.2 mm in length, made with a straight blade, immediately anterior to the peripheral vascular arcade after the dissection of the scleral flap.
- Capusulorhexis initiated with a bent needle and completed with a Masket forceps, having the anterior chamber fully filled with viscoelastic.
- Hydrodissection made by the injection of balanced salt solution (BSS) between the anterior capsule and the nucleus.
- Divide and conquer phacoemulsification. Depending upon the consistency of the nucleus, it was divided into two, three or four pieces, which were emulsified at the center of the pupillary area.
- Insertion of a three-piece foldable IOL. The models used in the present study were: SI30NB, SI18NB, SI26NB, SI19NGB and SI19NB, manufactured by Allergan Medical Optics (Table 34.1). The lenses were placed in the capsular bag using a Fine Folder I with the SI18NB, SI26NB, SI19NGB and SI19NB models and a Fine Folder II with the SI30NB model.
- A 1.5 × 3.0 mm section of trabecular meshwork was removed with a Kelly trabeculectomy punch.
- Injection of acetylcholine chloride into the anterior chamber.
- Peripheral iridectomy performed with forceps and Vannas scissors.
- The scleral flap was closed with two radial mononylon 10-0 sutures and the knots were buried.
- The conjunctival incision was repositioned using only bipolar cautery in all cases.

Patients were routinely examined 1 day, 2 days, 4 days, 1 week, 2 weeks, 1 month, 2 months, 3 months, 6 months and 1 year postoperatively.

On all visits except the first, refraction, visual acuity, applanation tonometry, a need for anti-glaucoma medication and the presence or absence of a filtering bleb were noted.

RESULTS

After the surgery, 12 eyes (14.8%) of the patients required topical medications for intraocular pressure control (Table 34.2). The number of medications used postoperatively ranged from zero to two (mean: 0.25).

Table 34.1
IOLs implanted.

SI30NB	35
SI18NB	22
SI26NB	10
SI19NGB	9
SI19NB	5

Table 34.2
Patients using medication.

Before surgery	81 eyes (100%)
After surgery	12 eyes (14.8%)

Table 34.3
Mean visual acuity.

Before surgery	20/80
After surgery	20/30

Table 34.4
Mean intraocular pressure.

Before surgery	19.29 mmHg
After surgery	13.88 mmHg

Table 34.5
Complications.

Posterior capsule opacification	18 eyes (22.22%)
Pigmentation on the IOL	15 eyes (18.51%)
Shallow anterior chamber during the immediate postoperative period	7 eyes (8.64%)
Hyphema	6 eyes (7.40%)
Pupillary membrane	5 eyes (6.17%)
Choroidal detachment	3 eyes (3.70%)
Cystoid macular edema	3 eyes (3.70%)
Ocular discomfort	2 eyes (2.46%)

The postoperative best-corrected visual acuity ranged from 20/200 to 20/20 (mean: 20/30). A comparison between the preoperative and the postoperative best-corrected visual acuity is shown in Table 34.3.

Postoperative intraocular pressure ranged from 10 to 18 mmHg (mean: 13.88 mmHg) (Table 34.4).

In 55 eyes (67.90%) examined at the slit lamp, a bleb was noted.

Causes of postoperative visual acuity less than 20/40 were present preoperatively: age-related macular degeneration (five cases) and glaucomatous visual field loss involving fixation (two cases).

There were no cases of retinal detachment, uveitis, endophthalmitis or corneal decompensation.

Table 34.5 shows the complications that occurred. The most frequent complication was posterior capsule opacification requiring neodymium:YAG laser capsulotomy, which occurred in 18 eyes (22%).

Twelve eyes (14.8%) presented pigment deposits on the surface of the IOL. Ten eyes (12.34%) responded well to topical medication and two eyes (2.46%) required neodymium:YAG laser cleaning of the anterior surface of the IOL.

Four eyes (4.9%) presented a shallow anterior chamber in the immediate postoperative period that responded well to the changing of the medication.

All other complications resolved well with clinical treatment.

DISCUSSION

Among the controversies related to silicone foldable lenses are discoloration[15] and some predisposition to develop pupillary capture of the IOL, particularly in the presence of hypotony and choroidal detachment.[18] In our study, none of the 81 IOLs examined by slit lamp showed any discoloration or other change since implantation; none of the three cases that presented choroidal detachment developed pupillary capture and all of them recovered well with clinical treatment.

Our results showed that the mean visual acuity of the patients improved from 20/80 to 20/30. Sixty-four eyes (79%) achieved a visual acuity of 20/40 or better, which is comparable to the results reported by Parker et al.,[15] Yang et al.[17] and Kosmin et al.,[19] considering trabeculectomy associated with phacoemulsification with foldable IOL implantation.

In our study, the mean intraocular pressure dropped from 19.29 to 13.88 mmHg, and in all patients it was 18 mmHg or less. our results compare favorably with those of other studies, using foldable and rigid IOLs.[15–17,19–21]

In the present study, only 12 eyes (14.81%) of the patients required one topical medication for intraocular pressure control. The mean 1.4 medications per eye dropped to 0.25 medications postoperatively. These results are also comparable to those in the existing literature.[12,15,16,21]

The comparison among different surgical techniques is always difficult because there are several factors that influence the results, including use of antimetabolites, criteria for success and follow-up time.

In the present study we chose not to use antimetabolites, because the series of patients operated on did not present a high risk for filtration failure. Besides that, we know that, in some patients, their use may increase the risk of complications such as hypotony maculopathy,[22] and their long-term adverse effects are still unknown.[17]

Although the results of our study can be considered satisfactory, we believe that a longer follow-up time will be necessary for a more complete evaluation of the surgical technique presented in it.

REFERENCES

1 Obstbaum AS. Combined surgery for glaucoma and cataract. *J Cataract Refract Surg* 1992; **18:** 539.

2 Gayton JL, Van Der Karr MA, Sanders V. Combined cataract and glaucoma procedures using temporal cataract surgery. *J Cataract Refract Surg* 1996; **22:** 1485–91.

3 Savage JA, Thomas JV, Belcher CD III, Simmons RJ. Extracapsular cataract extraction and posterior chamber intraocular lens implantation in glaucomatous eyes. *Ophthalmology* 1985; **92:** 1506–16.

4 Kooner KS, Cooksey JC, Perry P, Zimmerman TJ. Intraocular pressure following ECCE, phacoemulsification and PC-IOL implantation. *Ophthalmic Surg* 1988; **19:** 643–6.

5 Krupin T, Feitl ME, Bishop KI. Postoperative intraocular pressure rise in open-angle glaucoma patients after cataract or combined cataract-filtration surgery. *Ophthalmology* 1989; **96:** 579–84.

6 Zetterstrom C, Eriksson A. Changes in intraocular pressure following phacoemulsification and implantation of a posterior chamber lens. *Eur J Implant Refract Surg* 1994; **6:** 50–3.

7 McCartney DL, Memmen JE, Stark WJ, et al. The efficacy and safety of combined trabeculectomy, cataract extraction and intraocular lens implantation. *Ophthalmology* 1988; **95:** 754–62.

8 Stewart WC, Crinkley CMC, Carlson AN. Results of trabeculectomy combined with phacoemulsification versus trabeculectomy combined with extracapsular cataract extraction in patients with advanced glaucoma. *Ophthalmic Surg* 1994; **25**: 621–7.

9 Wishart PK, Austin MW. Combined cataract extraction trabeculectomy phacoemulsification compared with extracapsular technique. *Ophthalmic Surg* 1993; **24**: 814–21.

10 Wedrich A, Menapace R, Radax U, et al. Combined small-incision cataract surgery and trabeculectomy—technique and results. *Int Ophthalmol* 1992; **16**: 409–14.

11 Skorpic C, Paroussis P, Gnad HD, Menapace R. Trabeculectomy and intraocular lens implantation: a combined procedure. *J Cataract Refract Surg* 1987; **13**: 39–42.

12 Pasquale LR, Smith SG. Surgical outcome of phacoemulsification combined with the Pearce trabeculectomy in patients with glaucoma. *J Cataract Refract Surg* 1992; **18**: 301–5.

13 Menezo JL, Maldonado MJ, Muñoz G, Cisneros AL. Combined procedure for glaucoma and cataract: a retrospective study. *J Cataract Refract Surg* 1994; **20**: 498–503.

14 Shepherd JR. Induced astigmatism in small incision cataract surgery. *J Cataract Surg* 1989; **15**: 85–8.

15 Parker JS, Subba G, John G, Stark WJ. Combined trabeculectomy, cataract extraction and foldable lens implantation. *J Cataract Refract Surg* 1992; **18**: 582–5.

16 Mamalis N, Lohner S, Rand AN, et al. Combined phacoemulsification, intraocular lens implantation and trabeculectomy. *J Cataract Refract Surg* 1996; **22**: 467–73.

17 Yang KJ, Moster MR, Azuara-Blanco A, et al. Mitomycin-C supplemented trabeculectomy, phacoemulsification and foldable lens implantation. *J Cataract Refract Surg* 1997; **23**: 565–9.

18 Marcus DM, Azar D, Boerner C, Hunter DG. Pupillary capture of a flexible silicone posterior chamber intraocular lens. *Arch Ophthalmol* 1992; **110**: 609.

19 Kosmin AS, Wishart PK, Ridges PJG. Silicone versus poly(methyl methacrylate) lenses in combined phacoemulsification and trabeculectomy. *J Cataract Refract Surg* 1997; **23**: 97–105.

20 Gandolfi AS, Vecchi M. 5-Fluorouracil in combined trabeculectomy and clear-cornea phacoemulsification with posterior chamber intraocular lens implantation. *Ophthalmology* 1997; **104**: 181–6.

21 Shingleton BJ, Kalina PH. Combined phacoemulsification, intraocular lens implantation and trabeculectomy with a modified scleral tunnel and single-stitch closure. *J Cataract Refract Surg* 1995; **21**: 528–32.

22 Suner IJ, Greenfield DS, Miller MP, Nicolela MT, Palmberg PF. Hypotony maculopathy after filtering surgery with mitomycin C. *Ophthalmology* 1997; **104**: 207–15.

Chapter 35 **Antifibrosis agents and combined cataract/trabeculectomy**

Richard P Wilson

The prevalence of glaucoma rises dramatically with age, as does that of cataract. In a study in Oxfordshire, UK, diabetes was responsible for more than 11% of cataracts, but 5% of all cataracts were thought to be attributable to glaucoma. Indeed, the relative risk of cataract formation in patients with glaucoma was found to be 2.6 in men and 6.6 in women. The increased relative risk for the population as a whole was 2.9 for those younger than 70 years of age and 4.5 for those older than 70 years of age.[1] The coexistence of these diseases in an aging population will only increase.

The importance of this coexistence is that cataract surgery in glaucomatous eyes is much less satisfactory than that in non-glaucomatous eyes. Miotic pupils with posterior synechiae require stretching, which results in sphincter tears or cutting of the sphincter in multiple places. Both techniques produce an outpouring of serum into the anterior chamber which is made worse by the lowering of the blood–aqueous barrier resulting from chronic glaucoma medication usage. The resulting fibrin in the anterior chamber may glue the scleral flap down and the iris to the anterior capsule or lens. In addition, changes in the conjunctiva resulting from chronic topical medication usage result in an angrier eye postoperatively.

Glaucoma surgeons searching for improved results have moved past the use of corticosteroid and nonsteroidal agents to antifibrosis drugs. The first one of these in use in the USA was 5-fluorouracil (5-FU). This pyrimidine analog interferes with DNA and RNA synthesis, thereby reducing postoperative scarring by inhibiting fibroblast proliferation. The success of adjunct 5-FU in complicated trabeculectomy has been demonstrated in many studies.[2–4]

However, the use of 5-FU for combined trabeculectomy and cataract extraction has benefits that are far less certain. A case in point is the study by Hennis and Stuart on the effect of postoperative 5-FU injections subconjunctivally in patients undergoing combined trabeculectomy and extracapsular cataract extraction with posterior chamber lens implantation. The mean intraocular pressure at 3 months postoperatively in the patients who received 5-FU was 13.1 ± 3.2 mmHg. In the 17 control patients, the intraocular pressure was 13.0 ± 3.0 mmHg ($P > 0.05$). The mean number of postoperative medications in the study patients was 0.7 and in the control patients 0.8 ($P > 0.05$). The authors felt that their study did not support the routine use of 5-FU in patients for combined surgery.[5]

However, in a retrospective study by Cohen, 22 eyes undergoing combined extracapsular cataract extraction and intraocular lens implantation with filtering surgery and adjunctive subconjunctival 5-FU were compared to a similar group without 5-FU injections. There was an average 17.3 mg of 5-FU injected subconjunctivally over the course of the postoperative treatment in the 5-FU group. The intraocular pressure was controlled with fewer medications postoperatively than preoperatively in both groups. However, the 5-FU group demonstrated a statistically significant greater improvement in their intraocular pressure control than the control group ($P = 0.043$).[6]

A later study by Gandolfi and Vecchi, a prospective randomized controlled clinical trial that lasted 1 year, showed an intraocular pressure equal to or less than 15 mmHg at the end of 1 year in 10 of 12 eyes in the 5-FU group versus only 1 of 12 eyes in the control group (Fisher's exact test, $P = 0.00064$). The interesting thing about this study was that the 5-FU group had five subconjunctival injections of 5 mg of 5-FU starting on day 8 after surgery with one injection per week. Their conclusion was that 5-FU was helpful in obtaining lower intraocular pressures after combined cataract and glaucoma surgery.[7]

Mitomycin C was the next agent to become popular as an adjunct to filtering surgery. This alkylating agent inhibits DNA-dependent RNA synthesis and binds to cellular DNA and sites on cell membranes. The result is the formation of free radicals and/or chelating metals which inhibit fibroblast proliferation. Unlike that of 5-FU, however, the action is relatively cell-cycle non-specific. Studies by Chen et al.[8] and Palmer[9] showed mitomycin to be effective as an adjunct in complicated glaucoma filtering surgery. Kitazawa et al.[10] randomized patients to either ten 5-mg injections of 5-FU, or mitomycin at 4 mg for 5 min. At 1 year, the surgical success, which was defined as an intraocular pressure less than or equal to 20 mmHg without medications, was 88% in the mitomycin C eyes and 40% in the 5-FU eyes.

On the basis of these results, it was hoped that mitomycin C would be equally effective when combined with cataract surgery. However, a study by Shin et al. looked at 78 patients who were prospectively randomized to receive either no mitomycin C or a subconjunctival application of 1, 3 or 5 min of mitomycin C at 0.5 mg/ml. The average follow-up was 21 ± 7.7 months. There was no significant difference at each follow-up time in terms of intraocular pressure, medications or best-corrected vision among all four groups. Shin et al. had concluded that mitomycin C did not further improve the final intraocular pressure outcome of primary trabeculectomy combined with phacoemulsification and intraocular lens implantation in primary open angle glaucoma.[11] This was true of patients with uncomplicated primary open angle glaucoma. Patients in the same practice with more risk factors for filter failure have done better with mitomycin C in combined procedures (Shin DH, personal communication).

On the other hand, studies by Joos et al.[12] Costa et al.,[13] Belyea et al.[14] and Carlson et al.[15] indicated that the adjunct use of mitomycin resulted in lower intraocular pressure results. The only note of caution was sounded by Belyea et al., who felt that, although the intraocular pressures were significantly reduced after combined surgery, many of their patients showed visual fields which continued a diffuse glaucomatous progression for the year or two following glaucoma surgery. They also had the development of late endophthalmitis in two eyes. Their concern was that there might be a direct toxic effect of mitomycin on the intraocular contents, resulting in the continued diffuse reduction in retinal sensitivity. This concern is supported by an article by Kee et al. They showed that a 5-min soak on cynomolgus monkey eyes in all four quadrants at 0.5 mg/ml did result in reduced aqueous flow over the first 3 weeks after surgery. Aqueous production did return to

normal at 4 weeks, but their study suggests a toxic effect in the early postoperative period when mitomycin is applied directly to the sclera.[16] Although this dosage was at least four times or more what is used in human surgery, it does raise concern.

These studies suggest that antifibrosis regimens offer the surgeon performing combined cataract and glaucoma surgery both the potential for a higher success rate and a lower final intraocular pressure, as well as increased potential for short- and long-term complications. Mitomycin C carries with it an increased incidence of hypotony and wound problems, e.g. conjunctival wound dehiscence, and scleral wound slippage with secondary astigmatism, along with a long-term risk of bleb leaks and infection. The above studies support the use of mitomycin C for combined procedures. The lower intraocular pressures obtainable with mitomycin C allow the use of a combined procedure rather than doing the filtration surgery first, allowing the fistula to mature, and then removing the cataract through clear cornea. This latter technique, which was well entrenched for far-advanced glaucoma cases, is now rarely necessary. With this technique, a wait of 4 or more months was usually required to allow the filtering fistula to mature. During this period, the cataract usually progressed more rapidly, leaving the patient with poor vision in the eye. Subsequent cataract extraction often compromised bleb function. A combined cataract extraction with trabeculectomy using mitomycin C at a near-maximal dose has become the default procedure for these cases.

PRINCIPLES

One of the first principles of glaucoma surgery is to adjust the patient's expectations appropriately. A patient undergoing a cataract extraction with trabeculectomy and mitomycin C will not see as soon nor get their glasses as early in the postoperative period as a patient undergoing just a cataract extraction. The final result will be what the patient's glaucoma and retina allow. A patient who expects slow progress and many postoperative visits can be pleasantly surprised by a smooth, uneventful, postoperative course but will not be dismayed by a complicated one.

Preoperatively, discontinuing as many glaucoma medications as possible to minimize inflammation and maximize aqueous production in the early postoperative period is prudent. Clearly, too much of a preoperative pressure rise should not be tolerated and the preoperative taper of glaucoma medicines needs to be individualized for each patient. Phospholine iodide and carbachol need to be discontinued 2 weeks preoperatively, as they are the greatest offenders in terms of lowering the blood–aqueous barrier, causing more intraocular inflammation postoperatively. Pilocarpine may be substituted for either of these medications with a smaller overall drop in the blood–aqueous barrier. Steroids may need to be started for a period preoperatively to counteract any inflammatory stimulus and allow the eye to undergo surgery in as quiet a state as possible.

The less damaging the surgery, the better the intraocular pressure results are. A smaller wound gives less concern with wound problems when an antifibrosis regimen is used. It is possible that a large portion of the variability among the above studies concerning the use of 5-FU and mitomycin with combined cataract/glaucoma surgery is due to the changeover from extracapsular cataract extraction to phacoemulsification. The increase in success rate due just to the implementation of phacoemulsification makes it harder to single out and appreciate the effect of mitomycin.

ASPECTS OF SURGICAL TECHNIQUE

The conjunctival flap may be either limbus-based or fornix-based. A study by Berestka and Brown did not find any difference between these two techniques.[17] Many glaucoma surgeons prefer the limbus-based conjunctival flap with the conjunctival incision as high up in the superior fornix as possible. This technique takes longer for those who do not perform a large number of conjunctival closures but does minimize the risk of mitomycin C use, especially long-term leaks and corneal exposure. Digital ocular compression and laser suture lysis with the Hoskins or Ritch lenses on the day after surgery are not a problem. Other surgeons prefer fornix-based conjunctival flaps, as the flap does not get in the way during surgery and is often a quicker procedure. The conjunctival closure, however, requires great care to avoid leaks.

Theoretically, it would seem that mitomycin C applied over a small area of sclera would result in a small, ischemic bleb surrounded by a vascularized cicatrix that would dam the aqueous into a circumscribed area. Concentration of all the aqueous pressure in a small area would result in a much greater pressure per unit area than would a large area of mitomycin C soak resulting in a larger, more diffuse, ischemic bleb. The risk of bleb thinning and later leakage should be reduced with the larger bleb. Preliminary studies have also shown that lower intraocular pressures are achieved by a large area of soak. This is one more argument for the use of limbus-based conjunctival flaps, which allow a larger area of sclera to be soaked than fornix-based flaps.

Since we know from the study of Kee et al. above[16] and work ongoing in Germany that mitomycin C can penetrate through intact sclera, it makes sense that it would be safer to apply mitomycin C prior to any scleral incision. Often, an anterior scleral incision up to the limbus may be deep enough to cut into Schlemm's canal and allow possible reflux of mitomycin C into the anterior chamber. Although the study by Prata et al.[18] showed a greater success rate with trabeculectomy if mitomycin C was applied after the scleral flap dissection, i.e. under the trabeculectomy flap, than if it was applied before any scleral incision, further studies will be needed to elucidate the risk–benefit relationship. At this point, the use of mitomycin C before or after the scleral flap dissection is at the surgeon's discretion.

In addition to the limbus- versus fornix-based flap and whether to apply the mitomycin under the scleral flap, there are three variables: concentration of mitomycin, duration of application, and area of application. Most ophthalmologists use a concentration of 0.2–0.4 mg/ml for 2–3.5 min, depending upon the risk factors for filter failure. A usual application is a solution of 0.4 mg/ml for 2–3.5 min unless the conjunctiva is overly thin or the patient quite elderly. In these cases, I would use only a 1–2-min application. For a small area of application, a corneal light shield truncated on one side makes an excellent mitomycin applicator (Figs 35.1a,b). For a larger area, the Merocel instrument wipe makes an excellent application vehicle and can be cut to the exact size desired (Figs 35.2a,b). If neither is available, a Weck-cel sponge can be pulled apart to one-third thickness and then trimmed to fit over the proposed filtering site. The mitomycin C application should be centered more on the side of the trabeculectomy flap, where the aqueous flow will be directed.

After the mitomycin C application is completed, the area, including under the conjunctiva to each side, must be irrigated with at least one bottle of balanced salt solution (Fig. 35.3). The irrigating solution is

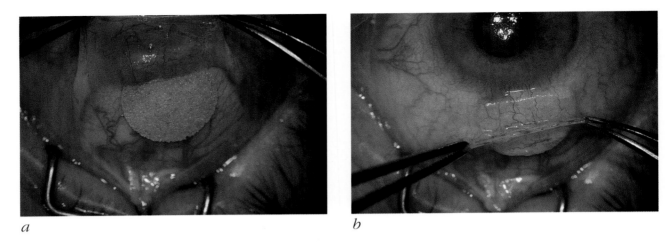

a *b*

Figure 35.1. *(a) A corneal light shield truncated on one side is soaked in mitomycin C and placed over the projected filtration site. (b) Same patient with the conjunctival Tenon's flap pulled back over the mitomycin C applicator. The cut edge of conjunctiva is rolled anteriorly away from contact with the mitomycin.*

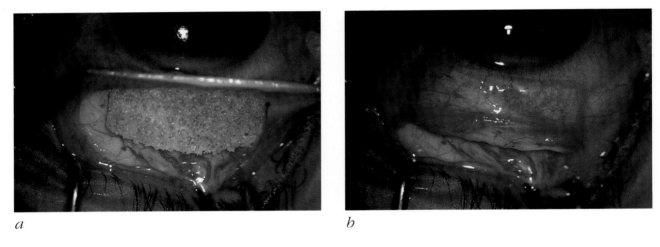

a *b*

Figure 35.2. *(a) In this patient, a Merocel instrument wipe is trimmed to fit the limbus and cover a much larger area. With the larger area of application, the exposure time is reduced. (b) The conjunctival Tenon's flap is pulled over the applicator with the edge rolled anteriorly to prevent contact of the cut edge with mitomycin C.*

collected and anything that has been in contact with the mitomycin C is disposed of in a container approved for chemotherapy waste. Instruments that were used to apply the mitomycin C also need to be rinsed.

If a buttonhole occurs after the application of mitomycin C, the site of filtration probably needs to be moved and mitomycin C applied at the new site. Buttonholes are always problematic but are far more serious after mitomycin C has been applied to the

area. With luck, there is a fairly good layer of Tenon's underneath the buttonhole to bolster it from the back as it is sewn watertight with 10-0 or 11-0 nylon. 11-0 Nylon, although more difficult to work with, is not as stiff and does not tug at the wound as much with blinking and saccades. If there is not much Tenon's to bolster the back of the buttonhole, it is best to excise a piece of Tenon's that has not come in contact with mitomycin C and use it to bolster the buttonhole from underneath. This provides live,

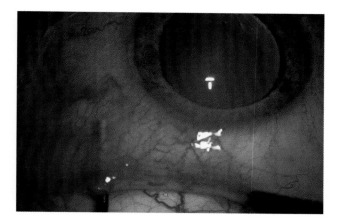

Figure 35.3. *A stream of balanced salt solution is used to rinse the area of mitomycin C contact, including under the conjunctiva to each side.*

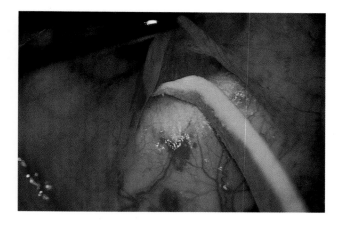

Figure 35.4. *A Weck-cel sponge is used to bluntly dissect the anterior attachments of the conjunctival Tenon's flap forward to the limbus.*

active cells to help with healing of the buttonhole. It is best, however, to use a meticulous technique to avoid buttonholes.

My approach is to use a Weck-cel sponge to bluntly dissect the limbus forward (Fig. 35.4), saving the 67 beaver blade only for patients who have tightly adherent Tenon's and conjunctiva. Tenonectomies are rarely indicated and then only if there is an extremely thick capsule that will prevent visibility of the flap sutures for later laser suture lysis.

Laserable sutures are usually preferable to releasable sutures in patients with the adjunct use of mitomycin C. This is because the use of mitomycin C delays the time that suture lysis will be needed from at the end of 1 week to 2 or 3 weeks after the procedure. If the pressure is quite low and the surgeon does not want to risk chronic hypotony, laser suture lysis may need to be put off for 6 weeks or more following surgery.

Releasable sutures for trabeculectomy all have at least one drawback. The suture described by Cohen and Osher[19,20] has a small loop underneath the conjunctiva. If it is left in place for long, fibrosis passes through the loop and prevents it from being released. The suture I developed[21,22] can be left for prolonged periods and then removed without difficulty. However, during the time this suture is in place, there is significant astigmatism. For these reasons, laser suture lysis is the preferred technique when used with mitomycin C. However, if no laser is available, or if there is excessive bleeding during surgery and blood may prevent the surgeon from accessing the scleral flap suture with a laser to cut it during the postoperative period, then a releasable suture becomes necessary.

If one reopens a working trabeculectomy years after the original surgery, one finds only one small fistula through which aqueous is filtering. This is true even if there was aqueous leakage on all three sides of the original trabeculectomy flap. Since the fistula is prevented from healing by the force of the aqueous going through it, it seems sensible to direct all the aqueous flow through one site. This allows the maximal amount of aqueous flow through this area in the early postoperative period.

Theoretically, forcing all aqueous through one filtration site should create the largest fistula possible. With the variable but often dramatic effect of mitomycin C, it is prudent to place two, long, easily lasered sutures to limit aqueous filtration in the early postoperative period. Having two sutures directly over the area of filtration allows a stepwise drop in intraocular pressure. This prevents a pressure of 18 mmHg dropping to 2 mmHg, as often happens with only one laserable suture in place. Fig. 35.5 shows one variation of a combined procedure. The use of a sliding knot on the sutures over the area of filtration allows fine adjustments to be made in the amount of filtering aqueous (Fig. 35.6a,b). A balanced salt solution is injected through the paracentesis to firm the eye, and the sutures are adjusted to achieve the desired filtration. Usually a slow ooze is required with an intraocular pressure in

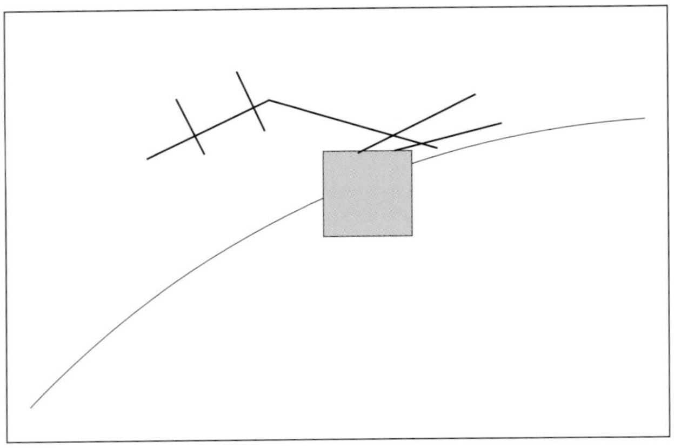

a

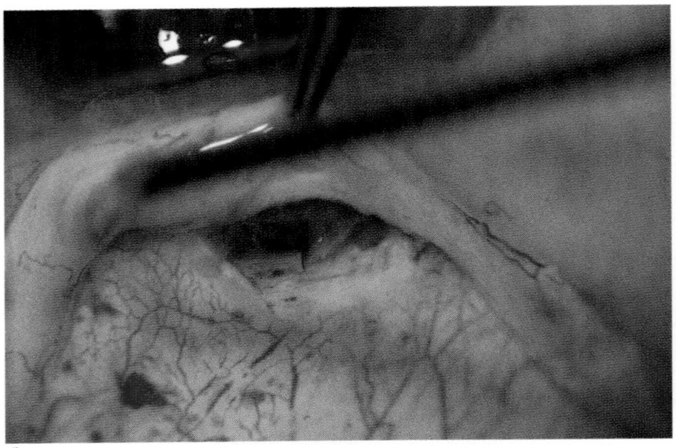

b

Figure 35.5. *A combined scleral tunnel and trabeculectomy wound with the trabeculectomy block displaced all the way to the edge of the scleral flap to achieve maximal flow with excellent control.*

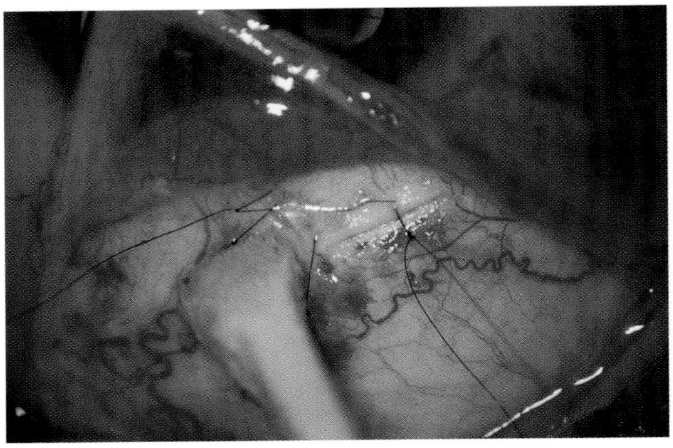

a

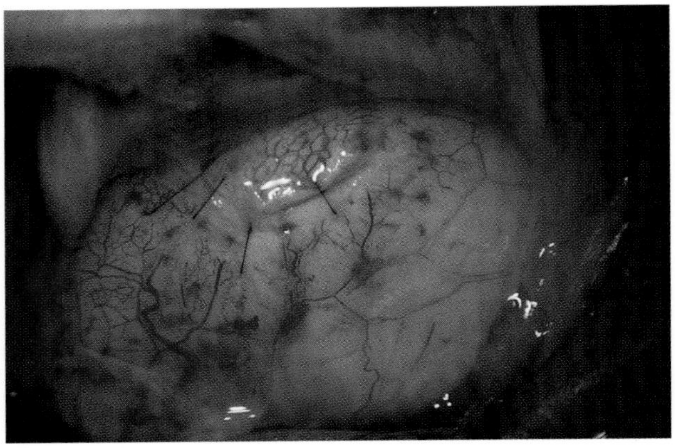

b

Figure 35.6. *After pressurizing of the globe with balanced salt solution through the paracentesis track, the sliding knot sutures overlying the point of filtration are adjusted to allow the desired amount of filtration. At that point the sutures are tied permanently and trimmed.*

the upper teens. Fluid is let out of the eye until the pressure is 10 mmHg or under, at which point there should be very little if any filtration. Taking the extra time to be certain the amount of filtration is the exact amount desired may often prevent problems in the postoperative period.

Whether there is a limbus-based or fornix-based flap, the conjunctival closure needs to be meticulous in the face of mitomycin C. My preference is a limbus-based conjunctival flap with 10-0 nylon, which is the least reactive and longest-lasting in case mitomycin C has come in contact with the conjunctival wound. I remove it when it starts to extrude. Fornix-based flaps can be closed with an X-suture at each end and, if

necessary, an additional horizontal mattress across the front.

Management of the patient following combined cataract trabeculectomy with mitomycin C is as important to the final outcome as the original surgery. Since mitomycin C cannot be titrated to effect as 5-FU can, the timing employed for lasering or releasing the flap sutures is critical to obtaining the desired intraocular pressures. The release of flap sutures too soon results in sudden hypotony leading to choroidal detachment formation and a shallow anterior chamber with limited aqueous production. If the sutures are released too late, the flap will have fibrosed and sealed, resulting in intraocular pressure that is too high.

Remember that a combined cataract and glaucoma operation is not nearly as sensitive to the effects of mitomycin C as a trabeculectomy, especially a primary trabeculectomy in a virgin eye. One must be much more aggressive in releasing sutures than one would be with trabeculectomy and mitomycin C. I release sutures as needed to keep the intraocular pressure in the middle teens for the first 2 weeks. If an intraocular pressure in single digits is required, I then cut more sutures to achieve the desired result at that time. Suture lysis needs to be individualized according to the desired intraocular pressure level, age of the patient, race, the number of topical medications and length of time the patient has been on them, any history of how the patient has reacted to previous surgery, and the amount of inflammation present. With a 3–4-mm wound, the posterior sutures, i.e. all flap sutures, can be cut if necessary without engendering excessive astigmatism. Digital ocular compression is often required and may be started on the evening of surgery if it is dangerously early to laser sutures.

My technique for digital ocular compression is to have the patient fixate directly in front of them with the contralateral eye, close the eye to be compressed, and, using the soft pad of the index or middle finger, press on the cornea through the lid directly towards the occiput with a firm, steady pressure. I do this technique myself in the office before prescribing and find out how many seconds it takes to achieve the desired drop in intraocular pressure. I never have them exert pressure for more than 10 s without releasing for 5 s. After several weeks, the usual frequency is, every 1–2 h, 10 s of pressure on, 5 s off, and 10 s on again. Between 3 and 6 months, I taper the digital ocular compression down slowly. In patients requiring extremely low intraocular pressures, it may be beneficial to continue them on digital ocular compression two to four times per day for the long term.

CONCLUSION

With less damaging surgery, refined techniques, and the use of evolving antifibrosis regimens, the results of combined cataract–trabeculectomy are improving steadily. Underlining these improved results continues to be attention to detail and extra visits and effort in the postoperative period.

REFERENCES

1 Harding JJ, Egerton M, van Heyningen R, Harding RS. Diabetes, glaucoma, sex, and cataract: analysis of combined data from two case control studies. *Br J Ophthalmol* 1993; **77:** 2–6.
2 Rockwood EJ, Parrish RK II, Heuer DK, et al. Glaucoma filtering surgery with 5-fluorouracil. *Ophthalmology* 1987; **93:** 1071–8.
3 Weinreb RN. Adjusting the dose of 5-fluorouracil after filtration surgery to minimize side effects. *Ophthalmology* 1987; **94:** 565–70.
4 Fluorouracil Filtering Surgery Study Group. Fluorouracil Filtering Surgery Study One-Year Follow-Up. *Am J Ophthalmol* 1989; **108:** 625–35.
5 Hennis HL, Stewart WC. The use of 5-fluorouracil in patients following combined trabeculectomy and cataract extraction. *Ophthalmic Surg* 1991; **22:** 451–4.
6 Cohen JS. Combined cataract implant and filtering surgery with 5-fluorouracil. *Ophthalmic Surg* 1990; **21:** 181–6.
7 Gandolfi SA, Vecchi M. 5-Fluorouracil in combined trabeculectomy and clear-cornea phacoemulsification with posterior chamber intraocular lens implantation. *Ophthalmology* 1997; **104:** 181–6.
8 Chen C-W, Huang H-T, Bair J-S, Lee C-C. Trabeculectomy with simultaneous topical application of mitomycin-C in refractory glaucoma. *J Ocul Pharmacol* 1990; **6:** 175–82.
9 Palmer SS. Mitomycin as adjunct chemotherapy with trabeculectomy. *Ophthalmology* 1991; **98:** 317–21.
10 Kitazawa Y, Kawase K, Matsushita H, Minobe M. Trabeculectomy with mitomycin. A comparative study with 5-fluorouracil. *Arch Ophthalmol* 1991; **109:** 1693–8.
11 Shin DH, Simone PA, Song MS, et al. Adjunctive subconjunctival mitomycin C in glaucoma triple procedure. *Ophthalmology* 1995; **102:** 347–8.
12 Joos KM, Bueche MJ, Palmberg PF, Feuer WJ, Grajewski AL. One-year follow-up results of combined mitomycin C trabeculectomy and extracapsular cataract extraction. *Ophthalmology* 1995; **102:** 76–83.
13 Costa VP, Moster MR, Wilson RP, Schmidt CM, Gandham S, Smith M. Effects of topical mitomycin C on primary trabeculectomies and combined procedures. *Br J Ophthalmol* 1993; **77:** 693–7.
14 Belyea DA, Dan JA, Lieberman MF, Stamper RL. Midterm follow-up results of combined phacoemulsification, lens implantation, and mitomycin-C trabeculectomy procedure. *J Glaucoma* 1997; **6:** 90–8.
15 Carlson DW, Alward WL, Barad JP, Zimmerman MB, Carney BL. A randomized study of mitomycin augmentation in combined phacoemulsification and trabeculectomy. *Ophthalmology* 1997; **104:** 719–24.

16 Kee C, Pelzek CD, Kaufman PL. Mitomycin C suppresses aqueous humor flow in cynomolgus monkeys. *Arch Ophthalmol* 1995; **113:** 239–42.

17 Berestka JS, Brown SVL. Limbus- versus fornix-based conjunctival flaps in combined phacoemulsification and mitomycin C trabeculectomy surgery. *Ophthalmology* 1997; **104:** 187–96.

18 Prata Jr JA, Minckler DS, Baerveldt G, Lee PP, Heuer DK. Site of mitomycin-C application during trabeculectomy. *J Glaucoma* 1994; **3:** 296–301.

19 Cohen JS. Removable suture technique for trabeculectomy. In: Minckler DS, Van Buskirk EM, eds. *Color Atlas of Ophthalmic Surgery, Glaucoma.* (Philadelphia: JB Lippincott, 1992) 91–9.

20 Cohen JS, Osher RH. Releasable suture in filtering and combined surgery. *Ophthalmol Clin North Am* 1988; **1:** 187–97.

21 Wilson RP. Technical advances in filtration surgery. In: McAllister JA, Wilson RP, eds. *Glaucoma* (Boston: Butterworths, 1986) 243–50.

22 Wilson RP, Steinmann WC. Use of trabeculectomy with postoperative 5-fluorouracil in patients requiring extremely low intraocular pressure levels to limit further glaucoma progression. *Ophthalmology* 1991; **98:** 1047–52.

Index